NEUROLOGY IN PRACTICE:

SERIES EDITORS: ROBERT A. GROSS, DEPARTMENT OF NEUROLOGY, UNIVERSITY OF ROCHESTER MEDICAL CENTER, ROCHESTER, NY, USA

JONATHAN W. MINK, DEPARTMENT OF NEUROLOGY, UNIVERSITY OF ROCHESTER MEDICAL CENTER, ROCHESTER, NY, USA

Emergency Management in Neurocritical Care

EDITED BY

EDWARD M. MANNO

MD, FCCM, FAAN, FAHA
Head, Neurological Intensive Care Unit
Cleveland Clinic
Cleveland, OH, USA

T0176358

WILEY-BLACKWELL

A John Wiley & Sons, Ltd., Publication

Contents

PART VI: ACUTE NEUROIMAGING AND NEUROMONITORING IN NEUROCRITICAL CARE

The color plate can be found facing page 54.

Contributors

Peter J.D. Andrews, MD, MB, ChB, FRCA
Centre for Clinical Brain Sciences
University of Edinburgh
Edinburgh, UK

Patrícia Canhão, MD, PhD
Department of Neurosciences
Serviço de Neurologia
Hospital de Santa Maria
University of Lisbon
Lisboa, Portugal

Jan Claassen MD, PhD
Division of Neurocritical Care and
the Comprehensive Epilepsy Center
Department of Neurology
Columbia University
New York, NY, USA

Maxwell S. Damian, MD, PhD
Department of Neurology and
the Neurocritical Care Unit
Cambridge University Hospitals
Cambridge, UK

Michael N. Diringer, MD
Neurology/Neurosurgery Intensive
Care Unit
Department of Neurology and
Neurological Surgery
Washington University School
of Medicine
Saint Louis, MO, USA

Ali E. Elsayed, MD
Mountainside Hospital
Montclaire, NJ, USA

José M. Ferro, MD, PhD
Department of Neurosciences
Serviço de Neurologia
Hospital de Santa Maria
University of Lisbon
Lisboa, Portugal

Jennifer A. Frontera, MD
Neuroscience Intensive Care Unit
Departments of Neurosurgery and Neurology
Mount Sinai School of Medicine
New York, NY, USA

James M. Gebel, Jr, MD, MS, FAHA
Cerebrovascular Center
Cleveland Clinic
Cleveland, OH, USA

Leonid Groysman, MD
Neurocritical Care and Stroke Division
University of Southern California
Los Angeles, CA, USA

Rishi Gupta, MD
Department of Neurology, Neurosurgery
and Radiology
Emory University School of Medicine
Marcus Stroke and Neuroscience Center
Grady Memorial Hospital
Atlanta, GA, USA

J. Claude Hemphill III, MD, MAS
Department of Neurology
University of California
San Francisco, CA, USA

Carlos Leiva-Salinas, MD
Department of Radiology
Neuroradiology Division
University of Virginia
Charlottesville, VA, USA

Karen J. McAllen, Pharm.D
Department of Pharmacy Services
Spectrum Health Hospitals
Grand Rapids, MI, USA

Iain J. McCullagh, MBChB, FRCA
Department of Anaesthesia, Critical Care
and Pain Management
University of Edinburgh
Edinburgh, UK

**Edward M. Manno, MD, FCCM,
FAAN, FAHA**
Neurological Intensive Care Unit
Cleveland Clinic
Cleveland, OH, USA

Laurie McWilliams, MD
Neurocritical Care Unit
Cerebrovascular Center
Department of Neurology and Neurosurgery
Cleveland clinic
Cleveland, OH, USA

Bharath R. Naravetla, MD
Department of Neurology
Neurovascular Service
University of California, San Francisco
San Francisco, CA, USA

Bartnett R. Nathan, MD
Departments of Neurology and Internal
Medicine
NeuroCritical Care and NeuroInfectious
Disease
University of Virginia
Charlottesville, VA, USA

Dennis Parker, Jr, Pharm.D
Eugene Applebaum College of
Pharmacy & Health Sciences
Wayne State University
Detroit, MI, USA

J. Javier Provencio, MD
Cerebrovascular Center
Cleveland Clinic
Cleveland, OH, USA

Alejandro A. Rabinstein, MD
Department of Neurology
Mayo Clinic College of Medicine
Rochester, MN, USA

**Denise H. Rhoney, Pharm.D,
FCCP, FCCM**
Eugene Applebaum College of Pharmacy &
Health Sciences
Wayne State University
Detroit, MI, USA

Tomoko Rie Sampson, MD, MPH
Neurology/Neurosurgery Intensive Care Unit
Department of Neurology and Neurological
Surgery
Washington University School of Medicine
Saint Louis, MO, USA

Cathy Sila, MD
Department of Neurology
Case Western Reserve University
School of Medicine
and Stroke & Cerebrovascular Center,
Neurological Institute
University Hospitals–Case Medical Center
Cleveland, OH, USA

Wade Smith, MD, PhD
Department of Neurology
University of California
San Francisco, CA, USA

Michael J. Souter, MB, ChB, FRCA
Department of Anesthesiology & Pain Medicine;
and Department of Neurological Surgery
University of Washington;
Department of Anesthesiology
Harborview Medical Center
Seattle, WA, USA

Gene Sung, MD, MPH
Neurocritical Care and Stroke Division
University of Southern California
Los Angeles, CA, USA

Muhammad A. Taqui, MD
Department of Neurology and Neurosurgery
The Ohio State University
Columbus, OH, USA

Michel T. Torbey, MD, MPH, FAHA, FCCM
Department of Neurology and Neurosurgery
The Ohio State University
Columbus, OH, USA

Max Wintermark MD
Department of Radiology
Neuroradiology Division
University of Virginia
Charlottesville, VA, USA

Series Foreword

The genesis for this book series started with the proposition that, increasingly, physicians want direct, useful information to help them in clinical care. Textbooks, while comprehensive, are useful primarily as detailed reference works but pose challenges for uses at the point of care. By contrast, more outline-type references often leave out the "hows and whys" – pathophysiology, pharmacology – that form the basis of management decisions. Our goal for this series is to present books, covering most areas of neurology, that provide enough background information to allow the reader to feel comfortable, but not so much as to be overwhelming; and to associate that with practical advice from experts about care, combining the growing evidence base with best practices.

Our series will encompass various aspects of neurology, with topics and the specific content chosen to be accessible and useful.

Chapters cover critical information that will inform the reader of the disease processes and mechanisms as a prelude to treatment planning. Algorithms and guidelines are presented, when appropriate. "Tips & Tricks" boxes provide expert suggestions, while other boxes present cautions and warnings to avoid pitfalls. Finally, we provide "Science Revisited" sections that review the most important and relevant science background material, and "Bibliography" sections that guide the reader to additional material.

We welcome feedback. As additional volumes are added to the series, we hope to refine the content and format so that our readers will be best served.

Our thanks, appreciation, and respect go out to our editors and their contributors, who conceived and refined the content for each volume, assuring a high-quality, practical approach to neurological conditions and their treatment.

Our thanks also go to our mentors and students (past, present, and future), who have challenged and delighted us; to our book editors and their contributors, who were willing to take on additional work for an educational goal; and to our publisher, Martin Sugden, for his ideas and support for wonderful discussions and commiseration over baseball and soccer teams that might not quite have lived up to expectations. We would like to dedicate the series to Marsha, Jake and Dan; and to Janet, Laura and David. And also to Steven R. Schwid, MD, our friend and colleague, whose ideas helped to shape this project and whose humor brightened our lives, but he could not complete this goal with us.

Robert A. Gross
Jonathan W. Mink
Rochester, July 2011

Preface

Since its beginning in the early 1980s the field of neurocritical care has expanded at a dramatic rate. In the last decade there has been the development of an international society with over 1000 members, a specialized journal with a growing impact factor, accredited fellowship programs, and a board certification process through the United Council of Neurological Subspecialties. To date there are close to 100 neurocritical care units in the United States, a similar number in Europe, and a growing presence in South America and Asia. The inclusion of a textbook of Neurocritical Care in the Neurology in Practice series is a testimony to the field's growing influence.

The rapid growth of neurocritical care has encouraged a commensurate growth of literature in the field. Interestingly, this has mostly taken the form of single author texts or handbooks primarily designed to disseminate information quickly and systematically to keep pace with this growing field.

This book, *Emergency Management in Neurocritical Care* is the first multi-authored textbook in the field since the first text, *Neurological and Neurosurgical Intensive Care,* was edited by Allan Ropper and Sean Kennedy in 1983. The primary aim is to provide a comprehensive guide to the management of acutely ill neurological or neurosurgical patients wherever they may be located in the hospital. The scope of the book will include basic principles in emergency neurology and critical care, which will review the underlying basic science and cerebrovascular physiology of the critically ill neurological patient. Later sections will focus more on the critical aspects of the neurologically ill. Specific sections dedicated to cerebrovascular disease, neuromuscular disorders, epilepsy, and neurological consultations in general intensive care unit are included. A final section on neuroimaging and neuromonitoring reflects the growing reliance on technology in neurological critical care.

The chapters are written by experts in their respective areas and represent a worldwide distribution of multidisciplinary authors. The book contains more detailed information than a handbook, but is presented in a concise and user-friendly manner to serve as a quick reference when needed. The "Tips & Tricks" and "Science Revisited" sections are designed to increase the readability of the chapters.

Endeavors of this size are not undertaken without help, and I would like to thank Jonathan Mink MD, one of the series editor, for including this topic. I would also like to thank Lewis O'Sullivan, Martin Sugden, Michael Bevan, and Lucinda Yeates at Wiley–Blackwell Publishing who were instrumental in guiding me through this process.

Finally, my father passed away during the editing of this text, and on retrieving his personal items I discovered a number of medals of valor he received during World War II. He never spoke of these and my family was unaware of his possessions. This book is dedicated to him and to all the physicians, nurses, and personnel in the neurological intensive care unit and elsewhere who perform daily acts of valor with no expectation of recognition.

Edward M. Manno
Cleveland

Part I

Acute Management of Neurological Emergencies

1

Hypertensive Emergency

Laurie McWilliams

Neurocritical Care Unit, Cerebrovascular Center, Department of Neurology and Neurosurgery, Cleveland Clinic, Cleveland, OH, USA

Introduction

Hypertension and neurologic disease coexist frequently, either as a cause or consequence of the underlying neurologic disease. In addition, the management of elevated blood pressures in this setting has significant impact on outcomes. Hypertension is defined as systolic blood pressure greater than 140 mmHg or diastolic blood pressure greater than 90 mmHg. The National Health and Nutrition Survey (NHANES) is conducted by the Centers for Disease Control and Prevention obtaining data from US household individuals regarding health and nutrition for the purpose of improving the US health through policy. The NHANES 2005 to 2006 data reported that 29% of the United States population 18 years and older are diagnosed with hypertension. Of the population with treated hypertension, greater than 64% has controlled hypertension. Men have a higher rate of hypertension until the age of 45 when the incidence of hypertension equalizes between men and women.

In 2006 the mortality from hypertension was reported in 56,561 individuals. Both the prevalence from hypertension and mortality has increased from the late 1990s to the 2000s. The estimated direct and indirect cost of hypertension for the year 2010 was 76.6 billion US dollars.

The sequelae of hypertension include strokes, myocardial ischemia, aortic dissection, and renal insufficiency. The remaining text of the chapter will focus on the management of blood pressure in the specified acute neurologic diseases.

Hypertensive crisis is defined as an abrupt elevation of blood pressure, to a point that the blood vessels are unable to maintain constant blood flow in the setting of increasing perfusion pressures to specific organs, also known as disruption of autoregulation. The end result leads to end-organ damage from ischemia or hemorrhage. The end result leads to end-organ damage from ischemia or hemorrhage.

Patients with blood pressure elevations greater than 180/110 mmHg are categorized into the following diagnoses:

1. Severe hypertension: no to mild symptoms and no acute end-organ damage
2. Hypertensive urgency: significant symptoms and mild acute end-organ damage. Mild end-organ damage is defined as dyspnea and headaches.
3. Hypertensive emergency: severe symptoms with life-threatening end-organ damage.

Life-threatening end-organ damage is defined as acute ischemic stroke, intracerebral hemorrhage, subarachnoid hemorrhage, acute aortic dissection, myocardial infarction, acute heart failure, eclampsia, renal insufficiency, and acute

Emergency Management in Neurocritical Care, First Edition. Edited by Edward M. Manno.
© 2012 John Wiley & Sons, Ltd. Published 2012 by John Wiley & Sons, Ltd.

pulmonary edema, to name a few. The first instinct when dealt with this situation as a practitioner is to acutely correct the problem. However, there are some considerations prior to acutely correcting the blood pressure in a hypertensive crisis. The remainder of the chapter will discuss these considerations in relation to neurologic emergencies.

Hypertensive urgencies include 25% of ED medical visits, while hypertensive emergencies are one-third of the cases. CNS complications are the most frequent of the hypertensive emergencies. The hypertensive emergent patient with neurologic sequelae needs urgent attention, with hourly blood pressure monitoring and neurologic examination in an intensive care unit. Prior to discussing blood pressure management, a discussion of cerebral autoregulation and the parental antihypertensive agents will be reviewed.

Cerebral Autogregulation

Cerebral blood flow (CBF) is tightly controlled under the normal conditions, with cerebral perfusion pressures (CPP) ranging from 50 to 150 mgHg. Cerebral perfusion pressures can be calculated from mean arterial pressure (MAP) minus jugular vein pressure (JVP). Intracracranial pressure (ICP) is substituted for JVP under conditions where the ICP is greater than the JVP. Cerebral autogregulation involves arteriole caliber changes in response to changes in the blood pressure; however, there are upper and lower limits that lead to a disruption of this system with resultant ischemia or cerebral edema (Figure 1.1).

The underlying mechanisms of autoregulation that allow for vessel caliber changes are myogenic and metabolic. When the MAP decreases, the arterioles constrict to increase the CBF; however, if hypotension persists beyond the lower limit threshold, resultant cerebral ischemia exists. If the blood pressure continues to increase above the higher limit threshold, the result is hyperemia and cerebral edema. However, in brain dysfunction, the blood–brain barrier and cerebral endothelium is disrupted, leading to leaky blood vessels with subsequent fibrinoid deposition into the cerebral vasculature. This results in vascular narrowing, with compensatory vasodilation. In these circumstances the autoregulation curve follows a more linear pattern with the CBF being dependent on perfusion pressures.

Normal CBF is 50 mL/100 g brain tissue per minute. Reversible injury, occurs at 15–20 mL/100 g/min, and irreversible injury is less than 15 mL/100 g/min. The occurrence of cell death is based on the product of the degree and length of time of ischemia. The ischemic penumbra is vulnerable tissue with impaired autoregulation and low blood flow despite high oxygen extraction. Therefore the tissue is salvageable but has a high risk of becoming ischemic if the blood flow is not recovered in a short period of time.

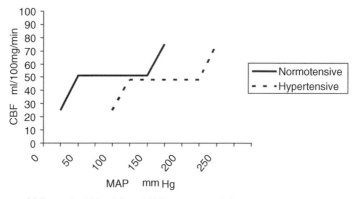

CBF=cerebral blood flow; MAP=mean arterial pressure

Figure 1.1. Autoregulation maintains cerebral blood flow relatively constant between 50 and 150 mmHg mean arterial pressure. The range is right shifted in chronically hypertensive patients. (Reproduced from Ruland and Aiyagari. *Hypertension* 2007; **49:** 978, with permission from Wolters Kluwer Health.)

An EEG is a useful tool for monitoring seizures, but also for detecting cerebral blood flow. In the operation room, older studies have shown that EEG can detect real-time ischemia. When cerebral blood flow reaches 25–30 mL/100 g/min, an EEG demonstrates a change in morphology, amplitude, and frequency. When the CBF decreases to less than 15 mL/1006/min, the EEG becomes isoelectric. The neurons that produce the excitatory post-synaptic potential (EPSP) and inhibitory post-synaptic potential (IPSP) for the electrodes are the same neurons (pyramidal neurons) that are sensitive to hypoxia.

Antihypertensive Agents

Hypertensive emergency can be fatal, and needs prompt treatment. The initial treatment is blood pressure control, in a reliable and controlled fashion, therefore oftentimes, requiring parental agents and arterial blood pressure monitoring. There are multiple classes of antihypertensives one has to choose from; however, there are also many factors to consider prior to administration. The most important factor to consider in neurologic damage is increased intracranial pressure. A few class of antihypertensive agents work via vasodilatory mechanisms, which can lead to further increases in intracranial pressure and potentially further worsening of neurologic injury. Another factor is the onset and duration of action. Rapid fluctuations of hypotension and hypertension can lead to worsening cerebral injury. An agent that can be turned off and out of the system quickly is more desirable in case of an acute hypotensive episode.

Preferred Agents for Hypertensive Emergencies with Brain Dysfunction

Beta Blockers

Labetalol is a selective alpha-1 and nonselective beta antagonist. The onset of action is 2–5 minutes with a peak effect seen in 5–15 minutes. The hypertensive effect can last for 2–4 hours. Beta action does cause a decrease in heart rate but maintains the cardiac output. Similarly, cerebral perfusion is maintained with the use of beta blockers.

Start with a loading dose of 20 mg, increasing subsequent doses from 20 to 80 mg every 10 minutes to the desired effect. In the author's institution, if repeat labetalol boluses do not result in the desired effect, an infusion is initiated starting at 1–2 mg/min.

Esmolol is a short-acting beta antagonist, with no direct affect on the peripheral vasculature. Decreased blood pressure is secondary by decreasing cardiac output. The onset of action is 60 seconds, with a duration of action of 10–20 minutes. esmolol has a unique metabolic profile, being metabolized by red blood cell (RBC) esterases. In the setting of anemia, Esmolol can have a prolonged effect. Due to its pure beta action, caution should be used in patients with COPD. Similarly it should be avoided in patients in decompensated heart failure, due to compromising myocardial function.

Start with a loading dose of 500–1000 µg/kg, with a continuous infusion at 50 µg/kg/min to a maximum of 300 µg/kg/min.

Beta blocker toxicity can present with bradycardia, hypotension, bronchospasm, and hypoglycemia. An ECG can be helpful with detecting PR prolongation. QT prolongation can sometimes be detected. It should be treated with atropine for bradycardia, intravenous fluids and vasopressors for hypotension. Glucagon is a well-known antidote for the treatment of beta blocker toxicity.

Calcium Channel Blockers

Three types of calcium channel blocker exist: dihydropyridines, phenylalkylamines, and benzothiapines. The two types of calcium channels that exist in the vasculature are L-type and T-type.

The action of calcium channel blockers on L-type channels decrease calcium influx, resulting in elevated GMP levels. The elevated GMP levels lead to vascular smooth muscle relaxation, vasodilation and decrease systolic blood pressure.

Nicardipine and clevidipine are the preferred parental calcium blocker agents for cerebrovascular hypertensive emergencies. Nicardipine crosses the blood brain barrier, leading to vasodilation of the small-resistance arterioles, with little to no increases in intracranial pressure. The infusion rate starts at 5 mg/h, with incremental increases 2.5 mg/h every 5 minutes for a maximum infusion 30 mg/h. The onset of action is 5–15 minutes, with duration of action 4 to 6 hours.

Of note, nicardipine has other properties that make it attractive in neurological diseases. It has a high affinity to ischemic cerebral tissue due to the acidic pH of ischemic tissue. Once in the cell, it is transformed to its active form, which may lead to a direct neuroprotective effect.

The effect of nicardipine on intracranial pressure has been studied. Narotam et al. (2008) performed a prospective case-control study of 30 patients with hypertensive emergencies in acute brain disease. Nicardipine was the first-line antihypertensive agent. The results supported the ability to maintain cerebral perfusion pressures above 70 with no increase in ICP and increased parenchymal brain tissue oxygenation.

Clevidipine is a third-generation dihydropyridine calcium channel blocker, recently used in a trial of blood pressure management in acute intracerebral hemorrhage. The drug acts by arteriole dilation, with an onset of action 2–4 minutes and a duration of action 5–15 minutes. It is metabolized by red blood cell esterases. Clevidipine has antioxidative properties as a free-radical scavenger. Continuous infusions start at 1–2 mg/h, and is increased every 90 seconds until blood pressure goals are attained. However, there are a few less attractive features of the drug: 1) infused in a lipid emulsion, requiring triglyceride monitoring during infusion, 2) contraindicated in patients with allergies to soy and egg products, and patients with lipid metabolism disorders, and 3) can develop microbial growth in solution.

Other Agents Used for Hypertensive Emergencies
Nitric Oxide Vasodilators

Sodium nitroprusside is a potent arterial and venous vasodilator, leading to significant preload and afterload reductions. However, ICP elevations can occur in patients with neurologic injury. The first studies were performed on neurosurgical patients under anesthesia revealing vasodilation of large-capacitance vessels leading to vasodilation and increased intracranial pressure. Another negative consequence is cyanide toxicity. Sodium nitroprusside contains 44% of cyanide, which is further metabolized to thiocyanate by the liver, and eliminated by the kidneys. There is an increased risk for cyanide toxicity in patients with liver and kidney dysfunction. Cyanide toxicity leads to cellular hypoxia with neurologic consequences and cardiac arrest. The neurologic consequences include encephalopathy, seizures, and coma. Thus, the use of sodium nitroprusside and other nitric oxide drugs are discouraged due to the potential for worsening intracranial pressures.

Diuretics have no role in the acute management of hypertensive emergencies in neurological and nonneurological disorders due to the increased frequency of volume depletion. Specifically in the neurological patient, altered mental status and dysphagia can further exacerbate volume depletion, leading to increased fluid administration in the acute setting to prevent further dehydration and kidney injury.

A list of medications used to treat acute hypertensive emergencies and the doses used are listed in Table 1.1.

Acute Ischemic Stroke

Blood pressure management in acute ischemic stroke is complex; lowering blood pressure could potentially worsen the infarct size and cause neurologic deterioration, while allowing blood pressures to remain elevated could lead to hemorrhagic transformation and worsening brain edema. If the patient is a thrombolytic candidate or received thrombolytics, pressures excessively elevated can also lead to hemorrhagic transformation. Retrospective analysis of outcomes post-thrombolysis has also shown a worse outcome in

Table 1.1. Antihypertensives and management of neurologic emergencies

Drug	Mechanism of action	Dosage	Onset	Duration	Contraindications
Labetalol	α1β antagonist	Loading doses 20 mg with repeated boluses every 10 min Infusion rates 1–2 mg/min for target blood pressure	2–5 min	2–4 h	Reactive airway disease COPD Decompensated heart failure Bradycardia Second or third degree heart block
Esmolol	β1 antagonist	Loading dose 0.5–1.0 mg/kg Infusion rates 50 ug/kg/min to max 300 ug/kg/min	60 s	10–20 min	Reactive airway disease COPD Decompensated heart failure Bradycardia Second or third degree heart block
Nicardipine	Dihydropyridine calcium channel antagonist	Initial infusion 5 mg/h, increasing 2.5 mg/h every 5 min. Maximum 15 mg/h	5–15 min	4–6 h	Severe aortic stenosis
Clevidipine	Dihydropyridine calcium channel antagonist	Initial infusion 1–2 mg/h, increasing the dose x2 every 90 s to max 32 mg/h	6 min		Defective lipid metabolism disorders
Enalaprilat	ACE inhibitor	Initial dose of 0.625 with repeated doses 1.25 mg every 6 h	15 min	12–24 h	Acute renal failure Acute MI Bilateral renal artery stenosis Pregnancy hyperkalemia
Sodium nitroprusside	Nitric oxide donor leading to vascular smooth muscle relaxation via intracellular second messenger systems	Initial dose of 0.3–0.5 µg/kg/min, increasing 0.5 µg/kg/min for desired effect, max dose 2 µg/kg/min.	1–3 min	1–3 min	Increased intracranial pressures Acute MI Hepatic or renal failure due to increase risk for cyanide toxicity

patients with a history of hypertension, despite the administration of thrombolysis. Studies focusing on blood pressure management in acute ischemic stroke have shown that patients with lower blood pressure on admission had poor outcomes. Vemmos and colleagues examined the mortality at 1 month and 12 months after ischemic and hemorrhagic strokes in relation to admission blood pressures. Their findings concluded that patients with ischemic strokes had the best outcomes with an admission systolic blood pressure of 120–140 mmHg, and patients with an admission systolic blood pressure less than 101 mmHg or greater than 220 mmHg had the highest mortality rates. Therefore, current guidelines recommend maintaining systolic blood pressure less than 220 mmHg and diastolic blood pressure less than 120 mmHg. The majority of patients will reset to normotensive days after their stroke.

In regards to blood pressure augmentation during an acute stroke, there are no good studies to date to support artificially raising blood pressures in an acute stroke. Current recommendations are to discontinue home blood pressure medications and allow the blood pressures to rise to their specific targets irrespective of thrombolysis. If thrombolytics have been instituted, patients need monitoring in an intensive care unit, preferably a neurocritical care unit, with the use of short-acting parental antihypertensives if patients' blood pressures are raised outside their specific targets.

Intracerebral Hmorrhage

Intracerebral hemorrhages represent 15% of all strokes. Despite more sophisticated medical interventions, neurological outcome and mortality continue to significantly impact patients with intracerebral hemorrhages. More specifically, patients with a decrease in the neurologic examination prior to hospital admission have a significantly greater mortality. The initial neurologic deterioration is frequently due to rebleeding of the initial hemorrhage.

There has been poor evidence for guiding blood pressure goals in intracerebral hemorrhages; however, the 2010 Stroke Guidelines has a new recommendation based on two clinical trials: INTERACT and ATACH. The new guidelines state that it is "probably safe" to lower systolic blood pressures less than 140 mmHg if presenting systolic blood pressures are less than 220 mmHg. However, there is insufficient data for a defined blood pressure target.

Kazui et al. (1997) examined the risk factors for hematoma enlargement. 83% of the subjects had a pre-existing diagnosis of hypertension and 76% of the hemorrhages were in classical, hypertensive locations. In their study population, Kazui et al. (1997) noted that admission systolic blood pressure greater than 200 mmHg was significantly associated with hematoma enlargement.

The INTERACT trial randomized 404 patients to intensive blood pressure control of systolic blood pressure less than 140 mmHg or guideline-based blood pressure control of systolic blood pressure less than 180 mmHg for the first 24 hours to 7 days after stroke onset. 296 patients had all CT scans available for full statistical analysis. Patients in the intensive blood pressure lowering group showed reduced hematoma volumes, 3.15 cc and 2.45 cc at 24 and 72 hours, respectively. However, the results have been questioned due to enrollment bias with patients with smaller hemorrhage volumes than previous trials, less acuity based on NIHSS and GCS: NIHSS ranged from 5 to 15 and GCS ranged 13 to 15. The patient population was more diverse due to hospitals located in Australia, China, and South Korea, with possible different etiologies and pathophysiologies involved.

The ATACH trial enrolled 60 patients to one of three tiers of blood pressure goals within 6 hours of symptom onset. The primary outcomes included neurologic deterioration and serious adverse events. They did not analyze hematoma growth or perihematoma edema. The most serious adverse events and neurologic deterioration occurred in the most intensive tier, systolic blood pressure less than 140 mmHg. There was no difference in mortality between the groups. The ATACH trial produced opposite results to the INTERACT trial, showing more negative outcomes in patients with systolic blood pressures less than 140 mmHG after stroke onset. However, as pointed out, ATACH did not analyze the hematoma volumes and both studies had different patient populations.

There is still no correct answer for the low end of systolic blood pressure in intracerebral hemorrhage, or if patients have a worse outcome with high or low blood pressure. We still need high-powered studies to assist with this fundamental management of intracerebral hemorrhage in the acute setting.

✷ TIPS & TRICKS

Elevated blood pressures in intracerebral hemorrhage are frequently seen. However, persistent elevated blood pressures hours after the initial insult can be an indicator of rebleeding or worsening edema. If blood pressures are not responding to antihypertensives, a dose of mannitol or hypertonic saline can be given with close blood pressure monitoring. If blood pressures decrease, the persistent hypertension is an indicator of a worsening edema.

Blood Pressure and Aneurysmal SAH

Subarachnoid hemorrhage is a devastating disease, with a high mortality depending on the severity of the hemorrhage. The risk factors for aneurysmal subarachnoid hemorrhage include hypertension, alcohol use, tobacco use, Adult Polycystic Kidney Disease, and connective tissue disorders. 30-day mortality from subarachnoid hemorrhage has been reported as high as 50% in the AHA guidelines, with the amount of blood, medical comorbidities, and time to treatment being important factors affecting the outcome. However, the goal of this chapter is to discuss blood pressure management in subarchnoid hemorrhage. Blood pressure goals depend on the state of the aneurysm – unsecured or secured.

Many factors are thought to contribute to the risk of rebleeding in the unsecured aneurysm and the literature is currently unsure of the role of blood pressure and rebleeding risk. However, most centers in America will maintain a systolic blood pressure of less than 160 mmHg. The current stroke guidelines do not give an absolute value for blood pressure control; however, they recommend that the blood pressure should be

controlled. For blood pressure management, the use of short-acting parental antihypertensive agents should be instituted.

After securing the aneurysm, the goal of blood pressure focuses on vasospasm management. Vasospasm is the arterial narrowing secondary to inflammatory changes from blood products from the initial subarachnoid hemorrhage. Vasospasm can lead to neurologic deficits by reduced blood flow and ischemic brain tissue, collectively termed "delayed cerebral ischemia." Nimodipine, a calcium channel blocker, is the only proven drug that improves the outcomes in patients with cerebral vasospasm in the context of subarachnoid hemorrhage. Detecting cerebral vasospasm will be discussed in another chapter of this textbook, and the hypertensive management of vasospasm will be discussed only briefly here.

The goal of management of vasospasm is optimizing oxygenation to the brain. During the management of vasospasm, patients require intensive care monitoring for arterial catheterization and triple lumen catheters. This is performed by reducing cerebral metabolism and intracerebral pressures, and optimizing cerebral perfusion. Blood pressure management is paramount in optimizing cerebral perfusion pressures, which is achieved through the use of hemodynamic augmentation. Considerable controversy exists as to the best method to achieve increased cerebral blood flow in the patient with severe vasospasm. However, it is known that during the acute period of vasospasm cerebral autoregulation is disturbed. Methods to induce hypertension or increased cardiac output have been advocated and may require additional intravascular monitoring. When these measures have not resulted in reversal of delayed cerebral ischemia, patients are referred for intra-arterial opening of the vessels.

Dysautonomia in Guillain–Barre Syndrome (GBS)

Dysautonomia is now one of the leading causes of increased mortality in GBS. It is a very common phenomenon in GBS, with increased risk when patients present with respiratory failure, tetraplegia, or bulbar involvement. It is defined as overactivity or underactivity of the sympathetic system, causing either extreme hypertension and tachycardia and/or extreme hypotension and bradycardia.

Cortelli et al. (1990) have found pathological lesions in the intermediolateral horns of the spinal cord, sympathetic chains of white rami, and involvement of glossopharyngeal and vagus nerves in patients with dysautonomia from GBS. Durocher et al. (1980) examined the catecholamine levels of patients with dysautonomia, resulting in the high urinary catecholamine secretion of VMA, HVA, and 5 HIA; high CSF dopamine and serotonin levels; and normal serum serotonin levels.

These studies provide evidence for the underlying sympathetic pathology presenting with the signs of dysautonomia; however, the literature is scarce in the management of dysautonomia. Due to concerns for hypotension, it has been recommended to allow patients to maintain elevated blood pressures unless end-organ failure proceeds. When patients do progress to hypotension, pressors are indicated, and with severe bradycardia, transcutaneous pacing may be indicated.

Hypertensive Encephalopathy

Hypertensive encephalopathy is an entity seen in patients with acute blood pressure elevations in the setting of many clinical scenarios. A later chapter will be dedicated to hypertensive encephalopathy, however, to initiate the discussion on blood pressure management, it should be understood that the parietal-occipital lobes are preferably involved due to the lack of sympathetic innervation in the posterior circulataion. Acute blood pressure elevations lead to hyperperfusion and blood–brain barrier dysfunction, with protein and fluid extravasation leading to vasogenic edema and, sometimes, intracerebral hemorrhage.

The clinical effects of hypertensive encephalopathy include, but are not limited to, headache, altered mental status, visual changes, seizures, and coma.

Blood pressure management needs careful attention, with acute lowering of the MAP by 25% of admission MAP or diastolic less than 100 mmHg within 1 hour, to prevent seizures and intracranial hemorrhage. Short-acting agents are a better choice for tighter blood pressure control.

Bibliography

Anderson CS, Huang Y, Arima H, et al. Effects of early intensive blood pressure-lowering treatment on the growth of hematoma and perihematomal edema in acute intracerebral hemorrhage: The intensive blood pressure reduction in acute cerebral hemorrhage trial (INTERACT). *Stroke* 2010; **41**: 307–312.

Anderson CS, Huang Y, Wang JG, et al. Intensive blood pressure reduction in acute cerebral haemorrhage trial (INTERACT): a randomised pilot trial. *Lancet Neurol* 2008; **7**: 391–399.

Antihypertensive Treatment of Acute Cerebral Hemorrhage (ATACH) investigators. Antihypertensive treatment of acute cerebral hemorrhage. *Crit Care Med* 2010; **38**: 637–648.

Bartynski WS. Posterior reversible encephalopathy syndrome, Part 2: Controversies surrounding pathophysiology of vasogenic edema. *Am J Neuroradiol* 2008; **29**: 1043–1049.

Bath P, Chalmers J, Powers W, et al. International Society of Hypertension (ISH): Statement on the management of blood pressure in acute stroke. *J Hypertens* 2003; **21**: 665–672.

Cortelli P, Contin M, Lugaresi A, et al. Severe dysautonomic onset of Guillain–Barre syndrome with good recovery. A clinical and autonomic follow-up study. *Ital J Neurol Sci* 1990; **11**: 159–162.

Durocher A, Servais B, Caridroix M, et al. Autonomic dysfunction in the Guillain–Barre syndrome. Hemodynamic and neurobiochemical studies. *Intens Care Med* 1980; **6**: 3–6.

Haas AR, Marik PE. Current diagnosis and management of hypertensive emergency. *Semin Dial* 2006; **19**: 502–512.

Hund EF, Borel CO, Cornblath DR, Hanley DF, McKhann GM. Intensive management and treatment of severe Guillain–Barre syndrome. *Crit Care Med* 1993; **21**: 433–446.

Kazui S, Minematsu K, Yamamoto H, et al. Predisposing factors to enlargement of spontaneous intracerebral hemorrhage. *Stroke* 1997; **28**: 2370–2375.

Lee KH, Lukovits T, Friedman JA. "Triple-H" therapy for cerebral vasospasm following subarachnoid hemorrhage. *Neurocrit Care* 2006; **4**: 68–76.

Mocco J, Rose JC, Komotar RJ, Mayer SA. Blood pressure management in patients with intracerebral and subarachnoid hemorrhage. *Neurosurg Clin N Am* 2006; **17** (Suppl 1): 25–40.

Morgenstern LB, Hemphill JC, 3rd, Anderson C, et al. Guidelines for the management of spontaneous intracerebral hemorrhage: A guideline for healthcare professionals from the American Heart Association/American Stroke Association. *Stroke* 2010; **41**: 2108–2129.

Narotam PK, Puri V, Roberts JM, et al. Management of hypertensive emergencies in acute brain disease: evaluation of the treatment effects of intravenous nicardipine on cerebral oxygenation. *J Neurosurg* 2008; **109**: 1065–1074.

Ntaios G, Bath P, Michel P. Blood pressure treatment in acute ischemic stroke: a review of studies and recommendations. *Curr Opin Neurol* 2010; **23**: 46–52.

Powers WJ, Zazulia AR, Videen TO, et al. Autoregulation of cerebral blood flow surrounding acute (6 to 22 hours) intracerebral hemorrhage. *Neurology* 2001; **57**: 18–24.

Qureshi AI. Antihypertensive Treatment of Acute Cerebral Hemorrhage (ATACH): rationale and design. *Neurocrit Care* 2007; **6**: 56–66.

Qureshi AI, Palesch YY, Martin R, et al. Effect of systolic blood pressure reduction on hematoma expansion, perihematomal edema, and 3-month outcome among patients with intracerebral hemorrhage: results from the Antihypertensive Treatment of Acute Cerebral Hemorrhage study. *Arch Neurol* 2010; **67**: 570–576.

Rincon F, Mayer SA. Clinical review: critical care management of spontaneous intracerebral hemorrhage. *Crit Care* 2008; **12**: 237.

Rose JC, Mayer SA. Optimizing blood pressure in neurological emergencies. *Neurocrit Care* 2004; **1**: 287–299.

Ruland S, Aiyagari V. Cerebral autoregulation and blood pressure lowering. *Hypertension* 2007; **49**: 977–978.

Talbert RL. The challenge of blood pressure management in neurologic emergencies. *Pharmacotherapy* 2006; **26**: 123S–130S.

Vemmos KN, Tsivgoulis G, Spengos K, Zakopoulos N, Synetos A, Manios E, Konstantopoulou P, Mavrikakis M. U-shaped relationship between mortality and admission blood pressure in patients with acute stroke. *J Internal Medicine* 2004; 255(2): 257–265.

Airway Management in the Neurological and Neurosurgical Patient

Michael J. Souter

Department of Anesthesiology & Pain Medicine, and Department of Neurological Surgery, University of Washington, Department of Anesthesiology, Harborview Medical Center, Seattle, WA, USA

Introduction

The term "airway" is an oversimplification of an anatomical canal that serves many functions. This anatomical and functional distribution of the oropharynx, nasopharynx, and larynx allow for communication, mastication, swallowing, and continuous respiration.

A set of complex interconnections and reflex arcs, located diffusely throughout the brain, control the musculature of the pharynx and larynx. The diffuse distribution of these control centers and the complexity of the integration needed to coordinate these centers provide insight into the ease with which the airway can be compromised.

⚜ SCIENCE REVISITED

A masticatory center is located in the dorsolateral and anterolateral frontal cortex. Reflex swallowing is mediated by the lateral precentral gyri, postcentral gyri, supplementary motor area, insular cortex, and basal ganglia. These areas modulate the activity of the cranial nerve nuclei in the pons and brain stem. The control of respiration itself is dynamically affected by mechanical receptors in the upper airways, as well as neurohumoral and chemoreceptor activation.

Airway difficulties are often encountered after traumatic brain injury with over 50–70% of head injuries experiencing associated facial injury. Airway compromise can arise from associated soft tissue swelling (often with frightening speed of onset), hemorrhage and secretions, and fractured teeth. Maxillary fractures are associated with facial edema and pharyngeal blood, but may also disrupt the skeletal support of the oropharyngeal musculature leading to reduced pharyngeal dimensions, and increased susceptibility to obstruction.

Focal neurological insults to the midbrain, cerebellum, or brain stem (injury, stroke, demyelination) can adversely affect airway control centers. More diffuse disease (injury, infection, inflammation, ischemia) can threaten consciousness with the consequent impairment of cough and swallow.

A decreased level of consciousness can lead to a reduction in airway muscle tone which may lead to airway obstruction. Obstruction of the airway results in hypoxia, hypercarbia, and

Emergency Management in Neurocritical Care, First Edition. Edited by Edward M. Manno.
© 2012 John Wiley & Sons, Ltd. Published 2012 by John Wiley & Sons, Ltd.

further diminishes airway control. Subsequent increase in respiratory effort will generate negative intrathoracic pressure and further collapse airways.

> ⚠ CAUTION
>
> Care must be taken when attempting to alleviate an obstructed airway. Intervention itself can create the possibility of iatrogenic injury to the airway. Lip laceration, bleeding, dental damage, and tongue edema can all result from the use of poor technique in airway instrumentation, while repeated unsuccessful attempts at intubation may induce edema of the pharynx, epiglottis, and cords.

Assessment

The urgency of intubation should consider the neurological condition of the patient and the potential effects of hypercarbia and/or hypoxia. Either will lead to cerebral vasodilation with subsequent increases in cerebral blood volume and intracranial pressure.

The need for intubation requires clinical judgment. Some indications for intubation are listed in Table 2.1. They can often coexist to amplify the urgency. Once the decision has been made to intubate the patient, a number of questions will need to be addressed.

- What precautions are required?
- How easy is it to maintain a patent airway?
- How easy is it to intubate the airway?

Preparation

In ideal circumstances endotracheal intubation should be a structured and orderly process. This requires a thorough preprocedural preparation that should include optimization of the environment, with suction equipment connected, tested, and immediately at hand. Oxygen, tubing, and an inflatable bag are essential, and a broad range of endotracheal tubes should also be available. A 7 mm tube will fit most adults and induce minimal flow restrictions. Larger tubes (8 mm),

Table 2.1. Indications for intubation

In the field *and* in hospital
• Immediate (life-threatening hypoxia likely)
o persistent airway obstruction despite airway insertion
o inability to bag/mask ventilate
• Urgent
o Glasgow Coma Scale < 8
o protection of the lower respiratory tract from aspiration
o anticipated occlusion by:
• edema (burns, angioedema)
• hematoma
• displacement of a laryngotracheal fracture
In-hospital
• control of intracranial pressure by controlling pCO_2
• therapeutic ventilation for hypoxemia/hypercarbia in:
o pulmonary contusion/edema/infection
o flail chest
• therapeutic and diagnostic procedures in combative or uncooperative patients
• high metabolic demand from work of breathing

however, do allow for easier suctioning and/or bronchoscopy if needed.

Removing the gastric content prior to intubation is desirable since most patients will not have been fasting in an emergency situation. Existing gastric tubes should be drained, but insertion at this point is not recommended. The operator should identify and assign assistants to pass equipment, to monitor vital signs and oxygenation, to immobilize the head in case of cervical spine injury (see below), or to apply cricoid pressure. This maneuver presses on the only competent cartilage ring in the trachea to compress and close the esophagus. Its utility is controversial with some arguing that it increases the difficulty of intubation without adding additional protection.

If cricoid pressure is to be utilized, the clinician should carefully inform the assistants (a) on exactly how and when to apply this pressure, and (b) to stop only when instructed. A rapid sequence induction should be the norm in most urgent or emergent cases, with good quality of sedation, facilitated by adequate muscle relaxation.

Induction drugs comprise hypnotics, analgesics, and paralytics. Their use should consider the desired speed of action, hemodynamic consequences, and side effects. For hypnotics, there is little to choose between thiopental (3–5 mg/kg) and propofol (2–3 mg/kg), as both cause similar degree of reduction in cardiac output. Etomidate (0.3 mg/kg) has the least hemodynamic effect while ketamine (1–2 mg/kg) will maintain or even increase blood pressure with attendant tachycardia. There is controversy regarding the effect of etomidate upon adrenal suppression, which tempers its use. Midazolam (0.3–0.4 mg/kg) may be used for induction, causing slight hypotension but less than propofol or thiopental. All agents will produce transient apnea but ketamine has the least effect, followed by etomidate. Fentanyl (1–2 μg/kg) can synergistically reduce hypnotic doses at induction and serves to decrease subsequent coughing, as well as respiration. It has the most favorable hemodynamic profile of the opiates, and is consequently the most useful at induction. Paralytic drugs provide the highest quality relaxation for intubation, but at the risk of significant apnea and hypoxia if the airway can be neither intubated nor ventilated. However, coughing or moving on intubation does have consequences and the risk/benefit must be carefully considered for each patient. The shortest duration of effect is 3–5 minutes for succinyl choline (1–1.5 mg/kg). This well established agent has the fastest overall onset (45 s) but does have limitations due to hyperkalemia seen in burns and the recently immobilized (more than 72 hours since burn/immobility). Vecuronium, rocuronium or cistracurium are acceptable alternatives, with rocuronium (1 mg/kg) swiftly working at 60 seconds post injection, but the effect lasting longest to 60 minutes. Cisatracurium (0.15 mg/kg) and vecuronium (0.1 mg/kg) take 2–3 minutes respectively to work, but effects last for 30–40 minutes. There is no evidence of any protective effect of any of the above agents upon the brain.

Support of the Airway

Supporting the airway with bag mask ventilation is a greatly undervalued skill which is intrinsic to intubation, and is lifesaving when done correctly. Its application allows for the collection of neces-

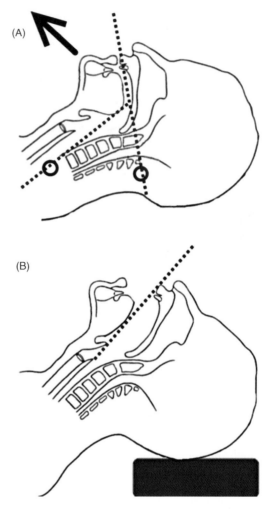

Figure 2.1. (A) Airway with oropharyngeal and tracheal axes, prior to positioning. Note the effect of gravity on the tongue. Axes will rotate around the lower cervical spine and atlanto-occipital joint (marked with circles). (B) Airway with orotracheal axis, after positioning.

sary resources and personnel to safely secure the airway. Competence requires frequent practice. An examination of Figure 2.1(A) illustrates that, in the supine position, there is a tendency for both the mandible and tongue to fall back against the posterior pharyngeal wall obstructing the airway. The application of jaw lift is achieved by applying upward pressure at the angle of the mandible, without moving the neck (crucial in circumstances of trauma without cervical spine clearance), or pushing the tongue into the pharynx. The insertion of an oropharyngeal airway will help to position the tongue anteriorly, particularly in the edentulous. An inexperienced provider can support the jaw with the fourth and fifth fingers of each hand, sealing the mask to the face with the thumb and first finger, while an assistant squeezes the bag. There are various bags available, but the easiest to use are the self-inflating types, e.g. Laerdal or Ambu.

Difficult Mask Ventilation

Difficult mask ventilation (DMV) can be defined as an unassisted provider being unable to keep the arterial pulse oximetry saturations above 92%, or to avoid and correct for signs of inadequate ventilation during positive-pressure mask ventilation. Identifying a potential DMV patient is an important step in addressing the adequacy of available resources and alternate strategies prior to any procedure.

A useful mnemonic to identify a possible DMV patient is O-B-E-S-E, where O = Obese patient (BMI > 26), B = Bearded patient, E = Elderly patient (age > 55), S = Snoring history of patient, and E = Edentulous patient. These factors have all been independently associated with DMV and may alert the clinician to possible difficulty. This can ensure the availability of adjunct devices or personnel prior to starting nonemergent intubation or before extubating patients with existing endotracheal tubes. Alternatively, it may indicate that difficult airway devices should be kept by the bedside if a need for airway support is anticipated later.

☠ CAUTION

Care should be taken with the insertion of any airway device since a rough technique can lacerate gums, tongue, and palate and cause bleeding which will exacerbate difficulty in any situation. Most oropharyngeal airways should be inserted with the end curving up, until the arch of the curve just enters the mouth, then rotated 180 degrees and

advanced. This helps to negotiate the tongue, which might otherwise obstruct the insertion.

Nasal airways can be used with caution, having a higher frequency of bleeding on insertion. They are relatively contraindicated in facial injuries or basal skull fractures.

In circumstances of difficulty in bag/mask ventilation, there are now a large variety of supraglottal airways, which all offer the ability to bring the airway closer to the epiglottis, and stay securely seated in the pharynx. These devices can be used for emergent support and ventilation, but should rarely be a first-line treatment. They do not protect the lungs from aspiration, and indeed may obscure the presence of vomitus in the pharynx.

Difficult Airway Intubation

Difficult intubation has a similar prevalence (1–8%) to that of difficult mask ventilation (3–8%). It has been defined by a need for more than three attempts at intubation or attempts that last longer than 10 minutes. This latter metric is more applicable to the elective pre-oxygenated patient in the operating room, as opposed to the emergent patient in the field, ER, or ICU.

Difficult intubation is usually associated with limited exposure of the glottis on direct laryngoscopy. In examining Figure 2.1(A and B), it can be seen that the degree of exposure correlates to the ability to align the pharyngeal, laryngeal, and oral axes.

The alignment involves a series of maneuvers, with the laryngeal axis moved "forward" by flexing the lower cervical spine, and the oral and pharyngeal axes moved "backward" by opening the mouth with an extension of the atlanto-occipital joint. Soft tissues can be managed by inserting a laryngoscope to displace the tongue to the left and, simultaneously, compressing the tongue into the submandibular space. The mandible is then lifted forward in the direction of the arrow. The final step is either (a) placement of the laryngoscope blade (Macintosh type) anterior to the epiglottis in

Table 2.2. Mallampati grading

Class I	visualization of the soft palate, fauces, uvula, and both anterior and posterior pillars
Class II	visualization of the soft palate, fauces, and uvula
Class III	visualization of the soft palate and the base of the uvula
Class IV (difficult)	the soft palate is not visible at all

the vallecula, which will exert pressure on the hyoepiglottic ligament lifting the epiglottis to expose the cords (in a manner akin to a stepping on a pedal bin to lift the lid), or (b) lifting the epiglottis with the laryngoscope blade itself (Miller type), to expose the cords directly. In this maneuver, the blade should *never* be used to lever the lower airways on the fulcrum of the upper jaw as this may induce trauma and does not improve the view.

A variety of clinical scoring assessments to predict the success of direct laryngoscopy have been described. The best known is the Mallampati score introduced in 1985. This requires patient cooperation, which limits its utility in the ICU, but may be available from a previous assessment. Classification from grade I to IV is associated with an increasing difficulty of intubation (and also of mask ventilation). Table 2.2 shows the scores obtained on examining the soft tissues of the pharynx in a seated patient with his mouth open and silent extension of the tongue.

Specificity and sensitivity for this scale range widely in the literature, from 40 to 60% and 70 to 95% respectively.

A number of other attributes have been identified to assess the patient for difficult intubation. These include decreased the thyromental distance (TMD), limited neck extension, the mentohyoid distance, the sternomental distance, the distance between incisors, and the inability to protrude lower incisors forward beyond the upper incisors (upper lip bite test). While this latter test has the highest sensitivity in recent studies,

the sensitivities and specificities for all these parameters vary widely.

★ **TIPS & TRICKS**

Finger width is not consistent! While 3 fingerbreadths has been a traditionally employed measure to define a "normal" thyromental distance, the variation in clinician finger size is considerable, and a better measure is to define a 6.5 cm distance as the threshold for normality. Some even suggest a height/TMD ratio (greater than 23.5) to offset size bias. This may also help with race and gender.

★ **TIPS & TRICKS**

The Upper Lip Bite Test (ULBT) classes are defined as:

Class I: Lower incisors can bite the upper lip above the vermilion line
Class II: Lower incisors can bite the upper lip below the vermilion line
Class III: Lower incisors cannot bite the upper lip; this correlates with difficult intubation.

Given the limitations of any single parameter, several authors have attempted to define composite scores based on an amalgam of physical and historical characteristics.

The LEMON score summates a variety of anthropometric features along with somatypic characteristics and neck mobility. It uses four "look" criteria, three "evaluate" criteria, the presence of airway obstruction, and neck mobility (Table 2.3). It has been evaluated in an emergency department setting.

If a test cannot be performed the patient receives a score of zero for that criterion.

The maximum airway assessment score possible is 10 and the minimum 0. In prospective studies, the "evaluate" criteria could be fully assessed in 90% of the emergency department

Table 2.3. LEMON score grading

Observation	Trigger	Point score
(L)ook externally	• facial trauma • large incisors • a beard or moustache • large tongue	0–4 points
(E)valuate the 3-3-2 rule	• Interincisor distance in fingers no less than three finger breadths (3) • Hyoid-mental distance no less than three finger breadths (3) • Thyroid notch to floor of mouth no less than two finger breadths (2)	0–3 points
(M)allampati score	Greater than 2	0–1 point
(O)bstruction?	e.g. epiglottis, peritonsillar abscesses, traumatic swelling	0–1 point
(N)eck mobility	Limited neck flexion or extension (includes cervical collar)	0–1 point

population and "Mallampati" was assessable in 57% of patients. Due to this limited utility a modification has been suggested to drop the Mallampati element and use a 9-point maximum. The designers of the LEMON score accept the inherent subjectivity of observations but stress the speed and sensitivity of the composite score.

The adequacy of any view itself should be recorded for future information. This can be expressed on the Cormack–Lehane scale – from 1 to 4 depending on the decreasing visualization of vocal cords past epiglottis or tongue (Figure 2.2).

Intubation itself should occur in an environment that has been as prepared as possible. There are a number of accessory devices that should be considered for inclusion in a "difficult airway kit" and it is the practice in many institutions to have one of these available in each unit or floor.

★ **TIPS & TRICKS**

SUGGESTIONS FOR A DIFFICULT INTUBATION KIT

Spare laryngoscope Handles (x 2)

Macintosh & Miller blades: sizes ranging through 2, 3, and 4

Eschmann "bougie" catheter or Cook Exchange catheter (not a ventilation device)

Laryngeal mask device: sizes ranging through 3, 4, and 5

McGill Forceps: for guiding tubes through the cords and/or removing obstructing foreign bodies

Spare CO_2 detector

The simple bougie is a straight catheter that can be used in circumstances where there is a restricted view of the glottis. The smaller size of

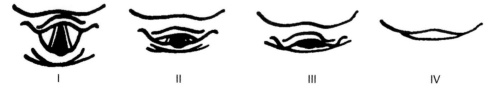

I II III IV

Figure 2.2. Cormack & Lehane classification of glottal view at intubation.

the Eschmann bougie allows placement through the glottis under direct vision, and an endotracheal tube can then be passed over the bougie. The Cook exchange catheter serves the same purpose but allows for a modest flow of oxygen. This flow is insufficient to allow ventilation but can maintain oxygenation in some circumstances. A malleable stylet inside the endotracheal tube can be molded to curve toward a larynx aligned anteriorly to the axis of view.

Other aids to difficult intubation range from articulated laryngoscope blades (McCoy) with the ability to exert more lift at the epiglottis, to video assisted laryngoscopes. The intubating laryngeal mask (ILMA) is a specially adapted supraglottic airway. When positioned above the glottis, an accompanying endotracheal tube can be inserted through the ILMA into the trachea. The ILMA can then be removed or remain in place.

Fiberoptic intubation is commonplace in the operating room and can transform an "impossible" intubation into a practical procedure. There are some caveats. There is a clear learning curve, which must be practiced in elective situations. Fiberoptic procedures require an anesthetized airway, by either local or general anesthesia, as their use in a poorly anesthetized airway can provoke secretions, bleeding, laryngospasm, coughing, and hypoxia. Fiberoptic visualization can also be compromised by the presence of secretions and/or bleeding. In these circumstances a "macroscopic" view of direct laryngoscopy is probably superior.

Once the endotracheal tube has been placed through the glottis, markers on some makes of tube signify an appropriate depth of insertion when positioned at the level of the vocal cords. The gold standard for tracheal placement is CO_2 detection. Portable devices are available that reflect either color change or display measured CO_2 concentrations as a waveform and/or numerical value. Relying on chest movement and breath sounds are inadequate and have fooled many experienced providers.

"When to Stop?"

This is an important question to ask during any difficult intubation. There are many case reports of experienced practitioners losing awareness of hypoventilation and hypoxia in the patient, in their desire to place an endotracheal tube. For

this reason, after three unsuccessful attempts to intubate, the ASA task force recommends proceeding through their difficult airway algorithm (*irrespective of the experience of the provider*).

A failure of intubation does not necessarily mean a failure to ventilate. A return to bag/mask ventilation may allow time for oxygenation to recover and accessory resources to be gathered. The intubator must acknowledge that repeated attempts will make airway edema, secretions, or bleeding more likely and could thus render ventilation difficult. While an experienced clinician may have more success at intubation than a novice, this advantage is eroded by increasing the number of attempts. For this reason, the intubator must give careful thought to stopping attempts while the situation is still under control. The intubator may want to seek assistance, while determining whether (a) changes in the patient's position may improve the intubating conditions; (b) the insertion of a supraglottic airway is appropriate; or (c) a cricothyroidotomy is required.

A modified difficult airway algorithm (adapted from the ASA version) is presented in Figure 2.3. Its utility outside of the operating room is to lead the clinician through a series of rescue maneuvers, with a clear indication for a surgical airway when required.

If the situation is uncontrolled (i.e. the patient's condition is deteriorating), there should be a low threshold to proceed straight to cricothyroidotomy. Since most providers are inexperienced in the surgical placement of cricothyroidotomy, an inexperienced provider should practice assembling the materials for this life-saving maneuver, and rehearse the practical steps below.

1. A 14 g intravenous cannula can be placed through the cricothyroid membrane into the trachea, the needle withdrawn and the catheter connected to the empty barrel of a 5 mL syringe with the plunger removed.
2. This syringe barrel will serendipitously connect to a 7 mm or 7.5 mm ET tube connector. This allows connection to a standard oxygen source for *small-volume ventilation*.
3. It is important to understand that this is a *life-saving maneuver* and will buy time in an extreme situation until a definitive surgical airway is secured.

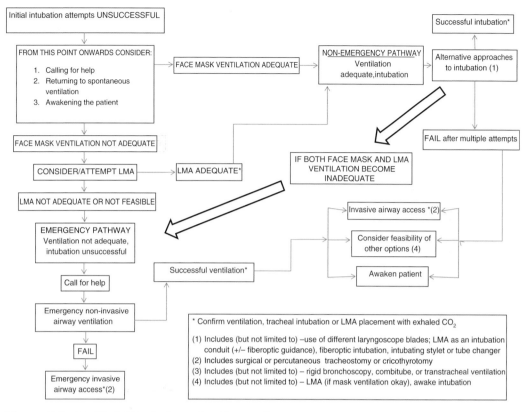

Figure 2.3. Modified difficult airway algorithm – reflecting urgent/emergent practice. (Modified from an report by the American Society of Anesthesiologists Task Force on Management of the Difficult Airway, 2003, with permission from Lippincott Williams & Wilkins.)

4. There are two important limitations to note:
   (a) This method will oxygenate but not ventilate;
   (b) To avoid the risk of barotrauma, insufflated gas must be allowed to escape from lungs through the trachea and mouth.

Suspected Cervical Spine Injury and Intubation

Trauma patients should always be considered to have a cervical spine injury until otherwise cleared. This requires immobilization of the neck during intubation by an assistant in either of two positions:

(a) stabilizing the head from "above" by crouching to the side of the intubator and support-ing the head between outstretched hands with the fingers stabilized on the patient's shoulders; or

(b) stabilizing from "below" with the fingers on the mastoid processes and the thumbs on the zygomas with wrist and forearms bracing the patient's neck on the shoulders.

Once the neck is supported, the front of the collar is removed to allow mandibular movement. There should be no flexion or extension of the neck, as this has been associated with iatrogenic spinal cord damage. The back of the collar may be left on. The head is left in a neutral position for laryngoscopy. Although this significantly adds to the difficulty of the procedure and increases the chances of failure, it is a necessary precaution against injury. Once the ET tube is placed, the collar is reassembled.

Extubation

We must briefly consider the appropriate circumstances for extubation. As most neurological patients will fail extubation due to airway issues, careful attention should be paid to the competency of the airway before extubating.

The possibility of swelling should be considered along with an assessment of the ability of cough and gag reflexes to protect the airway. This must be performed in the context of the overall neurological state of the patient. Swelling of the airway and cords is a noted problem that leads to secondary reintubation. A recent randomized trial demonstrated that steroids administered after an unsuccessful extubation, were clinically effective in facilitating subsequent extubation.

The question of how much reflex protection is required for the avoidance of aspiration is controversial. Giving a *trial* of extubation is important with appropriate warning to staff, patient, and family that reintubation may be required.

Conclusion

The ABCs must never be forgotten when supporting neurological function. The dependence on artificial airways and the potential complications demand significant expertise. The practitioner must take every opportunity to practice in elective circumstances, in order to be able to avoid insult and/or save lives in situations of urgency and stress.

References

Coplin WM, Pierson DJ, Cooley KD, et al. Implications of extubation delay in brain-injured patients meeting standard weaning criteria. *Am J Respir Crit Care Med* 2000; **161**: 1530–1536.

Cormac RS, Lehane J, Difficult tracheal intubation in obstetrics. *Anaesthesia* 1984; **39**: 1105–1111.

Khemani RG, Randolph A, Markovitz B. Corticosteroids for the prevention and treatment of post-extubation stridor in neonates, children and adults. *Cochrane Database Syst Rev* 2009 Jul **8**;(3): CD001000.

Langeron O, Masso E, Huraux C, et al. Prediction of difficult mask ventilation. *Anesthesiology* 2000; **92**: 1229–1236.

Levitan RM, Kinkle WC, Levin WJ, et al. Laryngeal view during laryngoscopy: a randomized trial comparing cricoid pressure, backward-upward-rightward pressure, and bimanual laryngoscopy. *Ann Emerg Med* 2006; **47**: 548–555.

Neilipovitz DT, Crosby ET. No evidence for decreased incidence of aspiration after rapid sequence induction. *Can J Anaesthesiol* 2007; **54**: 748–764.

Practice guidelines for management of the difficult airway: An updated report by the American Society of Anesthesiologists Task Force on Management of the Difficult Airway. *Anesthesiology* 2003; **98**: 1269–1277.

Ramachandran K, Kannan S. Laryngeal mask airway and the difficult airway. *Curr Opin Anaesthesiol* 2004; **17**: 491–493.

Reed MJ, Dunn MJ, McKeown DW. Can an airway assessment score predict difficulty at intubation in the emergency department? *Emerg Med J* 2005; **22**: 99–102.

Scrase I, Woollard M. Needle vs surgical cricothyroidotomy: a short cut to effective ventilation. *Anaesthesia* 2006; **61**: 921–923.

Yentis SM. Predicting difficult intubation – worthwhile exercise or pointless ritual? *Anaesthesia* 2002; **57**: 105–109.

Yildiz TS, Solak M, Toker K. The incidence and risk factors of difficult mask ventilation. *J Anesth* 2005; **19**: 7–11.

Traumatic Brain Injury and Intracranial Hypertension

Iain J. McCullagh[1] and Peter J.D. Andrews[2]

[1]Department of Anaesthesia, Critical Care and Pain Management, University of Edinburgh, Edinburgh, UK
[2]Centre for Clinical Brain Sciences, University of Edinburgh, Edinburgh, UK

Introduction

Epidemiology and Economic Assessment

The epidemiology of traumatic brain injury (TBI) is difficult to describe accurately due to inconsistencies in the definition and classification of the condition. It is estimated (2010) that there are more than 1.1 million new hospitalized cases of TBI per annum in the USA, Japan, France, Germany, Italy, Spain, and the UK. Cautious estimates show the incidence of hospitalized cases of TBI to be higher than the annual incidence of some cancers, epilepsy, HIV/AIDS, multiple sclerosis, and spinal cord injury. Importantly, there remains no treatment that is able to prevent the cascade of physiological events (known as the secondary injury process) that leads to neuronal cell death and is believed to result in poorer functional recovery. The overall annual incidence of TBI in the USA is 506.4 per 100,000, and each year approximately 50,000 patients die after TBI.

The major risk factors for TBI in the USA are age, gender, and low socioeconomic status. Persons at the extremes of age have the highest incidence rates, 900 and 659 per 100,000 for those younger than 10 and older than 74 years, respectively. The rate among men is nearly twice that of women.

The global extent of TBI is unknown, but the incidence of TBI that is severe enough to warrant medical attention or result in death is estimated to be more than 9.5 million (1990). Population-based studies from South Africa, India, and Taiwan suggest higher rates in developing countries, predominantly attributed to traffic injuries.

The consequences of TBI for patients, their families, and caregivers are financial, emotional, and psychological. Traumatic brain injury carries a high economic impact due to neurological deficit(s), including loss of memory and executive function, and behavioral disturbances that result in dependency and chronic disability necessitating lifelong care. It is estimated that 43.3% of TBI victims in the USA have residual disability one year after injury and recent estimates of the prevalence of US civilian residents living with disability following hospitalization with TBI is 3.2 million. The global burden of TBI approximates the combination of both cerebrovascular and depressive illness disorders. Though progress has been made to reduce the healthcare burden of TBI, including significant reductions in mortality over the last 20 years, it remains a major public health issue worldwide. For this reason

Emergency Management in Neurocritical Care, First Edition. Edited by Edward M. Manno.
© 2012 John Wiley & Sons, Ltd. Published 2012 by John Wiley & Sons, Ltd.

there has been a significant campaign to improve the outcomes of TBI patients, using evidence-based guideline management strategies developed by international panels of multidisciplinary experts. It is hoped that a review of the current evidence will focus research on those areas of TBI management that lack evidence-based guidelines. The primary responsibility of critical care physicians managing TBI patients is to minimize secondary brain injury. In this chapter we will explore the practical ways this may be achieved during the patient's journey from the prehospital arena, to recovery in a critical care unit.

Classification of Traumatic Brain Injury

The heterogeneity of TBI is considered to be one of the principal barriers to finding effective therapeutic interventions. In October 2007, the National Institute of Neurological Disorders and Stroke, with support from the Brain Injury Association of America, the Defense and Veterans Brain Injury Center, and the National Institute of Disability and Rehabilitation Research, convened a workshop to outline the steps needed to develop a reliable, efficient, and convincing classification system for TBI that could be used to link specific patterns of brain and neurovascular injury to appropriate therapeutic interventions.

Currently, the Glasgow Coma Scale (GCS) is the primary criterion for classification of TBI. While the GCS is extremely useful in the clinical management and prognosis of TBI, it does not provide specific information about the pathophysiological mechanisms that are responsible for neurological deficits and are targeted by interventions. Due to the limitations of the GCS, it has been proposed that a new, multidimensional classification system should be developed for TBI clinical trials.

In clinical practice, classification has generally been based on clinical indices of injury severity at presentation. The 15-point GCS (Teasdale et al., 1974) is the most commonly used neurological injury severity scale for adults, because of its high inter-observer reliability and generally good clinimetric and prognostic capabilities (Narayan et al., 2002). Mild injury is defined as GCS 15–13, moderate by GCS 12–9, and severe by GCS <9.

Development of Treatment Strategies

The goals of prehospital care for TBI are to stabilize patients for transport, to triage those with mass lesions and impending cerebral herniation, and to prevent secondary insults and injury. Increased intracranial pressure (ICP), cerebral edema, loss of cerebral autoregulation, and alterations in brain metabolism are inherent sequelae of the primary brain injury. External and/or iatrogenic events may exacerbate secondary injury processes. Patients with multiple trauma frequently incur injuries that compromise cardiopulmonary status, and they are therefore particularly vulnerable to secondary injury. These insults are common and are independent predictors of poor outcome in patients with TBI. Well-organized trauma systems with robust protocols for field resuscitation, transport, and trauma facility destination ensure reproducible high-quality prehospital care. Advances in prehospital practice are a key target for further improvements in long-term functional outcomes following TBI, not least because of the proximity to the time of impact.

Several guidelines for the treatment of TBI exist. The most frequently cited are those produced by a joint project of the Brain Trauma Foundation (BTF), the American Association of Neurological Surgeons and the Congress of Neurological Surgeons (AANS/CNS joint section on Neurotrauma and Critical Care). These evidence-based guidelines were first published in 1995 with the latest iteration published in 2007. The majority of the clinical trials reviewed were small and methodologically poor and therefore most guidelines are based on class II or III evidence with no *positive* level I recommendations. Despite these limitations, many experts regard them as a standard of care. It is hoped that adherence to a guideline-based approach for TBI care will improve outcomes through standardization; and this approach may also facilitate large-scale intervention trials in the future.

These guidelines support the monitoring and management of raised ICP in the intensive care unit. The influence of these guidelines is evidenced by the fact that between 1995 and 2005 the use of ICP monitoring has increased from 32 to 78%. This approach makes it possible to calculate, and subsequently manage, the cerebral perfusion pressure (CPP) which is an essential parameter in preventing secondary brain injury.

Intracranial Pressure and Cerebral Blood Flow

The understanding of a raised ICP originated from Scotland and is summarized in the principles credited to Edinburgh Professors Monro (1783) and Kellie (1824), which state that, once the fontanelles and sutures are closed:

1. the brain is enclosed in an inflexible case of bone of a fixed volume;
2. the brain parenchyma is nearly incompressible (80% of cranial contents are brain parenchyma, by volume approximately 1500 mL);
3. the volume of the fluid in the cranial cavity is therefore nearly constant (10% blood and 10% cerebrospinal fluid (CSF)); and
4. a continuous outflow of venous blood from the cranial cavity is required to make room for the continuous incoming arterial blood, keeping the overall cerebral blood volume (CBV) near constant.

The importance of these observations is that the skull cannot accommodate any additional volume and, therefore, when the system is challenged by additional volume, the displaceable contents (i.e. venous blood and CSF) are initially moved outside the skull by a process called compression elimination. When these physiological volumetric compensatory mechanisms become exhausted, the ability to accommodate any further new volume is impaired and intracranial compliance is reduced. The final effect is a raised ICP. The cranium can tolerate only a 25 mL rise in total volume acutely before the ICP rises sharply (Figure 3.1) but if the rise in volume is slow, it can tolerate up to 150 mL. The effect of any mass lesion is also strongly dependent on its site, with posterior fossa lesions causing obstruction of CSF flow and hydrocephalus, and subsequent brainstem compression with supratentorial lesions causing transtentorial herniation and uncal herniation (Figure 3.2).

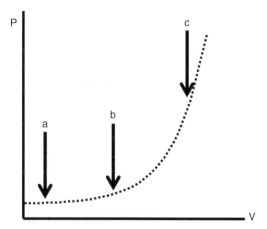

Figure 3.1. Intracranial compliance is the change in volume (δV) per unit change in pressure (δP). Compliance is the inverse of elastance ($\delta P/\delta V$) sometimes known as the volume-pressure response (VPR). *Compliance ($C = \delta V/\delta P$) = 1/Elastance = 1/VPR.* [a = normal intracranial compliance; b = reduced intracranial compliance; and c = exhaustion of volumetric compensatory mechanisms and critical reduction in compliance.] (Modified from Langfitt, 1964.)

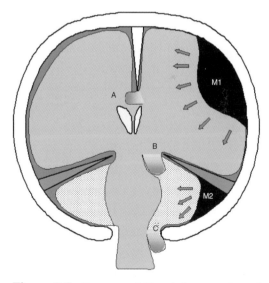

Figure 3.2. Transtentorial herniation (A) and uncal herniation (B) is produced by expanding supratentorial lesions (M1), as opposed to posterior fossa lesions (M2) which lead to both hydrocephalus via obstruction of CSF flow and tonsillar herniation (C) which will ultimately progress to brainstem death if no intervention occurs.

The relationship between intracranial pressure and volume is termed "compliance." Compliance varies with age, being higher in older patients due, in part, to a smaller volume of brain parenchyma. This may result in increased tolerance to space-occupying lesions, at least for a short period of time.

Cerebral Blood Flow

In healthly patients cerebral blood flow (CBF) is autoregulated and remains approximately 40–50 mL/kg/min between a mean arterial pressure (MAP) of 50–120 mmHg. Within this global measure, the metabolic demands of subregions of the brain create differential flow by several different mechanisms, generally termed "autoregulation." These mechanisms include metabolic feedback, with areas of high demand producing metabolites that increase the local blood supply. Neurogenic mechanisms probably play only a small role, via the autonomic nervous system, but autoregulation is not yet fully elucidated.

There is a near linear relationship between $PaCO_2$ and CBF within the physiological range. In TBI patients with raised ICP, an elevated $PaCO_2$ will result in an increase in CBF and CBV and a further rise in ICP. Loss of vasoreactivity to $PaCO_2$ is a poor prognostic sign. The relationship with oxygen tension is such that CBF is unaltered until a low PaO_2 threshold of approximately 50 mmHg is reached and arterial oxyhemoglobin desaturation occurs, thereafter vasodilation occurs to preserve the cerebral oxygen supply, potentially increasing CBV and ICP.

In the severely injured brain these autoregulation mechanisms function less efficiently and this has led to the modern practice of targeting a surrogate of global cerebral perfusion in an attempt to ensure an adequate cerebral oxygen supply.

Cerebral perfusion pressure (CPP) is equal to MAP minus ICP, and is a determinant of cerebral perfusion. Therefore, as ICP increases in the injured brain, MAP must also increase in order to maintain CPP. This relationship is fundamental principle of modern management of the injured brain. CPP is targeted in order to maintain the oxygen supply to the injured areas of the brain that have the potential to recover, and to prevent further damage. Areas of brain tissue adjacent to focal injury are especially vulnerable

to secondary injury. However, it is important to control both ICP and mean arterial pressure carefully within a balanced approach to CPP management.

Initial Management of TBI

All TBI patients are "trauma patients," including those thought to have an isolated brain injury. All should be assessed from head to toe, front and back, as a significant proportion of TBI patients will have multiple injuries that benefit from management in a systematic and appropriately triaged manner. This requires a team approach, with a team leader to coordinate their actions and prevent errors in prioritization. Most often this will involve a "trauma team" approach with appropriate early involvement of neurosurgery. The American College of Surgeons has developed a training program that guides therapy in this situation; the "Advanced Trauma Life Support" (ATLS) approach is now an international standard. The most life-threatening injuries are given an order of priority: airway, breathing, circulation, disability, and exposure. A detailed description is beyond the scope of this text but several important points should be made:

- All patients with a GCS score less than or equal to 8 (after resuscitation) should be intubated and mechanically ventilated (i.e. all severe TBI patients); many practitioners would recommend intubating all patients not obeying commands.
- *Avoidance of hypoxemia and hypoventilation is vital if secondary brain injury is to be avoided.*
- A primary survey (exposure) is undertaken early, identifying visible injuries and assessing carefully for concealed injuries in order to plan potential surgical management.

Management of the airway is inextricably linked to management of the cervical spine. In head-injured patients it should be assumed that the cervical spine is unstable until proven otherwise. This makes airway management in these patients potentially dangerous as movement of the cervical spine may result in catastrophic injury. Rapid sequence intubation with manual inline stabilization of the cervical spine is the recommended approach. This should be undertaken by experienced personnel with difficult airway equipment immediately available. An appropriately fitted cervical collar should be worn afterward and the patient "log rolled" until the cervical spine is "cleared." Direct laryngoscopy is likely to cause a significant and sudden elevation in blood pressure and heart rate, which leads to a rapid rise in ICP (as auto-regulation is impaired). If ICP is already elevated or unknown, then uncal herniation (coning) is a serious risk. Intravenous opiates (fentanyl/sufentanil/alfentanil) or lidocaine should be given prior to the anaesthetic induction agents as these can obtund this response. Induction agents should be chosen for hemodynamic stability and familiarity.

After intubation, prolonged hyperventilation may be harmful. It reduces CBF, by a combination of reduced venous return and cardiac output, and cerebral vasoconstriction. It is therefore important to use an end tidal carbon dioxide monitor both during and after the insertion of an endotracheal tube, and assess frequent arterial blood gas measurements. The BTF guidelines include a recommendation to administer two doses of broad spectrum antibiotics around the time of intubation to reduce pneumonia rates, but this is based on one small, single centre and unblinded study and many clinics do not perform this intervention.

Physiological Targets During and After Resuscitation

It is vital to maintain an adequate CPP and arterial oxygenation during resuscitation in order to ensure adequate cerebral oxygenation. PaO_2 greater than 100 mmHg or $SpO_2 > 90\%$ should be targeted. This SpO_2 target is included in the BTF guidelines but is based upon data from retrospective studies and the level of SpO_2 that harms the brain is unclear.

Volume resuscitation with 0.9% saline should occur concurrently with the initial assessment. The goal is to maintain a state of euvolemia. Assessment of volume status may be assisted by the insertion of a central venous catheter (CVC) but only a *dynamic* assessment of volume responsiveness is useful, e.g. after a fluid challenge. However, a CVC is also useful to deliver vasopressor agents such as norepinephrine (levophed), neosynephrine (phenylephrine), epinephrine, or vasopressin, though boluses of phenylephrine can be given peripherally. These agents may be

required to maintain the systolic blood pressure (SBP) above 90 mmHg, especially if sedative agents are being infused. This is a minimum SBP target in the initial phase even though it is likely that it will be associated with a MAP of less than 60 mmHg. Currently, there are no data to support a higher target, though many experienced clinicians will target a CPP of 60 mmHg (see below). Therapy may require some individualization when multiple trauma is evident and hemorrhage is not yet controlled.

☙ CAUTION

Evidence has clearly correlated that even short periods of hypotension worsen outcome. It is crucial that meticulous care be taken to avoid these episodes during all phases of resuscitation and subsequent management.

Indices of coagulation should be checked and actively treated, keeping the INR less than 1.4 and the platelets greater than $75 \times 10^3/mm^3$. The hemoglobin should also be maintained at a level greater than 8 gm/dL to ensure an adequate oxygen-carrying capacity. This is a controversial topic and many experts will target a higher hemoglobin level, particularly if monitors of cerebral oxygenation suggest an inadequate oxygen supply.

Finally, plasma glucose levels should be frequently checked to avoid even short periods of hypoglycemia (*ABC... Don't Ever Forget Glucose!*).

Decisions regarding non-neurosurgical surgical intervention should be made rapidly with the aim of terminating hemorrhage and managing any perforated viscus. Definitive surgery should be delayed until hemodynamic stability is present.

The surgical management of intracranial mass lesions depends on the nature of the lesion as defined by the initial CT scan, but does not generally take place until other hemorrhage has been controlled. Thereafter, the neurosurgical intervention will depend upon site, size, and mass effect of the lesion, and often includes placement of a ventriculostomy. Further guidance can be found in standard neurosurgical texts. Referral to neurosurgery should not be delayed longer than 2 hours from presentation. This is mandatory if the initial CT is abnormal or if an indication for ICP monitoring is present.

General ICU Care of TBI Patients

The intensive care management of TBI is a multidisciplinary process and high-quality nursing care is the cornerstone of this endeavor. Short periods of hypotension or hypoglycemia can be disastrous and can only be managed effectively by experienced and appropriately trained staff. The whole process is aimed at the prevention of secondary brain injury. It is vital that patients have the head of their beds elevated at least 30 degrees at all times and that a patient's head and neck are kept in a neutral position. Obstruction of jugular venous flow, including endotracheal tube ties, must be avoided (though internal jugular CVCs are acceptable) as this will lead to an increase in CBV and subsequent increases in ICP. Poorly fitted cervical collars can also cause this problem; the sizing and fitting of these should be meticulous, and their removal a priority if appropriate.

> ### ★ TIPS & TRICKS
>
> Family members of TBI patients come under unimaginable strain during the care of their close relative. Initial contact with medical staff should include a realistic and consistent assessment of potential positive or negative outcomes. One must not underestimate how long these conversations will be remembered by those who experience them. Above all remember to LISTEN attentively, and not simply pass on information.

Adequate nutrition should be provided, with nonpharmacologically paralyzed patients requiring around 140% of basal metabolic requirements (Harris Benedict Equation). Those who have received a muscle relaxant require 100% of basal metabolic requirements. Skin, bowel, and oral care should be meticulously managed, with oral care usually including antiseptic gel to reduce bacterial colonization. CVCs should be managed within strict local protocols to minimize infection.

Prophylaxis against deep venous thrombosis is important but minimal data are available to guide its use. The administration of subcutaneous heparin is delayed for at least 72 hours or more when intracranial hemorrhage is present, with some authors recommending a much greater delay of up to 14 days. Heparin is not normally used when an ICP monitor is in situ. Pneumatic sequential compression devices and TED stockings should be used in all patients unless contraindicated. Prophylaxis against stress ulceration is usually provided with ranitidine until patients are fully established on enteral nutrition.

Virtually all mechanically ventilated patients receive sedative and/or analgesic medications at some stage. Regimens for TBI patients generally include short-acting agents such as propofol in a dose of 2–5 mg/kg/h combined with an opiate such as fentanyl, alfentanil, or remifentanil. Shorter acting agents may reduce time to liberation from ventilation when elevated ICP has resolved. Most patients should have sedative infusions reduced or stopped at least daily to minimize drug accumulation and incidence of oversedation.

> ### ★ TIPS & TRICKS
>
> Propranolol reduces agitation in the post-sedation phase of care in the hyperadrenergic patient. It is the only intervention to reduce assaults on staff.

Early post traumatic seizures (PTSs) have not been definitively associated with worse outcomes, however TBI patients do have a relatively high incidence of PTSs. Consequently, the BTF guidelines recommend either phenytoin or valproate for at least 7 days. Regular monitoring of plasma levels is required to ensure therapeutic levels.

Monitoring of ICP

ICP Waveform. Brain tissue pressure and ICP increase with each cardiac cycle resembling an arterial pressure wave. The ICP pressure waveform has three distinct components that are related to physiological parameters (Figure 3.3). The first peak (P1) is the "percussive" wave and is due to arterial pressure being transmitted from the choroids plexus to the ventricle. It is sharply peaked and consistent in amplitude. The second wave (P2), called the "tidal" wave, is thought to be due to brain tissue compliance. It is variable, indicates cerebral compliance, and generally increases in amplitude as compliance decreases; if it elevates or exceeds the level of the P1 waveform there is a marked decrease in cerebral compliance. P3 is due to the closure of the aortic valve and therefore represents the dichrotic notch.

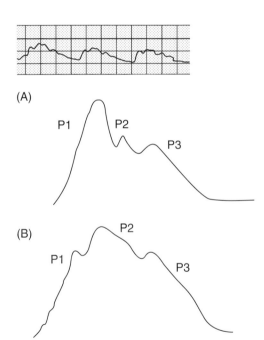

Figure 3.3. P1 is the "percussive" wave, due to arterial pressure transmitted from the choroids plexus to the ventricle. It is sharply peaked and consistent in amplitude. P2 is called the "tidal" wave, due to brain tissue compliance and generally increases in amplitude as compliance decreases; if it elevates or exceeds the level of the P1 waveform there is a marked decrease in cerebral compliance. P3 is due to the closure of the aortic valve.

Brain Distortion. There are several factors that have to be taken into consideration when a mass lesion within the cranial cavity starts to expand. One is distortion of the brain. Because of the viscoelastic properties of the brain, the tissues adjacent to the lesion will tend to flow away from it, with axial movement of the brain leading to brain displacement. Although the local properties of the brain are important, the major factor responsible for spatial compensation is a reduction in the volume of intracranial CSF. The progression is, therefore, local deformity with displacement of CSF, shift and distortion of the brain and, eventually, in the intact cranium, the appearance of internal herniation (Figure 3.2). This represents the displacement of brain tissue from one intracranial compartment to another or into the spinal canal. This herniation occurs due to the development of compartmentalized acute pressure gradients.

The BTF guidelines suggest that it is desirable to monitor ICP in the following patients: all patients with a GCS score of less than 8 and an abnormal CT scan (level II recommendation); patients with severe TBI and a normal CT who, if they are over 40, have (or have had) a blood pressure less than 90 mmHg systolic, or have unilateral or bilateral motor posturing (level III recommendation). These recommendations cannot be proscriptive to cover every clinical scenario. It is important to remember that a persistently raised ICP greater than 20 mmHg is associated with poor outcome, and this will not be detectable without ICP monitoring.

> ⋆ **TIPS & TRICKS**
>
> Never make assumptions about the quality of survival in the acute phase of care. Unless the injury is obviously unsurvivable (penetrating injury, etc.)

ICP Monitoring Device Technology

The ventricular fluid catheter attached to an external strain gauge is considered the gold standard. These devices can be re-zeroed at any time and can also be used to drain CSF, thus reducing raised ICP. These devices can be inserted at the time of surgery or in a separate procedure. They are accurate but carry an increased risk of infection. The zero reference for arterial and ICP transducers is the external auditory meatus, facilitating CPP measurement.

Intraparenchymal monitors, using micro strain gauge transducers or fibre optic technology, are commonly used and can be inserted at the bedside via an intracranial bolt. Several manufacturers produce them, and most manifest negligible drift which is independent of the duration of monitoring. This is important as they cannot be re-zeroed once inserted. There are several other invasive and noninvasive methods of measuring ICP available, and more information can be found in the Bibliography at the end of this chapter. However, the overall safety of ICP monitoring devices is excellent, with clinically significant complications (e.g. infection and hematoma) occurring infrequently.

Brain Oxygenation Monitors

It is possible to measure focal brain tissue PO_2, and have this measure guide care. The physiological concept behind cerebral oxygen monitoring is that the $P_{br}O_2$ value accurately represents the balance between oxygen delivery and oxygen consumption, and that changes in $P_{br}O_2$ will therefore reflect pathophysiological alterations. Five observational studies have reported that low $P_{br}O_2$ values in patients with TBI predict a poor outcome when an initial $P_{br}O_2 < 10\,mmHg$ for $\geq 30\,min$, and in those with $P_{br}O_2 < 15\,mmHg$ lasting $\geq 4\,h$. In addition, both the level and duration of low $P_{br}O_2$ correlated with mortality. The question whether these measurements can be used to improve outcome has not been well studied. When arterial oxygen tension is about 100 mmHg and the hemoglobin concentration is stable, these monitors provide data on cerebral perfusion (oxygen tension being the marker of perfusion). Manipulation of $PaCO_2$, CPP and hemoglobin can then be targeted to maintain an established perfusion or oxygenation goal.

ICP Monitoring and Management

There are no randomized-controlled trials comparing ICP treatment thresholds. Herniation and

pupillary changes are known to occur at levels as low as 18mmHg. The BTF guidelines suggest, in a level II recommendation, that an ICP of 20 mmHg should be the treatment threshold.

✋ CAUTION

In a patient with raised intracranial pressure, posture is all important. Never forget a neutral head position and head-up tilt, exaggeration of this tilt will often bring about rapid resolution of raised intracranial pressure. This position should be used in the patient that is considered euvolemic. If this position is used in the hypovolemic patient, cerebral vasodilation may occur in response to a drop in cerebral perfusion pressure. The supine position, e.g. for CVC insertion, may be hazardous especially if an intracranial pressure monitor is not in situ.

Cerebral Perfusion Pressure

The BTF guidelines recommend the avoidance of a CPP less than 50 mmHg, even for a brief duration. The sole RCT found no difference in outcomes in 189 adults with severe TBI treated according to either a CPP-based or an ICP-based algorithm. It should be noted that this study was neither blinded nor properly randomized and the groups were also managed differently in respect of $PaCO_2$. There was a significant increase in incidence of acute respiratory distress syndrome in the CPP > 70 mmHg group, partly due to excessive fluid administration, and this condition is associated with greater difficulty in arterial oxygenation and control of CO_2. This observation has led to concerns with targeting a higher CPP. The generally accepted CPP target is 60 mmHg and is pragmatically based on a 10 mmHg increase above a level thought to be harmful.

Treatment of Raised ICP

All patients with ICP monitoring and management following TBI will be mechanically ventilated and should receive comprehensive "Stage 1" interventions before considering any escalation of therapeutic intensity (Figure 3.4). Escalation to "Stages

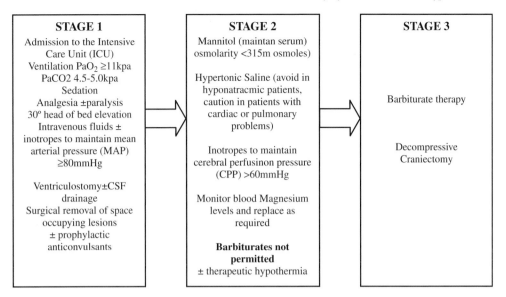

STAGE 1	STAGE 2	STAGE 3
Admission to the Intensive Care Unit (ICU) Ventilation PaO$_2$ ≥11kpa PaCO2 4.5-5.0kpa Sedation Analgesia ±paralysis 30° head of bed elevation Intravenous fluids ± inotropes to maintain mean arterial pressure (MAP) ≥80mmHg	Mannitol (maintan serum) osmolarity <315m osmoles) Hypertonic Saline (avoid in hyponatracmic patients, caution in patients with cardiac or pulmonary problems) Inotropes to maintain cerebral perfusinon pressure (CPP) >60mmHg	Barbiturate therapy Decompressive Craniectomy
Ventriculostomy±CSF drainage Surgical removal of space occupying lesions ± prophylactic anticonvulsants	Monitor blood Magnesium levels and replace as required **Barbiturates not permitted** ± therapeutic hypothermia	

Figure 3.4. Summary of tiered therapies to be used in control of raised ICP, as used in the Eurotherm3235 trial (ISRCTN 34555414). Tier one therapies must be provided meticulously until raised ICP is no longer a concern.

2 and 3" therapy is required in 10–15% of ICP-monitored patients after TBI (Eurotherm3235 Trial data). There are very few data to support any of the interventions listed, but evidence based medicine supports their *utility* for ICP reduction. A large RCT, www.Eurotherm3235Trial.eu, is examining titrated hypothermia in patients with TBI and raised ICP.

Hyperosmolar Therapy

The two commonly used agents are mannitol and hypertonic sodium chloride. Mannitol is a sugar alcohol molecule which is given in a dose of 0.25–1.0 g/kg intravenously over 15 minutes. It is believed to exert two separate effects. Firstly, it reduces blood viscosity and improves CBF (this effect is rapid). Secondly, there is an effect on cerebral water volume, reducing the water content of structurally normal brain and ICP. The evidence base for this therapy has been weakened by the recent withdrawal of a Cochrane systematic review due to concerns with trial data. Current recommendations remain that mannitol is an effective therapy to reduce ICP but the effect of long-term or high-dose therapy is not clear. If using this therapy, serum osmolality must be regularly measured (up to 4 times daily) and kept below 320 mOsm/L. Volume status must also be carefully assessed.

Hypertonic sodium chloride is widely used, but currently the BTF guidelines do not give any recommendations for this therapy due to a paucity of trial data. The dose is 250 mL of 3% saline over 30 minutes. Other centers have used varying concentrations of hypertonic solutions. Serum sodium should be kept below 160 mmol/L during therapy and it should not usually be used in patients who are hyponatremic.

Hyperventilation

Previously hyperventilation was seen as beneficial to TBI patients, but this is no longer accepted. The PaCO$_2$ should never be below 25 mmHg. This is a level II recommendation in the BTF guidelines, based on a single RCT that was underpowered and not blinded. Most consider that normocapnia is the accepted target (i.e. a PaCO$_2$ between 35 and 45 mmHg), especially in the early stages of injury, when CBF may already be substantially reduced. Hyperventilation should only be instituted in patients without ICP monitoring if signs of a critically raised ICP are seen, such as a dilating pupil or a Cushing response (sudden bradycardia or tachycardia and hypertension). In

ICP-monitored patients, hyperventilation may be used briefly for acute control of ICP where it is usually effective. However cerebral oxygen monitors such as brain tissue oxygen tension should be used if hyperventilation is considered for more prolonged periods.

Induced Hypothermia

Hypothermia is thought to be of benefit in reducing brain water content, modulation of cerebral repair mechanisms, and alterations in brain free-radical concentrations after injury. It also reduces global cerebral energy demands and may limit the production of excitatory neurotransmitters. The evidence in this area comes from six systematic reviews, two of which were positive ($n = 2096$ in total) and demonstrated a reduction in ICP during cooling.

☝ CAUTION

While hypothermia appears to be very effective in lowering ICP, the largest study to date did not demonstrate any benefit from hypothermia in a head trauma population. Clinical trials have not been able to demonstrate a benefit of hypothermia after head trauma even when hypothermia is applied soon after head trauma. However, subgroup analysis has raised the possibility that patients with hematomas removed surgically may benefit from hypothermia. More work with this subgroup will need to be performed.

Barbiturates

Patients in whom ICP is refractory to other therapies can be treated with barbiturates. This is a level II recommendation in the BTF guidelines. The long-term effect of these drugs is not clear and all the studies performed were in an era when prophylactic hyperventilation, fluid restriction, and steroids were routine therapies. They may provoke, or worsen, cardiovascular instability and are immunosuppressive. Barbiturates also reduce cerebral oxygen consumption significantly and may reduce cellular damage by a variety of mechanisms. Adequate volume status and careful monitoring of MAP is vital if this therapy is to be used and titration to EEG mandatory.

Neuromuscular Blocking Agents

These drugs can be used in patients with difficult to control ICP, and adequate levels of sedation must be assured prior to use. All will reduce muscle tone, prevent coughing, and respiratory efforts. This usually reduces ICP at least initially, but these agents also increase the risk of critical illness polyneuropathy which may have an effect on the long-term functional status. When used, a train of four monitor that assess muscle response to a standard stimulus should be used, and two twitches out of four should be seen.

Steroids

Steroid administration is controversial in many areas of critical care. Current evidence, based mainly on the 2004 Corticosteroid randomization after severe head injury (CRASH) trial is against therapy with steroids in TBI. This trial, which was stopped early (but still recruited >10,000 patients) demonstrated a mortality increase in the steroid-treated group (21% vs. 18%), but included moderate and even mild TBI.

Decompressive Craniectomy

Decompressive craniectomy is an option in treating refractory intracranial hypertension. No clear evidence exists regarding its utility, and although the procedure has been used for decades many questions have still to be answered. A most recent trial suggested that decompressive craniectomy was not useful for this population but has been criticized for its severe methodological limitations. Hopefully, ongoing randomized trials will help our understanding of the role and utility of this procedure in future. In the interim, when faced with refractory intracranial hypertension that is likely to produce a fatal outcome, clinicians should consider surgical decompressive craniectomy. Prior to making this decision, clinicians must have used all the medical therapies available against intracranial hypertension (in patients considered appropriate for surgical intervention.

Conclusion

It is to be hoped that, over the coming years, high-quality clinical trials will be conducted which clarify some of the contentious issues discussed above. Until then, as with all modern intensive care, outcomes are maximized when routine matters are attended to in detail, and adverse events are avoided.

Bibliography

Andrews PJ, Citerio G, Longhi L, et al. Neurointensive care and emergency medicine. (NICEM consensus on neurological monitoring in acute neurological disease. Section of the European Society of Intensive Care Medicine.) *Intens Care Med* 2008 Aug; **34(8)**:1362–1370. [Epub 2008 Apr 9.]

Andrews PJ, Citerio G. Intracranial pressure. Part one: historical overview and basic concepts. *Intens Care Med* 2004 Sep; **30(9)**:1730–1733. [Epub 2004 Jul 9.]

Cairns CB, Maier RV, Adeoye O, et al. (Roundtable External Participants and Roundtable Steering Committee and Federal Participants). NIH Roundtable on Emergency Trauma Research. *Ann Emerg Med* 2010 Nov; **56(5)**:538–550.

Citerio G, Andrews PJ. Intracranial pressure. Part two: Clinical applications and technology. *Intens Care Med* 2004 Oct; **30(10)**:1882–1885. [Epub 2004 Jul 9. No abstract available. PMID: 15243685.]

Clifton GL, Miller ER, Choi SC, et al. Lack of effect of induction of hypothermia after acute brain injury. *New Engl J Med* 2001 Feb; **344(8)**:556–563.

Langfitt TW, Weinstein JD, Kassell NF, Simeone FA. Transmission of increased intracranial pressure. I. Within the craniospinal axis. *J Neurosurg* 1964 Nov; **21**:989–997.

Maas AI, Roozenbeek B, Manley GT. Clinical trials in traumatic brain injury: past experience and current developments. *Neurotherapeutics* 2010 Jan; **7(1)**:115–126.

Narayan RK, Michel ME, Ansell B, et al. Clinical trials in head injury. *J Neurotrauma* 2002 May; **19(5)**:503–557.

Sahuquillo J, Arikan F. Decompressive craniectomy for the treatment of refractory high intracranial pressure in traumatic brain injury. *Cochrane Database Syst Rev* 2006 Jan; **25(1)**: CD003983.

Steiner LA, Andrews PJ. Monitoring the injured brain: ICP and CBF. *Br J Anaesthesiol* 2006 Jul; **97(1)**:26–38. [Epub 2006 May 12. Review.]

Teasdale G, Jennett B. Assessment of coma and impaired consciousness. A practical scale. *Lancet* 1974 Jul; **2(7872)**:81–84.

The Brain Trauma Foundation. The American Association of Neurological Surgeons. The Joint Section on Neurotrauma and Critical Care. Resuscitation of blood pressure and oxygenation. *J Neurotr* 2000 Jun–Jul; **17(6–7)**:471–478. Review.

Critical Care Management of Acute Spinal Cord Injury

Edward M. Manno

Neurological Intensive Care Unit, Cleveland Clinic, Cleveland, OH, USA

Introduction/Background

Acute spinal cord injury (ASCI) is a devastating injury with significant consequences. The most recent statistics for the United States estimate an incidence of 40 cases per million. Spinal cord injury mainly occurs in young men, who account for 81% of the presentations. The average age of injury has been slowly increasing with the aging of the population, and is now 40.2 years. Motor vehicle accidents are responsible for approximately 50% of the injuries. Falls and diving accidents contribute approximately 20% of injuries, while sports-related accidents and violence (mostly gunshot wounds) account for the remainder.

ASCI can be divided into primary and secondary injury. Primary injury represents damage to the spinal cord directly from cord compression. This occurs due to herniation from disks, bones, or ligaments. Forces that distract, or tear, local structures occur with flexion, extension, dislocation, and other rotational injuries. Secondary injuries represent changes that occur after the primary process. These injuries are attributed to secondary systemic and local vascular insults that lead to the development of focal edema and ischemia. The primary focus of acute care for spinal cord injury patients is to limit the amount of secondary damage. It is estimated that up to 25% of the final neurological deficit can be attributed to changes that occur after the initial insult.

An initial assessment requires a thorough neurological examination and documentation of the level of injury. Several grading systems exist for defining the location and severity of neurological injury after spinal cord injury. The most common classification system employed is the American Spinal Injury Association (ASIA) grading scale. This classification of impairment is based on the assessment of the neurological level that is involved and whether the injury is complete or incomplete. An ASIA impairment classified as an A represents no motor or sensory function in the sacral segments S4–5; B is an incomplete lesion that maintains normal sensation but no motor function below an identified level and includes the sacral S4–5 segments; C is an incomplete lesion with preserved motor function (identified as at least antigravity strength in more than half of the muscles) below an identified neurological level of injury; D is a similar incomplete lesion but has only half of the muscles below the lesion with preserved antigravity muscle strength; and E represents normal muscle and sensory function.

Emergency Management in Neurocritical Care, First Edition. Edited by Edward M. Manno.

Initial Assessment, Stabilization, and Transport

Spinal cord trauma is oftentimes accompanied by head or multisystem trauma. In 20% of patients, spinal cord injury occurs over multiple and often noncontiguous levels. This mandates that immediate immobilization must happen at the scene of the accident. Emergency personnel should assess the need for immediate spine immobilization based on several potential risk factors for cervical spinal injury in a trauma patient. These include patients with an altered mental status, evidence of intoxication, a suspected fracture or distracting injury, a focal neurological deficit, and spinal pain or tenderness.

Immobilization is accomplished through the use of a cervical collar and support blocks to prevent appendicular movements with restraints. The patient must be placed on a rigid backboard for stabilization and all transportation on and off of this backboard must include inline stabilization and maintenance of spinal alignment. This is accomplished through the technique of "log rolling" a patient, but as this maneuver places the patient at risk for pressure ulcers and aspiration, care must be taken to monitor respiratory function and skin breakdown. Measures should be initiated to prevent skin breakdown if prolonged immobilization is anticipated.

Guidelines should be developed to triage patients to centers with the most experience of treating ASCI patients. A growing body of evidence and opinion suggests that secondary complications due to ASCI are decreased in centers that are experienced in caring for these patients. Transfer to a level I trauma center (as defined by the American College of Surgeons) should be strongly considered, particularly in patients with multisystem trauma.

In patients with documented ASCI, neuro-imaging should be performed based on the resources of the institution and the ability to perform testing safely. Most institutions will start with a three-view cervical spine series. To increase the sensitivity for detecting subtle lesions or in areas difficult to visualize with plain imaging, many centers will include CT imaging of the spine. Spiral or helical CT is commonly used in the setting. If a cervical fracture is identified the entire spine should be imaged. Magnetic resonance imaging (MRI) is performed in areas of the spine that are known to be, or are suspected of being, injured. MRI is also used to identify ligamentous, disk, or bony injury in the obtunded or ventilated patient. In a patient with focal tenderness a fracture should be suspected and imaging should be focused on this area. Spinal clearance of the spine is left to the neurosurgeon or attending physician responsible for the acute trauma. In patients with potential or confirmed ASCI, a comprehensive trauma survey should be performed. When screening for cerebrovascular injury in a patient with ASCI, the use of CT or MR angiography should be considered.

Acute Management

Any trauma patient should have an immediate trauma assessment and survey. Any trauma patient that needs endotracheal intubation should be considered to have a cervical neck injury.

The level of injury will have a significant influence on the respiratory pattern of the patient. Patients with high cervical spinal cord injury will only be able to use their spinal accessory muscles to initiate respiration. These patients will almost always require emergent endotracheal intubation. Patients with injury below cervical levels 3–5 will leave phrenic innervation to the diaphragm variably affected, as this respiratory pattern may be more stable. These patients may have a particular respiratory pattern where the abdominal contents move outward with inspiration while the chest wall moves inward. This unique respiratory pattern represents the normal movement of the diaphragm; however, due to loss of thoracic intercostal muscle innervation, the chest will move inward with inspiration. The resultant tidal volume that is generated will be limited. Subsequently, these patients may require endotracheal intubation.

★ TIPS & TRICKS

Body positioning of the patient may assist respiration, depending upon the level of cervical spine injury. Patients with high cervical spine injuries should be sitting up (once the neck is stabilized). In this position the accessory muscles are best positioned to generate whatever small tidal volumes are possible.

Patients with lower cervical spinal cord damage and intact diaphragmatic movement will breathe easier when supine. This allows the abdominal contents to compress the dome of the diaphragm upward, which can increase air exchange. Patients that are awake and alert can often vocalize the position that is best for them.

The endotracheal intubation of patients with cervical neck injury requires considerable skill and expertise. Care must be taken to limit movement of the cervical spine. Awake, fiberoptic intubation is the preferred method if time and facilities allow. If fiberoptic equipment is not available, intubation should occur with rapid sequence induction and manual inline stabilization.

Careful consideration must be given to both the induction agent and the neuromuscular blocking agent. Propofol is commonly used for induction, however this may aggravate hypotension in the setting of ACSI. Etomidate, which has less hemodynamic effects but suppresses cortisol release, has been associated with acute adrenal crisis and some authors have suggested using supplemental corticosteroids with its use. Succinylcholine is the preferred neuromuscular blocker if used within the first 48 hours of injury, but it should be avoided if significant muscle damage is suspected due to the possibility of developing life-threatening hyperkalemia. Nondepolarizing neuromuscular blockers should be used in these circumstances. It is important that a complete neurological assessment be performed prior to using nondepolarizing neuromuscular blockade. If the patient does not require mechanical ventilation, it is prudent to obtain baseline pulmonary function tests that can be used for comparison during later studies.

Many patients after ASCI will develop hypotension. There are multiple possible etiologies that must be initially evaluated, including acute hemorrhages, aortic dissections, pneumothorax, adrenal insufficiency, pericardial tamponade, sepsis, etc. Evaluation may prove difficult since the ACSI patient may not be able to localize or identify the pain. Most patients will require imaging of the chest, abdomen, and pelvis to evaluate for these possibilities.

A significant number of ASCI patients will develop hypotension secondary to neurogenic shock. Sympathetic denervation to the vasculature is the responsible mechanism for neurogenic shock after ASCI. It is common in quadraparesis/plegia or in high-level paraparesis/plegia. Loss of sympathetic innervation to the peripheral circulation leads to arteriolar vasodilation and venous pooling of blood. In addition loss of cardiac sympathetic innervation (T1–4), results in unopposed parasympathetic-induced bradycardia and decreased systemic vascular resistance. Higher cord levels involved after ASCI appear to be related to worse hypotension.

Experimental data strongly suggests that hypotension is deleterious to spinal cord perfusion and worsens outcomes, therefore the aggressive treatment of hypotension after ACSI is warranted. The initial treatment for ASCI is fluid resuscitation. Vasodilation, which is common after ASCI, will require fluid resuscitation to maintain intravascular volume. Care must be taken to avoid overresuscitation since there are some concerns that this may aggravate spinal cord edema. Swan Ganz intravascular monitoring may be helpful in selected circumstances. An initial base deficit or lactate level can also be uses to assess the initial degree of shock and response to fluid resuscitation.

Vasopressors will often be needed to maintain adequate blood pressure and spinal cord perfusion, and the choice of vasopressor agent will depend upon the clinical situation. Phenylephrine is a pure alpha agonist and will lead to peripheral vasoconstriction. It is a good choice if vasodilation is the main source of hypotension as it will increase central venous pressures and increase venous return. Norepinephrine and dopamine possess both alpha and beta adrenergic qualities that will increase peripheral vascular resistance and cardiac rate and contractility. They are the preferred agents when symptomatic bradycardia or cardiac involvement occurs post-ACSI.

The use of corticosteroids as a neuroprotective agent post-ASCI have been controversial. There are three prospective randomized double-blind trials that have evaluated the use of high-dose methylprednisolone infusion after ASCI. Initially there was great enthusiasm for the use of corticosteroids since later trials seemed to suggest an improved one-year outcome. The initial enthusiasm waned, however, with closer scrutiny of the data and statistical methods, and concerns over medical complications with steroid use. Advocates against the use of steroids point out that the utility of steroids remains unproven and that the risks of medical complications should negate their use. Advocates for the use of steroids suggest that concerns over medical complications are overstated with close attention to medical detail, and that the current data, while not conclusive, continues to support its use.

There are several other neuroprotective agents that have been studied in ASCI and include tirilizad, naloxone, aspartate agonists, and the neuroganglioside GM-1. Unfortunately none to date has proven to be effective.

The timing of surgical decompression is controversial and variable. A majority of spine surgeons in one survey prefer to decompress ASCI within the first 24 hours. Surgery may be entertained earlier for patients with incomplete lesions. Central cord syndromes are usually managed nonoperatively initially.

Management in the Intensive Care Unit

There are several critical care issues that need to be evaluated and followed in the patient after ASCI. Most are related to the mechanism of the initial injury, loss of autonomic innervation, and care for the immobilized patient. Most patients with cervical neck injury will need to be admitted to an intensive care unit.

The first role in the intensive care unit is to maintain adequate oxygen delivery to the injured cord. Various modes of mechanical ventilation may be needed to provide adequate oxygenation in the multisystem trauma patient. In addition, maintenance of adequate blood pressure is needed to maintain appropriate spinal cord perfusion. A series of noncontrolled studies have supported the use of vasopressors to maintain a mean arterial blood pressure between 85 and 90 mmHg.

This is maintained for the first week post-ASCI. Similarly, bradycardia may need to be treated with atropine or glycopyrrolate. In recalcitrant cases a temporary and occasionally permanent pacemaker may be needed.

Patients with high cervical spine injury are likely to need mechanical ventilation for an extended period of time. In these circumstances the initiation of early tracheostomy can facilitate both pulmonary toilet and mobilization. Patients with lower cervical neck injuries may be able to come off mechanical ventilation over a period of 1 to 2 weeks. Vital capacities will improve as spasticity of the chest wall develops. A patient with an intact diaphragmatic function may be able to be successfully weaned from the ventilator. Patients after spinal cord injury or surgery will need to lie flat initially. Protocols to prevent aspiration pneumonia require raising the head of the bed to at least 30 degrees, and in such a situation reverse Trendelenburg may be used. Patients with neurogenic shock may develop symptomatic bradycardia in response to either internal or external stimuli. Endotracheal suctioning can commonly initiate this response.

Early nutrition is important to avoiding protein malnutrition. Many ASCI patients will develop a significant ileus early in their clinical course, which may make enteral nutrition difficult. Placement of a nasogastric tube for both decompression and early nutritional support is important. Enternal nutrition is preferred over parenteral nutrition. If a nasogastric tube is used, the head of the bed must be elevated and gastric residuals followed. A feeding tube placed into the duodenum may facilitate nutrition and is preferred for long-term treatment. Stress ulcer prophylaxis, as well as a bowel regimen, should be initiated in the intensive care unit as soon as feedings are started. The swallowing function prior to oral feeding should be evaluated in any patient with cervical spine surgery, prolonged intubation, tracheostomy, or halo fixation.

An indwelling urinary catheter should be placed during the initial assessment. It should be maintained until the patient is hemodynamically stable and strict control of the patient's fluid balance is no longer considered necessary.

A number of complications can be anticipated in patients with prolonged immobilization. Skin breakdown is common and must be evaluated frequently; patients should be placed on a pressure reduction mattress as soon as is feasible. Prophylaxis to prevent deep venous thrombosis should similarly be started as soon as feasible. Mechanical compression devices can be started early. Low molecular weight heparin or an un-fractionated heparin can be started once a concern for bleeding has abated. Early mobilization in a rotating bed may decrease the incidence of deep venous thrombosis.

✫ TIPS & TRICKS

A rotating bed can sometimes help with fluid mobilization. Patient with ASCI often receive large amounts of fluids - either during initial resuscitation or when returning from surgery. Many will have significant peripheral edema. In some cases the use of a rotating bed can mobilize fluid without the need for pharmacologic diuresis.

Psychological support is important for the patient with significant spinal cord injury, and frequent evaluation and support groups may be helpful. Consider the use of antidepressants in patients with early signs of depression. Similarly, pain can be underestimated in the patient with spinal cord injury, and pain should be evaluated using a rating scale. Methods to improve a patient's communication should also be initiated.

Conclusions

Patients after ASCI present a challenge to the critical care system. Acute stabilization of the injury and maintenance of adequate oxygen delivery to the spinal cord are paramount to improving long-term neurological function. An initial assessment and stabilization are required prior to a decision for surgery. The use of steroids remains controversial and a growing number of centers are not using this in routine practice. The optimization of spinal cord perfusion focuses on maintaining adequate mean arterial pressures, while the intensive care unit management focuses on preventing secondary complications and initiating early nutrition and mobilization.

Acknowledgment

The author would like to acknowledge Ed Benzel, MD, for his review of this chapter.

Bibliography

Berlly M, Shem K. Respiratory management during the first five days after spinal cord injury. *J Spinal Cord Med* 2007; **30:** 309–318.

Cohen-Gadol A, Pichelman MJ, Manno EM. Management of head and spinal cord trauma in adults. In: *Neurological Therapeutics Principles and Practice* (Noseworthy JH,ed.) Martin Dunitz Ltd, London, UK 2002 (2nd Edition, 2005), pp. 1221–1237.

Consortium for Spinal Cord Medicine. Early acute management in adults with spinal cord injury: a clinical practice guideline for healthcare professionals. *J Spinal Cord Med* 2008; **31:** 403–479.

Fehlings MG, Rabin D, Sears W, et al. Current practice and timing of surgical intervention in spinal cord injury. *Spine* 2010; **215:** S166–S173.

Hurlbert RJ. Strategies of medical intervention in the management of acute spinal cord injury. *Spine* 2006; **11** (Suppl): S16–S21.

Miko I, Gould R, Wolf S, Afifi S. Acute spinal cord injury. *Internat Anesthesiol Clin* 2009; **47:** 37–54.

Miller SM. Methylprednisolone in acute spinal cord injury: a tarnished standard. *J Neurosurg Anesthesiol* 2008; **20:** 140–142.

National spinal cord injury statistical center. Spinal cord injury Stats and figures. Updated June 2009. http://www.fscip.org/facts.htm.

Ploumis A, Yadlapalli N, Fehlings MG, et al. A systemic review of the evidence supporting a role for vasopressor support in acute SCI. *Spinal Cord* 2010; **48:** 356–362.

Rozet I. Methylprednisolone in acute spinal cord injury. Is there any other ethical choice? *J Neurosurg Anesthesiol* 2008; **20:** 137–139.

Subarachnoid Hemorrhage

Muhammad A. Taqi and Michel T. Torbey

Department of Neurology and Neurosurgery, The Ohio State University, Columbus, OH, USA

Introduction

The occurrence of subarachnoid hemorrhage (SAH) is almosy 3% of all strokes and one-third of hemorrhagic strokes. Aneurysm rupture is the most common cause of spontaneous SAH. The most common locations for an aneurysm include the anterior communicating artery, posterior communicating artery, bifurcation of the middle cerebral artery, tip of the basilar artery, and posterior inferior cerebellar artery origin. The incidence of SAH is between 6 and 8 per 100,000 population, with a mortality ranging between 32 and 67%.

Presenting Symptoms and Signs

The classic "worst headache of my life" presentation occurs in more than 80% of patients with aneurysmal SAH (aSAH). It is important to mention that only 1% of all headaches that present to the ED are SAH. Milder headaches associated with a sentinel bleed can be easily missed. Other common symptoms of SAH include nausea, vomiting, neck stiffness, focal neurological deficits, and/or brief loss of consciousness. Ocular hemorrhages (subhyloid, retinal, or vitreous) are present in up to one-fourth of the cases. The presence of risk factors such as like hypertension, smoking, and a family history of cerebral aneurysm, should raise suspicion for the diagnosis of SAH. Table 5.1 reviews the clinical Hunt and Hess grading of SAH.

Brain Imaging

The initial step in the diagnosis of a suspected SAH includes a CT scan of the head. The sensitivity immediately after the bleed is 98% within 12 hours and declines with time to 57% after day 6. With the advent of new proton density sequences like gradient echo (GRE), MRI use has been gaining popularity especially when the clinical suspicion of SAH is high and a CT scan is negative. Fisher grades and modified Fisher grades (Figures 5.1 and 5.2) are used to describe the extent of SAH on a CT scan (Table 5.2). The Fisher grade helps to predict the risk of cerebral vasospasm.

The next step after confirming the diagnosis of SAH is to identify the etiology. Traumatic SAH is mostly cortical with associated contusions, skull fractures and subdural/epidural hematomas. It is often difficult to conclude that the causal relationship between the trauma is the *result* of SAH or the *cause* of SAH, and concomitant injuries can therefore be deceiving. A diffuse SAH without evidence of trauma and contusions is very suggestive of an aneurysmal bleed.

Emergency Management in Neurocritical Care, First Edition. Edited by Edward M. Manno.
© 2012 John Wiley & Sons, Ltd. Published 2012 by John Wiley & Sons, Ltd.

Table 5.1. Hunt and Hess grade

Grade	Description
I	Asymptomatic, or mild headache and slight nuchal rigidity
II	CN palsy, moderate to severe headache, nuchal rigidity
III	Mild focal deficits, lethargy or confusion
IV	Stupor, moderate to severe hemiparesis, early decerebrate rigidity
V	Deep coma, decerebrate rigidity, moribund appearance

Add one grade for severe systemic disease(HTN, DM, COPD or severe atherosclerotic disease)

The location of bleed can be helpful in localizing the aneurysm. The following patterns correlate well with specific aneurysm locations:

- Interhemispheric fissure or gyrus rectus: Acomm
- Predominantly in one sylvian fissure: MCA or Pcomm

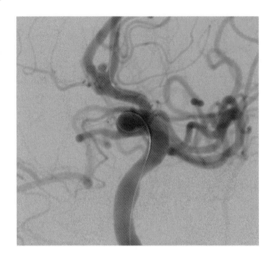

Figure 5.2. An associated Acomm aneurysm.

- Prepontine or peduncular: Basilar tip, Pcomm, PICA, or SCA
- Isolated or predominantly IVH: Depending on the ventricle could be PICA, vertebral artery, or basilar.

★ TIPS & TRICKS

- CT head can be negative in up to 2% of the acute bleed (within 12 hours) and up to 57% of subacute bleeds.
- Lumbar puncture is most sensitive for ruling out acute SAH, and MRI is most sensitive for detecting subacute SAH.

Cerebrospinal Fluid Studies

A negative CT scan does not exclude the diagnosis of SAH. Cerebrospinal fluid (CSF) evaluation is the most sensitive test to exclude SAH. However, a traumatic spinal tap could create a diagnostic dilemma, and the following steps may help further in the differentiation between a traumatic and an aneurysmal SAH:

- Test RBC in all four tubes: A decremental trend in RBC suggests a traumatic tap.
- Centrifuge immediately and observe the supernatant fluid by eye exam: yellow is suggestive of hemorrhage.

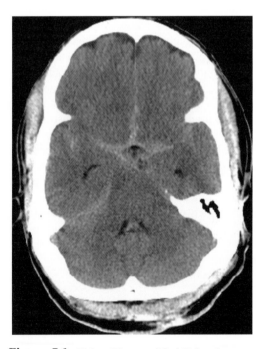

Figure 5.1. Fisher III or modified Fisher I aneurysmal SAH.

Table 5.2. Fisher grades

Grade	Description per Modified Fisher scale	Description per original Fisher scale
0	No blood	—
I	Thin cisternal blood without IVH	No blood
II	Thin cisternal blood with IVH	Diffuse or vertical layer < 1 mm thick
III	Thick cisternal blood without IVH	Localized clot or vertical layer >1 mm
IV	Thick cisternal blood with IVH	Intracerebral or intraventricular hemorrhage with or without SAH

- Spectrophotometry: The presence of only oxy-hemoglobin without bilirubin is suggestive of traumatic tap; the presence of erythrophages confirms nontraumatic hemorrhage.

It takes around 6 hours for red blood cells to lyse and release the product, therefore xanthochromia can be absent in the initial 6 hours post bleed. In some studies a visual inspection has been shown to provide a better assessment than spectrophotometry. Visual inspection against a white background is more specific, while spectrophotometry is more sensitive.

★ TIPS & TRICKS

In all CT negative thunderclap headaches with no other obvious etiology, lumbar puncture should be performed to rule out a sentinel bleed.

Vascular Imaging

Once aneurysmal SAH (aSAH) is suspected the next step is to identify the aneurysm by vascular studies. Available studies include CT angiogram, MR angiogram, and digital subtraction angiogram (DSA), which is the gold standard. The sensitivity

and specificity of CT angiogram has been reported to be between 80 and 90%. In a recent paper by Zhang et al. (2010), the sensitivity and specificity of dual energy CT angiogram (CTA) was 95% and 100%, respectively for aneurysms less than 6 mm. The sensitivity and specificity of an MR angiogram (MRA), according to Wilcock et al. (1996), is 81% and 100% respectively. In general, for aneurysms of less than 5 mm, the sensitivity of both CTA and MRA is suboptimal.

Management of Early Complications

The initial ABC management is crucial and should always be followed with any critically ill patient (Figure 5.3). This chapter will focus only on SAH-related management issues prior to surgical or endovascular treatment. The early specific complications of SAH are as follows, and warrant detailed discussion:

1. Rebleeding
2. Seizures
3. Hydrocephalus
4. Neurocardiogenic shock (Takotsabu cardio-myopathy)

Rebleeding

The mortality associated with rebleeding is 70%. It is one of the most preventable causes of poor outcome after aSAH. The risk of rebleeding is 4% on day 1 and 1–2% every day for 4 weeks. The risk of rebleeding decreases significantly after the first month to 3% per year. Recent studies have shown that ultra-early bleeds are more common in the first 2 hours. Factors associated with rebleeding are:

- Elevated blood pressure.
- Delay in securing an aneurysm.

Elevated Blood Pressure

There are no randomized trials to demonstrate that elevated blood pressure can lead to aneurysm re-rupture, but theoretically higher pressure can exert a pounding effect on the wall of recently ruptured aneurysm and potentially

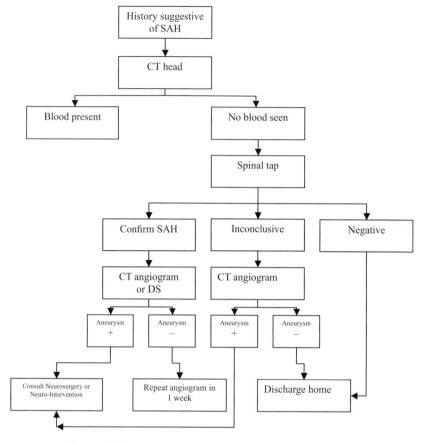

Figure 5.3. A flow chart for the initial evaluation of a SAH.

disrupt the clot covering the dome of the aneurysm. Fujii et al. (1996) demonstrated a correlation between rebleed and elevated blood pressure and found that a cutoff of systolic blood pressure (SBP) >150 was associated with a higher risk of rupture. In another study, a cutoff of SBP >160 was identified. Few studies found no correlation between the two. In our center a SBP cutoff of >140 is used to treat elevated blood pressure (Figure 5.4).

Commonly intravenous nicardipine drip or intermittent labetolol boluses are used to control blood pressure. Nitroprusside is avoided due to the potential effect of elevated ICP. Any procedure that can transiently elevate the blood pressure such as the placement of an arterial line, central line, intubation, or external ventricular drain (EVD) should be performed after optimal sedation and pain control. The American Stroke Association guidelines recommend the control of blood pressure to avoid rebleeding and to maintain optimal cerebral perfusion pressure. No specific target range is defined.

★ TIPS & TRICKS

Systolic blood pressure should be kept at least below 150–160 mmHg. If an ICP monitor is available, cerebral perfusion pressure (CPP) should be above 60.

Antifibrinolytics. Multiple randomized clinical trials have been performed using either tranexemic acid or aminocaproic acid with mixed results. Adam et al. (1981) published a meta analysis of three such trials showing reduction

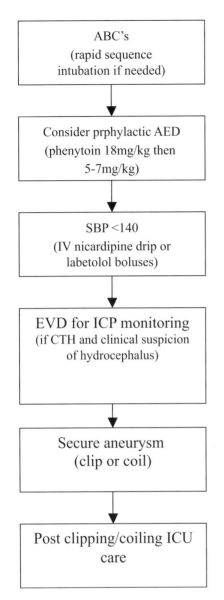

ABC's
(rapid sequence
intubation if needed)

↓

Consider prphylactic AED
(phenytoin 18mg/kg then
5-7mg/kg)

↓

SBP <140
(IV nicardipine drip or
labetolol boluses)

↓

EVD for ICP monitoring
(if CTH and clinical suspicion
of hydrocephalus)

↓

Secure aneurysm
(clip or coil)

↓

Post clipping/coiling ICU
care

Figure 5.4. Management of aSAH

★ TIPS & TRICKS

The use of antifibrinolytics may be helpful in selected circumstances where treatment is delayed and there appears to be little risk for developing delayed vasospasm. It can also be used in a situation where securing an immediate aneurysm is not possible due to an unstable medical condition.

Delay in Securing an Aneurysm

- *Lack of awareness*: No major studies have been performed to evaluate the awareness of SAH in the general community, but from acute ischemic stroke studies, it is well known that a lack of education regarding symptoms of acute stroke can cause significant delays. Although the symptoms of SAH are more robust and are more comparable with acute coronary syndrome, lack of awareness of the disease can result in significant delays in calling 911.
- *Delay in the emergency medical service (EMS)*: Although there is no way to definitely diagnose SAH without a brain-imaging study, a high suspicion based on the history and examination and subsequent triage to a comprehensive stroke center, helps significantly in achieving early intervention and proper management of an aSAH. The classic symptom "worst headache of life" along with complaints of neck stiffness, altered mental status, focal neurological deficits and/or loss of consciousness, should alert the EMS person for an aSAH. On site and prehospital management include ABC's, rapid sequence intubation if required and close monitoring of the blood pressure during the transfer.
- *Delay in the emergency room (ER)*: According to one study, the average ER door to CT scanner time is around 50 minutes. An early recognition of the above symptoms and appropriate report to the hospital in advance can expedite the process and confirm diagnosis. After confirming the diagnosis, consulting the neurosurgery or neurology service, managing ABCs, strict blood pressure control, and initiating seizure prophylaxis play an important role in avoiding rebleeding and other complications.

in the rate of rebleeding in patients using antifibrinolytics. Other studies have shown that the overall outcome is not changed, or even worse, which can be explained by the high risk of ischemic strokes with the use of antifibrinolytics. In particular, if the patient is to undergo endovascular treatment of an aneurysm, the use of antifibrinolytics can significantly increase the risk of thromboembolic complications.

- *Early clipping or coiling*: Multiple studies have shown the benefit of early treatment to secure an aneurysm by surgical or endovascular means. The mortality of aSAH has been reduced significantly in the past decade mainly due to early securing of an aneurysm.

Seizures

The incidence of seizures after SAH varies between 2 and 11%. No definite mechanism of seizure is known but theoretically it is related to the irritation of the cortex from the breakdown product of blood. This would suggest that patients with more cortical blood are at higher risk of seizures. None of the studies has actually demonstrated the detrimental effects of seizures in SAH patients. Other than the potential neuronal damage from prolonged seizure, the other potential effects include:

- Sudden increase in the intracranial pressure with seizures that could reduce the already compromised cerebral blood flow and cause brain ischemia. Elevated ICP can also result in central brain herniation.
- Increase cerebral blood flow related to hyperactive brain due to seizures can result in re-rupture of the aneurysm.
- Subclinical status can falsely present as a higher Hunt–Hess grade that might result in alteration of the treatment options, as most Hunt–Hess grade V patients are not taken to surgery due to poor prognosis.

The recommended treatment of seizures include loading with antiepileptic, the most commonly used is phenytoin. A comparison between a long-term phenytoin treatment (until discharge) versus a 3-day course of phenytoin has shown that patients with a prolonged hospital course had more side effects and no added benefit. Levicetracam has recently been studied for the prophylaxis in SAH and has shown promising results. Due to minimal drug interactions and less side effects, this might become the drug of choice in future. Other options include depakote and phenobarbital.

Later monitoring for subclinical seizures in SAH patients is controversial. Studies have reported an incidence of up to 28% in combined ICU populations, but the specific incidence of subclinical seizures in SAH patients on anticonvulsants is unknown. Mayer and colleagues (2005) showed the benefit of continuous EEG in this population for the detection of both vasospasm and seizure in a small number of patients. Clinical judgment should be used; if there is no evidence of significant hydrocephalus and the patient is a Hunt–Hess grade IV or V, an EEG to rule out subclinical status is not unreasonable.

☆ TIPS & TRICKS

The prophylactic use of anticonvulsants after subarachnoid hemorrhage is controversial. Traditionally, patients were loaded with phenytoin to prevent seizure activity which could potentially lead to an increased rate of rebleeding. Epidemiologic studies however have shown worse outcome in patients maintained on phenytoin. If anticonvulsant use is entertained then a loading dose of phenytoin 18 mg/kg should be considered in all suspected aSAH patients. Therapy should be continued for at least 3 days.

Hydrocephalus

The incidence of hydrocephalus after SAH has been reported using different definitions and ranges from 6 to 67%. The timing can vary from a few hours post-bleed to a few days. Hydrocephalus plays a significant role in the morbidity and mortality associated with SAH. Either a CT of the head or a MRI of the brain can be used to diagnose hydrocephalus. Several methods are available but most commonly a bicaudate index criterion is used for radiological diagnosis. This calculates the ratio of the frontal horns of lateral ventricles at the level of the caudate head to the distance between the inner tables of the frontal bone from side to side. The following cutoff values are used for different ages: < 36 years (0.16), 36–45 years (0.17), 46–55 years (0.18), 56–65 years (0.19), 66–75 years (0.20), and 76–85 years (0.21). An index more than or equal to these age-specific values suggests hydrocephalus.

⚛ SCIENCE REVISITED

- Hydrocephalus after SAH occurs as a result of malabsorption of the CSF through the

arachnoid villi or impedance of flow through the cerebral aqueduct.
- The amount of ventricular blood grade on presentation is a major predictor of the development of hydrocephalus, although there are a number of other variables that have been shown to be associated with hydrocephalus.
- Symptoms of hydrocephalus include headache, diplopia, nausea, vomiting, decreased level of consciousness and/or bilateral sixth nerve palsy.

Hydrocephalus after SAH represents a problem in either reabsorption of the CSF or impedance in the flow of the CSF due to high protein and blood products. In the acute phase, the hydrocephalus may be noncommunicating and hence should be treated with an external ventricular drainage.

In any patient with a Hunt–Hess grade greater than or equal to 3, and evidence of early hydrocephalus on CT, we recommend the placement of an EVD.

☝ CAUTION

Lumbar puncture in the setting of an acute noncommunicating hydrocephalus can lead to brain herniation and should be avoided.

Neurocardiogenic Shock (Takotsubo Cardiomyopathy)

Also known as broken heart syndrome, apical ballooning syndrome, Gebrochenes–Herz syndrome or stress cardiomyopathy, this is a cardiac dysfunction due to a nonischemic cause. Patients with aSAH can develop this stress-induced cardiomyopathy and it is frequently a cause of cardiogenic shock.

Stress-induced cardiomyopathy has been described with other acute neurological illnesses such as ischemic stroke and even psychological stress. It is more common in post-menopausal women. SAH patients presenting with hemodynamic instability require close cardiac monitoring. A Swan–Ganz catheter helps to diagnose and treat patients with hypotension and suspected

shock. After other potential causes of shock (septic/hemodynamic) are ruled out, the patient should be evaluated for causes of cardiogenic shock. The diagnosis of stress-induced cardiomyopathy is usually based on echocardiograph findings, which may include:

- *EKG findings*: Multiple EKG abnormalities have been reported with this kind of cardiomyopathy and include prolonged PR or QTc interval, focal or diffuse ST elevations, and pathological Q waves.
- *Cardiac enzymes*: Most of the patients have mild elevation of troponins and normal CK-MB.
- *Echocardiogram*: The classic echo findings of Takotsubo cardiomyopathy are apical akinesia with mid-ventricular dyskinesia and normokinesia of the heart base. The name Takotsubo derived from the word "octopus trap" which corresponds to the shape of the heart seen on the echo. This is usually reversible after few days.

⚛ SCIENCE REVISITED

The pathophysiology of a neurocardiogenic shock state is not very well understood. It is generally agreed that a strong sympathetic stimulation leads to myocardial stunning, but the mechanics of this is not clear. There are three proposed mechanisms:

- *Spasm of coronary arteries*: This has been led down by the fact that cardiac angiography even during the period of active ST elevations has been negative, except in one case series of Takotsubo cardiomyopathy.
- *Microvascular spasm*: Bybee et al. (2004) has demonstrated that the coronary flow can be abnormal even with normal coronary arteries in these patients.
- *Direct myocyte injury*: High levels of catecholamine can decrease the viability of myocyte through stress and calcium overload. Contraction band necrosis and inflammatory infiltrates have been described on the pathology of cardiac muscle in these patients.

Management

The first line of treatment is intravenous crystalloid or colloid fluids to maintain a CVP goal of

8–10 mmHg. Persistence hypotension after achieving optimal CVP requires cardiac output augmentation. This can be achieved with any inotropic/chronotropic agent. Dopamine helps to achieve this goal but has two potential disadvantages: (1) it increases the after load and can make the cardiogenic shock worse, and (2) since this is a hyper-adrenergic state, the addition of another catecholamine can potentially deteriorate the cardiac function by promoting the stunning phenomenon. Milrinone is better in this regard and has an altered mechanism of action through the phosphodiesterase pathway. It can potentially augment the cardiac output without any further increase in cardiac stress. Vasopressors, like norepinephrine or phenylephrine, should be avoided due to the fact that increasing the after load can actually worsen the cardiac output. Patients with hemodynamic instability should be stabilized prior to surgery or endovascular intervention.

★ TIPS & TRICKS

In a nutshell, the aim of the acute management of subarachnoid hemorrhage is to prevent rebleeding, to prevent global ischemia due to elevated intracranial pressure, and to manage the ABCs.

Bibliography

Adams HP Jr, Nibbelink DW, Torner JC, Sahs Al, Antifibrinolytic therapy in patients with aneurysmal subarachnoid hemorrhage. A report of the cooperative aneurysm study. *Arch Neurol* 1981 Jan; **38(1):** 25–9.

Buruma OJ, Janson HL, Den Bergh FA, Bots GT. Blood-stained cerebrospinal fluid: traumatic puncture or haemorrhage? *J Neurol Neurosurg Psychiat* 1981; **44:** 144–147.

Bybee KA, Prasad A, Barsness GW, Lerman A, Jaffe AS, Murphy JG, Wright RS, Rihal CS, Clinical characteristics and thrombolysis in myocardial infarction frame counts in women with transient left ventricular apical ballooning syndrome. *Am J Cardiol* 2004 Aug 1; **94(3):** 343–6.

Chumnanvej S, Dunn IF, Kim DH. Three-day phenytoin prophylaxis is adequate after sub-

arachnoid hemorrhage. *Neurosurgery* 2007 Jan; **60(1):**99–102.

Frontera JA, Claassen J, Schmidt JM, Prediction of symptomatic vasospasm after subarachnoid hemorrhage: the modified fisher scale. *Neurosurgery* 2006 Jul; **59(1):**21–27.

Fujii Y, Takeuchi S, Sasaki O, Ultra-early rebleeding in spontaneous subarachnoid hemorrhage. *J Neurosurg* 1996; **84:** 35–42.

Laidlaw JD, Kevin H, Siu KH. Ultra-early surgery for aneurysmal subarachnoid hemorrhage: outcomes for a consecutive series of 391 patients not selected by grade or age. *J Neurosurg* 2002; **97(2):**250–258.

Lee VH, Connolly HM, Fulgham JR, Takotsubo cardiomyopathy in aneurysmal subarachnoid hemorrhage: an underappreciated ventricular dysfunction. *J Neurosurg* 2006 Aug; **105(2):**264–270.

Mayer SA, Claassen J, Hirsch LJ, Continuous EEG monitoring in patients with subarachnoid hemorrhage. *J Clin Neurophysiol* 2005 Apr; **22(2):** 92–8.

Ohkuma H, Tsurutani H, Suzuki S. Incidence and significance of early aneurysmal rebleeding before neurosurgical or neurological management. *Stroke* 2001 May; **32(5):**1176–1180.

Szaflarski JP, Sangha KS, Lindsell CJ, Shutter LA. Prospective, randomized, single-blinded comparative trial of intravenous levetiracetam versus phenytoin for seizure prophylaxis. *Neurocrit Care* 2010 Apr; **12(2):**165–172.

Van der Wee N, Rinkel GJ, Hasan D, van Gijn J. Detection of subarachnoid haemorrhage on early CT: is lumbar puncture still needed after a negative scan? *J Neurol Neurosurg Psychiat* 1995; **58:** 357–359.

Wilcock D, Jaspan T, Holland I, Cherryman G, Worthington B, Comparison of magnetic resonance angiography with conventional angiography in the detection of intracranial aneurysms in patients presenting with subarachnoid haemorrhage. *Clin Radiol* 1996 May; **51 (5):** 330–4.

Zhang LJ, Wu SY, Niu JB, Dual-energy CT angiography in the evaluation of intracranial aneurysms: image quality, radiation dose, and comparison with 3D rotational digital subtraction angiography. *Am J Roentgenol* 2010 Jan; **194(1):**23–30.

Acute Management of Cerebral Ischemia

Leonid Groysman and Gene Sung

Neurocritical Care and Stroke Division, University of Southern California, Los Angeles, CA, USA

Introduction

Stroke is the third leading cause of death and the leading cause of disability in the United States. As with a lot of different nosological entities, the best treatment is primary prevention. But in case prophylaxis fails, the authors hope that this chapter will be of assistance in the acute management of cerebral ischemia.

There are two major categories of stroke: ischemic (~80%) and hemorrhagic (~20%), with further subdivision of the first one into three main etiologic subtypes: large-artery atherosclerotic, cardioembolic, and lacunar. However, at presentation, the main common treatment goal is reperfusion regardless of the etiology of the ischemic stroke. As with any emergency, ACLS goals (think ABC) should be met before any further steps are undertaken. Prehospital steps are outside the scope of this chapter, but the important points of stroke system activation require patients to call 911 with the first symptoms of neurological compromise. Expedited patient delivery to the hospital by the EMS with advance warning to the destination emergency room (ER) is of paramount importance in order to avoid unnecessary delays and meet ER "door-to-needle" time requirements of less than 60 minutes.

The First Hour

The availability of revascularization treatment modalities changed the practice of neurology from "diagnose and adios" to "time is brain." Once a patient arrives at the emergency department (ED), the stopwatch is started. The American Heart Association (AHA) guidelines prioritize the initial management before making decisions regarding treatment. The suggested "door-to-needle" time should be less than 60 minutes.

In the first 15 minutes in the ED, the patient should be screened by appropriately trained personnel and triaged accordingly. After initial cardiopulmonary stabilization (once again, remember ABC for Airway, Breathing, Circulation), the neurological deficit can be safely addressed.

In emergency settings, the most pertinent parts of the medical history include the history of baseline impairments, new symptoms, time of symptom onset, history of previous trauma, surgeries, strokes, cardiovascular events, intracranial hemorrhages, other comorbidities (notably hypertension, diabetes, and bleeding disorders), medication list (use of hypoglycemic, anticoagulant, or antiplatelet agents), and drug abuse. One of the paramount questions in obtaining the history is the time of symptoms onset, defined as "last seen normal." The patient may not be the

Emergency Management in Neurocritical Care, First Edition. Edited by Edward M. Manno.
© 2012 John Wiley & Sons, Ltd. Published 2012 by John Wiley & Sons, Ltd.

best source of information, and interviewing witnesses and family as well as confirmation of an estimated time of onset against verifiable time points, is essential.

> ★ TIPS & TRICKS
>
> One way to help toidentify the exact time on onset may include identifying the program the patient was viewing on the television. Clues in the household may include whether meals were being prepared or the patient was making plans for bed.

Obtaining vital signs, drawing blood for laboratory tests, and performing diagnostic tests may overlap with history-taking and examination. Physical and neurological exam may be limited and directed toward acute management and stroke evaluation (see NIH Stroke Scale below). General laboratory tests like Complete Blood Counts, coagulation panel, glucose, chemistry panel, and pregnancy tests (when appropriate) should be sent to the laboratory at the highest level of priority even before the arrival of the stroke team. Having a predefined stroke-related order sheet may help to significantly shorten the time to treatment. It is expected that assessment for anemia, thrombocytopenia, coagulopathy, electrolyte disorder, glucose level abnormality, or cardiac ischemia/arrhythmia (troponin and EKG) will be started immediately upon the patient's arrival in the emergency department. However, it is the ultimate responsibility of the managing physician to ensure the availability of this information at the time the decision for revascularization is made.

> ★ TIPS & TRICKS
>
> Symptoms associated with extremely high or low blood glucose level are the most frequent stroke mimics and should be ruled out early in the evaluation.

After the initial screening, a call to a neurologist should be started. It is advisable that the individual asking for assistance should err on the side of high sensitivity when deciding to activate the stroke team.

At this point an imaging study should be performed to help with the decision regarding eligibility for reperfusion. While there is significant data for use of MRI in this situation, the universal availability of computed tomography (CT) scanners and speed of performing CT makes this test the first choice in the majority of institutions. Imaging must be completed before the 30-minute time point after arrival in the ED. Availability of the creatinine/BUN level may assist in carrying out safely a contrast-based CT study (see the imaging section below). Anticipatory orders to the pharmacy to prepare a tissue plasminogen activator (tPA) may also expedite door-to-needle time.

Blood pressure management is still a subject of significant controversy. If the pressure is above 185/110 mmHg and the patient is eligible for tPA, lowering the pressure below the above level with labetalol boluses is mandatory to decrease the possibility of hemorrhagic complications. Failure to control the blood pressure with labetalol boluses, or the continuous infusion of nicardipine, is a contraindication for IV tPA. If the patient is not a candidate for IV tPA and does not have an intercerebral haemorrhage (ICH), we utilize permissive hypertension with blood pressure goals below 220/120 mmHg unless contraindicated.

In order for clinical, radiologic, and laboratory data to be available by the ~45-minute time point, collaboration of different teams and preemptive training of personnel are crucial. When the necessary diagnostic data is available, a brief discussion among involved teams and the patient's family should lead to a decision in support of or against tPA administration (see indications and contraindications in Table 6.1). Alteplase total dose is calculated as 0.9 mg/kg (maximal dose 90 mg). The first 10% is given as a bolus over 1 minute, and the remaining 90% is infused over 1 hour.

The First 24 Hours

If the patient is not eligible for IV tPA treatment (for example, in case the time of symptom onset

Table 6.1. Indications/contraindications to IV tPA

Indications
1. Age >18 years old
2. Clinical diagnosis of ischemic stroke with a measurable neurologic deficit
3. Exact time of onset established to be <180 minutes before treatment
Contraindications
1. Evidence of intracranial hemorrhage on pretreatment HCT
2. Minor or rapidly improving symptoms
3. Presentation suggestive of SAH even with normal HCT
4. Seizure at onset of stroke (relative)
5. Platelet count <100,000
6. Received heparin within 48 hours and with elevated PTT
7. Known history of intracranial hemorrhage
8. Other stroke or serious head trauma within past 3 months
9. Major surgery within the last 14 days
10. Sustained systolic BP>185 mmHg
11. Sustained diastolic BP >110 mmHg
12. Aggressive treatment necessary to lower BP
13. Gastrointestinal or urinary tract hemorrhage within 21 days
14. Arterial puncture at noncompressible site within 7 days
15. Serum glucose <50 mg/dL or >400 mg/dL

is beyond 4.5-hour window) or has demonstrable tissue at risk (so-called penumbra, see the imaging section), further consultation with the interventional team is recommended. Intra-arterial (IA) tPA may be beneficial if the patient angiographically demonstrates a middle cerebral artery occlusion and no major early infarct signs on the baseline head CT scan within 6 hours of symptom onset in selected cases. Emergency angioplasty and stenting or mechanical extraction of an occlusive clot are also available options in centers with the appropriate neurologic and interventional expertise. Mechanical thrombectomy may be used up to 6–8 hours after symptom onset. Mechanical thrombectomy is indicated for those patients where the IV tPA has not resolved a visible clot or the neurological examination has not improved with a residual clot visible on imaging and a diffusion–perfusion mismatch is present on MR or CT perfusion studies. The decision to try to remove a clot mechanically should be made on a patient-to-patient basis depending on the NIHSS score, underlying medical history, age, imaging data, and risk-benefit assessment.

Indications for Admission to the Neurocritical Care Unit (NCCU)

Patients with AIS may be admitted to the NCCU for neurologic or medical reasons (Table 6.2). Patients treated with IV tPA are at risk of intracranial hemorrhage and require close monitoring for at least 24 hours. Frequent neurology checks should be performed to assess for any worsening in a clinical examination. The presence of intracranial hemorrhage after thrombolytics requires the aggressive management of blood pressure (while maintaining proper cerebral perfusion) and the reversal of coagulopathy to prevent expansion of the hematoma. The presence of a massive middle cerebral artery (MCA) infarct as determined by an NIHSS >18, and >50% of the MCA territory involved on CT imaging is an indication for close monitoring in the NCCU. These patients may develop malignant cerebral edema in the first 3–5 days poststroke. The development of malignant cerebral edema carries a high mortality rate and has a high frequency of cardiac and pulmonary complications.

Table 6.2. Indications for admission to the NCCU after AIS

Neurologic
1. Post-thrombolysis
2. Massive cerebral infarction
3. Intracranial bleeding
4. Crescendo transient ischemic attacks
5. Progressive worsening of neurologic symptoms
6. Arterial dissection
7. Post-endovascular treatment
8. Cerebral vasospasm after subarachnoid hemorrhage
Non-neurologic
1. Respiratory failure
2. Mechanical ventilation for airway protection
3. Persistent hypotension
4. Intravenous drug management for hypertension
5. Aggressive pulmonary therapy
6. Cardiac infarction or arrhythmias
7. Severe systemic bleeding

The Brain Attack Coalition: tPA Stroke Study Group Guidelines.
http://www.stroke-site.org/guidelines/tpa_guidelines.html

Other neurologic conditions that warrant admission to the NCCU or stroke unit include crescendo transient ischemic attacks (TIAs) or limb-shaking TIAs (has a high incidence of ischemic stroke if untreated), progressive worsening of neurologic deficit (may benefit from the use of vasopressor agents to induce hypertension increased perfusion to brain), arterial dissection (requires hypervolemia and close blood pressure control), and post-endovascular therapy (high risk for embolization and re-occlusion).

Non-neurologic reasons for admission to the NCCU are those with respiratory failure, mechanical ventilation, vasopressor administration for hypotension, IV therapy for hypertension, cardiac abnormalities (i.e. infarction, ischemia, or arrythmias), severe systemic bleeding following thrombolytic therapy, and need for aggressive pulmonary therapy.

National Institute of Health Stroke Scale

The most widely accepted method to evaluate a patient with acute neurological deficits consistent with stroke is the National Institute of Health Stroke Scale (NIHSS). This scale evaluates different aspects of the neurological examination, including consciousness, language, sensorimotor systems, visual fields, speech, and inattention. A high score (maximum possible is 42) indicates significant neurological impairment. It is important to perform the NIHSS in the acute setting because it helps to screen patients who are eligible for aggressive medical management, facilitates communication between different teams, and aids the assessment of the evolution of stroke symptoms. Interviewing the patient and establishing an NIHSS score should not delay laboratory and radiological evaluations that are important for further interventions.

Stroke Imaging

Several imaging modalities are available for use in the AIS patient. These include head CT, CT angiography, CT perfusion, magnetic resonance imaging (MRI), magnetic resonance angiography (MRA), and transcranial doppler (TCD).

Head CT is the fastest scan to obtain to differentiate acute ischemic strokes from hemorrhagic strokes, subarachnoid hemorrhages, subdural hematomas, hydrocephalus, and cerebral edema. The presence of hypodense areas affecting more than one-third of the MCA territory within 3 hours of symptom onset may be a contraindication for administering IV tPA due to the increased risk of hemorrhagic conversion. Involvement of the entire MCA territory 24–48 hours after stroke onset is highly predictive of poor outcome and death in 80% of these patients. The visualization of a hyperdensity in one of the MCA lumens on a CT scan may signify a clot. This has been labeled the "hyperdense MCA sign." This sign, however, has low sensitivity and specificity and should not guide further management. A CT angiography of the head and neck can be administered and evaluated in a timely manner and can assess the vasculature of the head and neck for an obstruction amenable to intervention.

MRI is another imaging modality that has revolutionized the evaluation process of patients with AIS. Such techniques include diffusion-weighted imaging (DWI) and perfusion-weighted imaging (PWI). DWI measures the diffusion of water molecules in the brain tissue which can be quantified by the calculation of the apparent diffusion coefficients (ADCs). DWI is more sensitive than conventional MRI sequences to detect ischemic tissue within minutes after stroke onset in both animal and human studies. Abnormal areas appear hyperintense compared to normal brain tissue. The addition of PWI gives a better understanding of the hemodynamic characteristics of the ischemic brain. A MRA of the head and neck is also used to assess the vasculature, though it is less specific than a CT angiography in the evaluation of a vascular obstruction.

Cerebral angiography is considered to be the "gold standard" radiological method of choice to detect cerebral vessel occlusion and delineate the vascular anatomy. The advantages of this technique are the possibility of intra-arterial administration of medications (i.e. thrombolytic agents), and the performance of endovascular treatments (i.e. angioplasty or stent placement of stenosed arteries).

Transcranial dopplers (TCDs) are useful in the evaluation of vessel stenosis or occlusion. They may prove to be indispensible in the estimation of collateral circulation, the origination of micro-emboli in the heart or proximal arteries, and be particularly useful as a safe bedside test when following patients before and after treatment with thrombolytic agents to gauge recanalization success.

Subsequent Management of Acute Ischemic Stroke (AIS) in the Neuroscience ICU

Blood Pressure (BP) Before and After IV/IA tPA

The management of arterial hypertension remains controversial. The goal of maintaining adequate cerebral perfusion must be balanced by minimizing the complications of hypertension. The blood pressure (BP) before administering IV tPA should be systolic BP <185 mmHg or diastolic DB <110 mmHg. The guidelines recommend labetalol, nitropaste, or nicardipine infusions to help to lower the BP to less than 185/110 mmHg. The goal for blood pressure management post-IV/IA tPA or other acute reperfusion interventions should be systolic BP <180 and diastolic BP<105 for at least the first 24 hours. Blood pressure should be measured every 15 minutes for the first 2 hours and subsequently every 30 minutes for the next 6 hours, then hourly until 24 hours after treatment. If, during or after IV tPA, the systolic BP ranges from 180 to 230 mmHg, or the diastolic BP ranges from 105 to 120 mmHg, then labetalol should be given. If the systolic BP >230 mmHg, or the diastolic BP is between 121 and 140 mmHg, then labetalol or nicardipine IV drip may be used. If the BP remains uncontrolled with the use of the aforementioned agents, then one may consider the use of nitroprusside. As nitrates and nitroprusside can lead to cerebral vasodilation, and can increase intracranial pressures, they should be used with caution.

Failure to meet the BP parameters after administration of tPA is associated with an increased risk of symptomatic hemorrhagic transformation and poor neurological outcome. The lower limit of blood pressure should be adequate to keep the cerebral perfusion pressure (CPP) >70 mmHg. CPP is a derived measure of cerebral blood flow (CBF). It is a function of both systemic BP and intracranial pressure (ICP) and is estimated using the following equation:

$$CPP = MAP - ICP$$

No antiplatelets or antithrombotics should be given for 24 hours after receiving tPA. One should also avoid placing nasogastric tubes, indwelling bladder catheters, or intra-arterial pressure catheters for 24 hours. Many patients have a spontaneous decline in BP within the first hours of stroke, even without treatment. This may be facilitated when, in a less stressful environment (out of the ED, in a quiet room), the bladder is emptied and pain is controlled.

There is a need for large, well-designed trials to clarify the management of arterial hypertension after an acute stroke. Lowering the blood pressure post-stroke may be beneficial in that lowering pressures reduces the formation of brain edema, lessens the risk of hemorrhagic transformation of infarction, prevents further vascular damage, and forestalls early recurrent strokes. However, Castillo et al. (2004) noted that the aggressive treatment of BP (>20 mmHg) may lead to worsening of the neurological examination, higher rates of poor outcomes or death, and larger infarct volumes by reducing the perfusion pressures to infracted areas of the brain. A trial testing the utility of antihypertensive therapy in the setting of stroke – Controlling Hypertension and Hypotension Immediately Post-Stroke (CHHIPS) – showed that stroke patients who were treated for hypertension had lower mortality after 3 months than patients who received placebo. BP reduction was not associated with deterioration in neurological status at 72 hours and treatment did not alter death or disability at 2 weeks. The CHHIPS pilot data emphasizes the need for a full-scale trial to see if these encouraging preliminary results can be reproduced. Pending ongoing trials on whether the acute lowering of BP or keeping BP high in the acute setting is better, the consensus is that emergency administration of antihypertensive agents should be withheld unless the diastolic BP is >120 mmHg or the systolic BP >220 mmHg. Lowering the BP should be done cautiously. A reasonable goal would be to lower the BP by 15–25% within the first day (post-24 hours tPA). No data supports the administration of any specific antihypertensive agent and the treating physician should select medications for lowering the BP in the acute stroke setting on a case-by-case basis, based on any underlying medical conditions that would prohibit certain BP medications (i.e. using beta blockers in asthmatics).

Glucose Control in the NCCU

When being evaluated, all suspected acute stroke patients should get their blood glucose checked since hypoglycemia may mimic symptoms of ischemic stroke and may also lead to brain injury. The glucose level at presentation predicts symptomatic intracerebral hemorrhage as well as mortality and functional outcomes on 12-month modified Rankin scales and NIHSS scores. Most patients who present to the ED with stroke symptoms usually have moderate elevations of glucose in their serum. This is most likely a reflection of the hyperadrenergic state encountered post-stroke. The effect of high blood sugar in acute stroke patients is not completely understood but may have to do with increasing tissue acidosis from anaerobic glycolysis, lactic acidosis, and free radical production. It may affect the blood–brain barrier and the development of brain edema. Baird et al. (2003) found that the effects of hyperglycemia (blood glucose level > 200 mg/dL) during the first 24 hours after stroke independently predicted the expansion of the volume of ischemic stroke and poor neurological outcomes. Also reported was a 25% symptomatic hemorrhage rate in ischemic stroke patients who received tPA and whose serum glucose was >200 mg/dL. The desired level of blood glucose is in the range of 80–140 mg/dL.

In the NCCU, the serum glucose should be monitored every 4 hours and a sliding scale of insulin or insulin drips started if glucose is >140. In patients who received tPA, admission glucose levels of 140 mg/dL were associated with poor outcomes. Until more conclusive evidence is found, avoiding both hypoglycemia and hyperglycemia in acute stroke patients should continue. A serum glucose level >140 mg/dL will trigger the administration of an insulin drip at our institution, with close monitoring of the serum glucose to avoid hypoglycemia.

Temperature Management in the NCCU

Fever in the setting of an acute ischemic stroke is associated with an increased risk of morbidity and mortality by increasing the metabolic demands of the brain (releasing neurotransmitters) and the production of free radicals. When a patient becomes febrile, the source of fever should be investigated by obtaining blood cultures, urine cultures, chest radiograph, and assessing line status (i.e. when lines were placed and whether that could be a nidus for infection). Patients are placed on acetaminophen 650 mg every 4–6 hours by mouth, per rectum, or by nasogastric tube when the temperature is >38 °C. If the temperature is > 38.5 °C, a cooling blanket and ice packs may also be used on top of acetaminophen to lower the temperature to less than or equal to 37 °C. There have been several studies in the past with using either aspirin or acetaminophen to achieve normothermia. To date, there is no data demonstrating that lowering body temperature among febrile or afebrile patients improves neurological prognosis after a stroke. The goal in the NCCU is to maintain normothermia in the AIS patient.

Hypothermia has been shown to be neuroprotective in experimental and focal hypoxic brain injury models. It is thought that cooling the brain delays the depletion of energy stores, lessens intracellular acidosis, slows the influx of calcium into ischemic cells, suppresses the production of oxygen free radicals, and lessens the impact of excitatory amino acids. Hypothermia has been shown to reduce mortality and improve neurological outcomes among patients with cardiac arrest (ventricular fibrillation). Hypothermia on the central nervous system may decrease ICP by cerebral vasoconstriction and an associated decrease in blood volume. It may also act as an anticonvulsant.

Studies using induced hypothermia in patients with malignant ischemic strokes in improving neurological outcome have been mixed. Reith et al. (1996) prospectively enrolled 390 patients within 6 hours of stroke onset. They found that an association exists between body temperature and initial stroke severity, infarct size, mortality, and outcome. Mortality rates and neurological outcome improved in the hypothermic group. For every 1 °C increase in temperature, the risk of poor outcome doubled. Only randomized-controlled trials of hypothermia can prove whether this relation is causal.

The COOL AID (Cooling for Acute Ischemic Brain Damage) trial tested whether endovascular cooling combined with meperidine, buspirone, and surface warming could achieve hypothermia

rapidly in AIS patients. Induced moderate hypothermia was feasible using an endovascular cooling device in most patients with AIS. Further studies are still needed to determine if hypothermia improves neurological outcome in AIS patients.

There are several methods of cooling down the body as well as the brain. Cooling blankets are available but do not efficiently cool the body down in a controlled manner, as is the case of other traditional methods such as ice water baths and fans. Newer methodologies utilize computer-regulated cooling units that circulate cool water through an endovascular device or superconductive gel pads that circulate to effectively cool patients down to 33 or 34 °C over a 24-hour period. The endovascular cooling devices have been used effectively to cool patients in a controlled fashion but require the placement of a large-bore catheter in the inferior vena cava via a femoral vein. The machine allows for the controlled rewarming of a patient no greater than 0.3 °C/hour up to 36.5–37 °C to prevent the risk of cerebral edema. The use of paralytics and sedative agents are indicated to help to prevent shivering during the cooling process and prevent the body from increasing its core temperature. The patient should be placed on a deep venous thrombosis (DVT) prophylaxis 12 hours after the removal of the catheter. A lower extremity doppler ultrasound may be obtained if a DVT is suspected since the use of an intravascular device predisposes one to DVTs (because of the large size of catheter). Some of the side effects to therapeutic hypothermia are hypotension, cardiac arrythmias, and infections. An intranasal cooling device is under development that may effectively cool the brain and avoid some of the side effects, and deliver a perfluorochemical spray via nasal tongs within minutes. The nasal cavity is cooled down to 5 °C, thus cooling the brain by conduction.. Exciting devices are being developed and hopefully larger well-designed trials will prove that hypothermia is safe and effective in the treatment of acute ischemic strokes.

Fluid Status Management and Nutrition in AIS

The goal in the NCCU for AIS patients is to maintain euvolemia. Systemic dehydration may reduce cerebral edema but may worsen cerebral perfusion. The average maintenance fluid is 1 ml/kg/hour, which is approximately 2000–2500 mL/day for adults. Normal saline is the intravenous fluid of choice in the NCCU. Hypotonic solutions can worsen cerebral edema and are avoided. Dextrose-containing solutions are also avoided in that glucose is metabolized to lactic acid in the ischemic tissue by anaerobic metabolism and worsens cerebral injury. An ongoing trial ALIAS (albumin therapy for neuroprotection in AIS) is currently enrolling patients to determine if human serum albumin at 2 g/kg given over 2 hours to ischemic stroke victims within 5 hours of stroke onset, results in improved outcome at 3 months. If the results are significant when the trial is completed, it would be the first neuroprotective agent to improve outcome in AIS patients.

Nutrition considerations in the NCCU are important. Metabolic activity and nutritional demands are increased post-stroke. Early institution of nutrition is associated with improved outcomes. A formal swallow evaluation should be done to assess whether or not the patient has difficulty swallowing and is at risk for aspiration. Patients who have a decreased level of consciousness or fail their swallow study should have a nasogastric tube placed, nutritional consultation, and nutritional preparations started. A good bowel regimen should also be implemented since delayed gastric emptying is common in the NCCU. The use of narcotic agents for pain may also delay bowel movements and laxatives should be started. A gastrointestinal prophylaxis should also be started in NCCU patients.

DVT and PE Prophylaxis

Deep venous thrombosis (DVT) and pulmonary embolism (PE) are frequent complications in stroke patients. Stroke patients with restricted movement because of weakness, and are bedridden, should receive SC (subcutaneous) low-dose heparin or SC low molecular weight heparins. PREVAIL (Prevention of Venous thrombo-embolism after AIS) was an open-label, randomized comparison of either enoxaparin 40 mg SC once a day or unfractionated heparin (UFH) at 5000 units SQ every 12 hours in patients with ischemic stroke. The risk of both symptomatic intracranial bleeding and major extracranial bleeding was similar in both groups. There was, however, a reduction seen of asymptomatic DVTs in the enoxaparin group but this was matched to an increase in major extracranial bleeding.. Low molecular weight heparins have been found to be equivalent to, or better than, UFH in preventing DVT.

In patients with an acute intracerebral hemorrhage or any contraindication to anticoagulants, intermittent pneumatic compression (IPC) devices or elastic stockings should be used initially. In stable patients with intracerebral hemorrhage, the use of low-dose SC heparin can be started as soon as the second day post-hemorrhage. This recommendation is based on one study that emphasizes the risk reduction of thromboembolism compared to minimizing the risk of cerebral rebleeding.

Management of Intracranial Bleeding After Thrombolytic Therapy

The major risk of thrombolytic therapy is intracranial hemorrhage. If bleeding occurs, infusions of a thrombolytic should be stopped immediately. A head CT without contrast is ordered immediately if intracranial hemorrhage is suspected. Hemorrhagic transformation (petechial hemorrhage within an infarct) and parenchymal or symptomatic hemorrhage should be differentiated. Poor compliance with national guidelines for the administration of thrombolytic therapy increases the incidence of intracranial bleeding.

If bleeding is suspected, blood should be immediately drawn to measure the patient's hematocrit, hemoglobin, partial thromboplastin time (PTT), prothrombin time (PT), international normalized ratio (INR), platelet count, and fibrinogen. Blood should also be typed and cross-matched if transfusions are needed (at least 4 units of packed red blood cells, 5–6 units of fresh frozen plasma, or 6–8 units of cryoprecipitate and 1 unit of donor platelets). These blood products should be available for emergent administration. Neurosurgery should also be consulted if evacuation is a consideration. Surgical evacuation of an intracerebral haemorrhage can be carried out once the coagulopathy is corrected, the size of hematoma is assessed, and the location of the hematoma is determined. Cerebellar hematomas that are > 3 cm, or larger (>60 cc) lobar hematomas with mass effect, should be evacuated emergently.

Management of Malignant Hemispheric Ischemic Strokes with Cerebral Edema and/or Elevated Intracranial Pressures

Cerebral edema in acute ischemic infarcts usually peaks in 48–72 hours and starts to resolve by day 5. The treatment of cerebral edema is primarily medical and overlaps with that of elevated intracranial pressure (ICP). First and foremost, one must assess the patient's ability to protect hisairway if he starts to become less responsive. Endotracheal intubation should be initiated if the patient appears to be in respiratory distress and if his Glasgow Coma Scale (GCS) score is <8. Short-acting medications should be used for intubation such as etomidate, thiopental, propofol, or lidocaine. Once controlled, hyperventilation to a $PaCO_2$ of <25 should be avoided because of the possibility of cerebral vasoconstriction and ischemia. At the same time, MAP should be maintained with intravenous isotonic fluids and vasopressors if necessary to keep CPP >70 mmHg, and head of the bed elevated about 30 degrees. The use of an intracranial pressure (ICP) monitoring device should be implemented, especially when using osmotic agents to help decrease ICP. Several devices are available for ICP monitoring: intraventricular catheters (IVCs), subarachnoid bolts, and fiberoptic transducers.

Osmotic agents such as mannitol are used to reduce the cerebral water content. It also decreases the viscosity of blood in the cerebral arterioles and induces vasoconstriction leading to reduction in ICP. The initial dose is 0.5–2.0 g/kg and maintenance dose of 0.25 g/kg every 4–6 hours to keep serum osmolality between 310 and 320 mOsm/L. Serum sodium and osmolalities are usually checked every 6 hours when mannitol and/or hypertonic saline is used to help to keep ICP <20 mmHg. 3% hypertonic saline boluses may also be used to help to lower ICPs as well. A bolus of 250 cc every 6 hours, needed to keep the serum osmolality in the 310–320 mOsm/L range, can be given while trying to maintain euvolemia. Barbiturate coma can be instituted once all other medical maneuvers have failed, but it is important to anticipate possible complications from this therapy. These include: cardiac and blood pressure depression, diminished interstitial peristalsis, sepsis, pneumonia, poikilothermia, and coagulopathies. Maintaining normothermia and euglycemia are also important in these patients. Decompressive hemicraniectomy by neurosurgery can also be considered on a case by case basis in those patients >50 years of age that were otherwise healthy with large territory infarcts that are unresponsive to maximal medical management. Patients age 50 or younger with a decreased level of consciousness and infarction involving >50% of MCA territory are at risk of developing malignant edema. In those patients that desire aggressive therapy, decompressive hemicraniectomy may be offered.

Conclusion

The close attention that a neurocritical care unit provides for an AIS patient is important in the long- term prognosis and recovery from this devastating illness. The importance of BP control before and after IV tPA, maintaining euglycemia, normothermia, euvolemia, and following cerebral edema can all be monitored in the NCCU. Exciting new therapies such as induced hypothermia in AIS and whether or not blood pressure lowering in AIS is beneficial will be determined in the near future. As time goes on, many new options will be available for treating AIS patients in the NCCU, which will get them out of the acute phase and on the road to rehabilitation.

Bibliography

Adams HP, Jr., Bendixen BH, Kappelle LJ, et al. Classification of subtype of acute ischemic stroke. Definitions for use in a multicenter clinical trial. TOAST. Trial of Org 10172 in Acute Stroke Treatment. *Stroke* 1993; **24:** 35–41.

Ahmed N, Wahlgren N, Brainin M, et al. Relationship of blood pressure, antihypertensive therapy, and outcome in ischemic stroke treated with intravenous thrombolysis: retrospective analysis from Safe Implementation of Thrombolysis in Stroke–International Stroke Thrombolysis Register (SITS–ISTR). *Stroke* 2009; **40:** 2442–2449.

Baird TA, Parsons MW, Phanh T, et al. Persistent poststroke hyperglycemia is independently associated with infarct expansion and worse clinical outcome. *Stroke* 2003; **34:** 2208–2214.

Castillo J, Leira R, García MM, et al. Blood pressure decrease during the acute phase of ischemic stroke is associated with brain injury and poor stroke outcome. *Stroke* 2004; **35:** 520–526.

Flint AC, Duckwiler GR, Budzik RF, et al. Mechanical thrombectomy of intracranial internal carotid occlusion: pooled results of the MERCI and Multi MERCI, Part I Trials. *Stroke* 2007; **38:** 1274–1280.

Gruber A. Interventional management of stroke. *Stroke* 2008; **39:** 1663–1664.

Hacke W, Kaste M, Bluhmki E, et al. Thrombolysis with Alteplase 3 to 4.5 hours after acute ischemic stroke. *New Engl J Med* 2008; **359:** 1317–1329.

Latchaw RE, Alberts MJ, Lev MH, et al. Recommendations for imaging of acute ischemic stroke: a scientific statement from the American Heart Association. *Stroke* 2009; **40:** 3646–3678.

Lyden P, Brott T, Tilley B, et al. Improved reliability of the NIH Stroke Scale using video training. NINDS TPA Stroke Study Group. Stroke 1994; **25:** 2220–2226.

Reith J, Jørgensen HS, Pedersen PM, et al. Body temperature in acute stroke: relation to stroke severity, infarct size, mortality, and outcome. *Lancet* 1996; **347:** 422–425.

Sung GY. *Emergency and Critical Care Management of Acute Ischemic Stroke.* American Academy of Neurology, 2008.

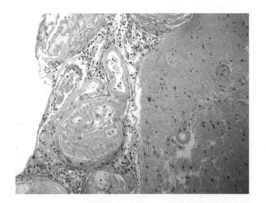

Plate 7.1 Congo red staining of cerebral amyloid angiopathy showing thickened sub-cortical arteriole wall (left) which demonstrates apple green birefringence (right) which is neuropathologically diagnostic of the condition.

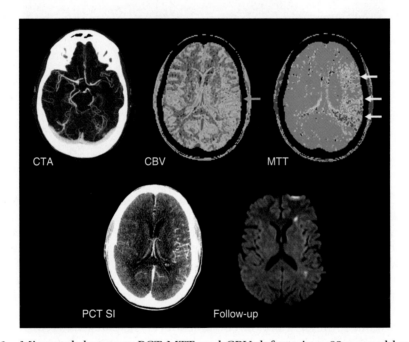

Plate 23.1 Mismatch between PCT MTT and CBV defects in a 63-year-old man evaluated 3 hours after sudden onset of right face-arm-leg weakness. CTA images show occlusion of the distal M1 segment of the left middle cerebral artery. CTA curved multiplanar reconstruction shows a calcified plaque at the origin of the left internal carotid artery (arrowhead) with a bypass from the left common carotid artery to the distal left internal carotid artery. PCT parametric maps show a mismatch between the region with prolonged MTT (white arrows) and the absence of decreased CBV (CBV is increased) (gray arrow). PCT source images (PCT SI) show good collateral flow in the tissue with prolonged MTT and no area showing paucity of vessels. The patient was treated with intravenous tPA. Follow up DWI image performed 12 hours later (Follow-up) show two small infarcts in the watershed territories, represented by the small foci of restricted water diffusion (purple arrows).

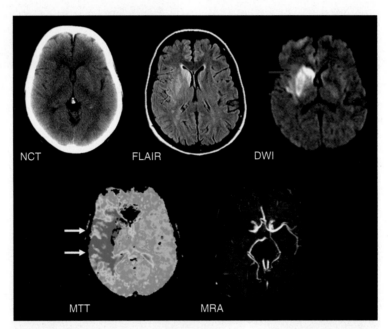

Plate 23.2 Example of obscuration of the lentiform nucleus sign, and mismatch between PWI and DWI in a 66-year-old woman evaluated for left face-arm-leg weakness. NCT of the brain obtained 4 hours after symptom onset show obscuration of the right lentiform nucleus. MRI was performed 4.5 hours after symptom onset. There is a mismatch between the region with prolonged MTT (involving the entire right MCA territory) (white arrows) and the region of DWI abnormality (limited to the head of the caudate and lentiform nuclei) (purple arrows), which represents the infarct core. Note how the DWI abnormality in not completely apparent on FLAIR sequence. MR angiography (MRA) shows occlusion of the M1 segment of the right middle cerebral artery. The patient was treated with intravenous tPA. The final infarct volume on the follow up MRI performed 24 hours later corresponded to the area of baseline restricted diffusion (not shown).

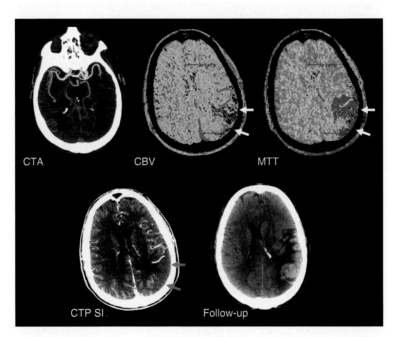

Plate 23.3 MTT-CBV match in a 62-year-old man evaluated after sudden onset of right face, arm and leg weakness consistent with acute ischemic stroke. CTA images (CTA) show occlusion of the M1/M2 junction segment of the left MCA. PCT parametric maps (CBV and MTT) show a complete match between the areas of prolonged MTT and decreased CBV (involving the posterior superficial right MCA territory), consistent with infarcted tissue (white arrows). CTA and PCT source images (PCT-SI) show poor collateral flow an area of paucity of vessels that outlines the infarct core (purple arrows). Follow-up NCT (Follow-up) show that the final infarct corresponds to the area of predicted infarct core as represented by the area of decreased CBV. Hemorrhagic transformation was present.

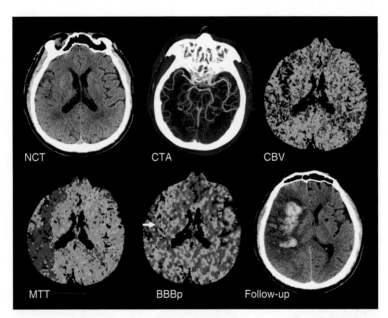

Plate 23.4 Imaging for Blood-brain permeability in a 73-year-old man with acute ischemic stroke and hemorrhagic transformation. Non-contrast CT (NCT) of the brain acquired 2 hours after symptom onset show slight obscuration of the right insular ribbon. CTA images acquired at that time (CTA) show occlusion of the distal M1 segment of the right middle cerebral artery. CBV ant MTT parametric maps (CBV and MTT) show a mismatch between the region with prolonged MTT and the absence of decreased CBV. The map of microvascular permeability (BBB) shows a region of blood brain barrier disruption involving the right insula (white arrow). The patient was treated with intravenous rt-PA. Follow-up NCT (Follow-up) obtained 24 hours later show hemorrhagic transformation. Note how the intracranial hemorrhage is centered in the predicted region of blood brain barrier permeability disruption.

Neurocritical Care of Intracerebral Hemorrhage

James M. Gebel Jr

Cerebrovascular Center, Cleveland Clinic, Cleveland, OH, USA

Introduction

Background

Intracerebral hemorrhage (ICH) is the most common form of hemorrhagic stroke in the United States and is twice as common as subarachnoid hemorrhage. Although ICH represents only 10–15% of all strokes, it has a higher mortality, particularly in certain ethnic groups. For instance, African American men ages 35 to 54 in the United States have quadruple the stroke mortality attributable to ICH than comparable age Caucasian men. ICH mortality rates range from 25 to 50% in most series, with only 25% recovering without death or permanent significant neurological disability. Thus, by definition, most ICH patients are neurologically critically ill. Furthermore, a substantial proportion of hyper-acute ICH patients who, upon initial presentation, appear neurologically and medically stable deteriorate within minutes or hours secondary to rebleeding, intraventricular extension, acute obstructive hydrocephalus, or airway compromise. Others suffer from delayed neurological deterioration due to perihematomal edema. Therefore, the best approach is to assume that any hyper-acute or acute ICH patient is critically ill. This requires that the patient is triaged to an area in the hospital that has the resources to monitor and proactively address potential medical and neurological complications.

Pathophysiology

The most common cause of spontaneous ICH is uncontrolled hypertension, which leads to the rupture of deep penetrating arteries and explains why hypertensive ICHs are most often located in the basal ganglia (putamen, thalamus, internal capsule, caudate), subcortical white matter, cerebellum, and brainstem. In fact, approximately one quarter of all ICHs in hypertensive patients would be eliminated if hypertension were treated. Charcot–Bouchard micro-aneurysms are believed to be the direct pathophysiological substrate of these vessels rupturing, with lipo-hyalinosis preceding the formation and rupture of these micro-aneurysms. Fisher, however, was able to identify these aneurysms in only about 10% of patients after ICH (Figure 7.1).

Cerebral amyloid angiopathy (CAA) is the second most common cause of ICH and affects the lobar regions preferentially due to its underlying pathological substrate of amyloid deposition predominantly in small cortical arterioles in this region (Plate 7.1). It mainly affects elderly individuals and is also associated with Alzheimer dementia. A more recently described variant of

Emergency Management in Neurocritical Care, First Edition. Edited by Edward M. Manno.

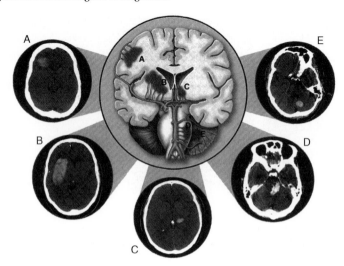

Figure 7.1. Location and computed tomographic correlates of intracerebral hemorrhages attributed to chronic hypertension. Chronic hypertension leads to pathological changes in the perforating arteries of the large basal cerebral arteries leading to hemorrhages commonly found in the (A) deep white matter, (B) basal ganglia, (C) thalamus, (D) pons, and (E) cerebellum. (Reproduced from Manno et al. (2005), with permission from Elsevier.)

this disorder is CAA with cerebral edema. Individuals with this variant suffer sustained perihematomal edema out of proportion to the hematoma's size due to ongoing inflammatory reaction to adjacent tissue. Coagulopathy (especially warfarin-associated ICH) is another common and important cause of spontaneous ICH. Its risk and severity increase with higher PT/INR values, especially once the PT/INR exceeds 4.0, after which risk exponentially increases. Underlying structural lesions causing ICH include neoplasms, vascular malformations, and infections (especially so-called "mycotic" aneurysms due to subacute bacterial endocarditis-related septic cerebral emboli, and aspergillosis, which affects immunocompromised individuals). Primary or secondary CNS angiitis and Moya Moya disease/syndrome rarely cause ICH.

Presenting Clinical Features

The "classic" presentation of ICH is abrupt onset of headache, often with nausea +/– vomiting and smoothly progressive focal neurological deficits attributable to the anatomical location where the hematoma develops. A diminished level of consciousness (LOC) out of proportion to the expected anatomical size and location often clinically differentiates ICH from ischemic stroke of a similar anatomical location. Progressive or abrupt decline in the LOC is also characteristic of ICH as compared to ischemic stroke. Despite these classic differentiating features, the clinical presentation should never be relied upon as the means of diagnosing ICH, which can only be reliably ascertained by obtaining a noncontrast head CT scan (or MRI). (Figure 7.2).

Neurocritical Care of ICH

Neurocritical care of ICH begins with the ABCs –airway, breathing, and circulation. ICH patients are often obtunded, stuporous, or comatose upon or shortly after initial presentation, rendering them unable to adequately protect their airway and increasing their aspiration risk. This is often compounded by dysphagia due to their associated focal neurological injury. Timely elective intubation assures adequate gas exchange and minimizes the risk of precipitous respiratory failure and aspiration pneumonitis. Intubation should occur by experienced clinicians, with special care to avoid acute increases in intracranial hypertension (see Chapter 2).

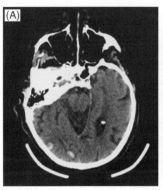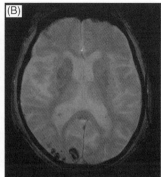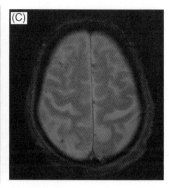

Figure 7.2. Patient with multiple post-thrombolytic ICHs following IV tPA therapy for acute ischemic stroke on their 24-hour post-IV tPA CT scan (A) determined to be due to underlying cerebral amyloid angiopathy as evidenced by visualization of low signal microbleeds on axial gradient echo MRI images (B and C).

A history should be obtained whenever feasible, with special attention to whether or not the patient became unresponsive, had or had not seizure activity, has a known history of hypertension, diabetes, or uses anticoagulant or antiplatelet medications.

Initial Medical Critical Care of ICH

The initial vital sign assessment should focus on uncontrolled hypertension which, in addition to its own independent adverse effects on cardiac output and function, may, if not treated, increase the risk of rebleeding during the first 24 hours of clinical presentation. Furthermore, a Cushing's response (hypertension, bradycardia, and widened pulse pressure) may indicate markedly increased intracranial pressure. Erratic and irregular heart rhythms can occur and may indicate catecholamine-induced cardiac arrhythmias.

The first major medical critical care issue that needs to be emergently treated when present is hypertension. Studies suggest, but do not prove, that uncontrolled hypertension during the first 24 hours post-ICH onset is associated with a worse clinical outcome and increased risk of rebleeding. Two important pilot studies, INTERACT and ATACH, have preliminarily investigated whether aggressive early therapeutic blood pressure (BP) lowering in hypertensive ICH patients is safe and feasible. INTERACT open label randomized 404 ICH patients who could be evaluated and treated with any available intravenous antihypertensive

medication within 6 hours of clinical ICH onset. Patients were randomized to a more aggressive BP reduction strategy of a systolic BP < 140 mmHg within 1 hour as compared to systolic BP < 180 mmHg. The results suggested a trend toward better outcome in those patients assigned to the < 140 mmHg arm, but this difference was not statistically significant. ATACH used a nicardipine drip to lower systolic BP in hypertensive ICH patients to one of three target ranges: 100–139, 140–169, and 170–199. Current AHA clinical practice guidelines (CPGs) provide no definitive or high evidence level specific BP management targets.

Rebleeding, defined as at least a 33% increase in hematoma volume from baseline noncontrast head CT, occurs in up to 28% of hyperacute (presenting within 3 hours of clinical onset) ICH patients within the first hour and 38% within the first 24 hours of presentation.

The second major medical critical care issue that needs to be emergently treated is correction of coagulopathy in patients with thrombolysis or coagulopathy-associated ICH (TICH), especially in those with warfarin- and heparin-related ICH. TICHs on average have three times greater volume than noncoagulopathic ICH, and are more likely to extend into the subarachnoid, subdural, and intraventricular spaces. They are associated with a very high mortality rate, ranging from 70% to >90% in most series. TICHs may be radiologically differentiated from non-TICHs by the frequent presence of a blood-fluid level and lack of early perihematomal edema, both of which indicate unclotted blood within the hematoma.

★ TIPS & TRICKS

It is important to note that whereas the window for risk of rebleeding essentially ends at 24 hours in patients with noncoagulopathic ICH, by contrast those with TICH are at indefinite duration risk of rebleeding until the coagulopathy has been adequately reversed. This is true even for patients with initially small TICHs whose clinical and radiological presentation appears benign, but whom have high risk of subsequent or ongoing bleeding until their coagulopathy is adequately corrected.

Some studies suggest that patients treated with antiplatelet medication are also at increased risk of rebleeding and death due to ICH, but at present there is no evidence supporting the efficacy of empiric platelet transfusion to reduce THE risk of ICH-related morbidity or mortality.

For patients with warfarin-associated ICH, administration of recombinant factor VIIa (rfVIIa) in a dose of 20 to 80 µg/kg is recommended to immediately reverse warfarin coagulopathy, though its effects are only temporary, lasting from 4 to 12 hours on average in this dosing range. Emergent administration of prothrombin complex concentrate (PCC) is an alternative and possibly more effective strategy for immediate temporary reversal of the warfarin anticoagulant effect. Dosing for reversal of the warfarin effect is not well established, but a dose of 50 u/kg would raise levels of factors II, IX, and X by approximately 50% of the normal levels, and raise factor VII levels by a small amount.

After administration of an immediate reversal agent, fresh frozen plasma (2 to 8 units depending on initial PT/INR value and subsequent follow-up values) should be transfused to maintain a more durable reversal of anticoagulation, as well as 3–10 mg of IV vitamin K. This infusion must be given slowly since anaphylaxis occurs in

1 of 10,000 patients given IV vitamin K. For heparin-associated ICH, rapid reversal is accomplished with protamine sulfate. One milligram of protamine reverses per 100 units of unfractionated heparin, 1 mg of enoxaparin, or 100 u of antifactor Xa activity for daltaparin or tinzaparin. Maximum dose is 50 mg. It should also be administered slowly as an intravenous pyelogram (IVP) over 10 minutes and the patient should be carefully observed for anaphylaxis. A STAT repeat PT/INR should be obtained 5 minutes after initial reversal agent for warfarin, with follow-up PT/INR levels every 4 hours until two consecutive normal values are obtained.

It should be noted that empiric treatment of patients with spontaneous, noncoagulopathic ICH with rfVIIa was shown to have statistically significantly less hematoma expansion in both phase IIb and phase III clinical trials (FAST trial). Unfortunately, this reduction of rebleeding did not translate into any improvement in clinical outcomes, though median hematoma size in these trials was small. Use of rfVIIa for spontaneous, noncoagulopathic ICH is currently not recommended.

Initial ICH care should also include proactive measures to prevent deep venous thrombosis (DVT) formation, pressure ulcer formation, and aspiration. All ICH patients should be considered NPO until an initial swallow screen is performed (followed by full speech pathology and a dysphagia evaluation) to assess the patient's aspiration risk. Pneumatic compression devices and elastic stockings should both be applied to ICH patients and remain in place until the patients are fully active and ambulatory. Pharmacological DVT prophylaxis with DVT prophylaxis dose subcutaneous (SQ) unfractionated heparin (5000u SQ every 8 to 12 hours) or low molecular weight heparinoids (enoxaparin 40 mg SQ daily) can be initiated 48 hours post-ICH onset in patients with noncoagulopathy-related ICH. The PREVAIL trial proved the superiority of enoxaparin 40 mg SQ daily over unfractionated heparin 5000u SQ every 12 hours in stroke patients in preventing lower extremity DVT and pulmonary embolism, but enoxaparin was also associated with an increased risk of major bleeding events as well.

Initial Neurological Assessment and Treatment of ICH

Initial neurological assessment should include a complete neurological examination (or coma examination in unresponsive patients) to establish a baseline against which future assessments can be compared. This should particularly focus on the LOC, signs of increased intracranial pressure such as sixth nerve palsies and papilledema, signs of hydrocephalus such as impaired upgaze or forced downgaze, degree of dysphagia, and presence of significant motor deficits that would predispose to DVT formation.

★ TIPS & TRICKS

The performance and careful documentation of this initial assessment is particularly important because most ICH patients who suffer early neurological deterioration do so within the first 3 to 6 hours post-clinical onset.

If the patient's neurological examination has significantly deteriorated since arriving at the ED (or outside hospital ED if transferred), a STAT repeat head CT should be obtained as soon as feasible.

In addition to rebleeding, other important acute neurological complications include: (1) the development of intraventricular extension (IVH); (2) the development of acute obstructive hydrocephalus which is often secondary to the intraventricular extension of ICH; (3) herniation due to increasing mass effect; and (4) increased intracranial pressure (ICP).

IVH is most common in deep hypertensive ICHs and most often presents as abrupt deterioration in the LOC. Those who remain lucid will usually complain of abrupt onset of or abrupt worsening of headache, accompanied by nausea and vomiting. Treatment may include temporizing measures to reduce the ICP, such as osmotic diuretics (mannitol), hyperventilation, or hypertonic saline, but the definitive treatment of symptomatic IVH is placement of an extraventricular drain (EVD). The development of IVH is a poor prognostic feature for ICH.

Acute obstructive hydrocephalus usually presents as acute to subacute worsening of headache, a declining LOC, and loss of upgaze (or, in more severe cases, forced downgaze) with acute papilledema and loss of venous pulsations on fundoscopic examination when it is sufficient to increase the ICP. As with IVH, although medical therapy measures may temporarily ameliorate its effects, EVD placement is the definitive therapy to effectively and durably alleviate ICP elevation and herniation due to this complication. Intraventricular (intrathecal) administration of tissue plasminogen activator (tPA) is being tested as a novel therapeutic approach in the CLEAR-IVH trial, but is not presently routinely recommended in clinical practice. The development of hydrocephalus is also a poor prognostic feature for ICH.

Herniation and consequent irreversible brainstem compression, resulting in coma and death, is the most feared complication of ICH. Measures to reduce the mass effect of the hematoma may include the administration of mannitol (0.25 to 1g/kg IV every 4 to 6 hours and as needed) and other osmotic diuretics, hypertonic saline (1.5, 2, or 3%) titrated to desired ICP or mass effect/shift reduction. These work subacutely over 15 to 30 minutes.

CAUTION

Great care must be taken to maintain intravascular volume when administering osmotic diuretics. Otherwise, precipitous diffuse cerebral arteriolar dilatation, which abruptly increases intracranial volume occupied by these vessels may be provoked and precipitate a dangerous or fatal spike or so-called "plateau wave" of increased ICP.

Hyperventilation to a pCO_2 of 20–25 produces an almost immediate reduction in cerebral volume and ICP but is short-lived and not a viable long-term solution. Surgical evacuation of hematoma was first tested in four small clinical trials, only one of which (by Auer et al., 1989, which involved endoscopically guided hematoma evacuation) showed any potential benefit.

The definitive surgical management of an ICH clinical trial was the ISTICH trial, which randomized 1033 patients to early craniotomy (empiric evacuation of the hematoma prior to any clinical evidence of herniation or significant neurological deterioration) versus delayed craniotomy (craniotomy only when marked clinical deterioration/herniation was occurring despite initial conservative care). No significant difference in good outcome was observed between the early craniotomy group (26%) and the delayed craniotomy group (24%, $p = 0.41$). A trend toward improved outcome was noted in young patients with lobar ICH within 1 cm of the cortex. This group is now being studied in the STICH II trial. STICH I, like other trials of surgery for ICH, only included patients with supratentorial ICH.

The benefit of the surgical evacuation of cerebellar ICH causing actual or threatened hydrocephalus or brainstem compression is well established. The MISTIE trial is investigating whether or not stereotactically guided sequential intrahematomal administration of tPA with sequential aspiration of a liquefied clot is of benefit as a minimally invasive procedure for hematoma evacuation.

This trial has recently been completed and revealed a significant improvement in outcome in patients (defined as a Modified Rankin Score of 0-3) that had at least 15 ml of blood removed. A phase III trial has been submitted for funding. If the phase III trials can verify these findings, this will have a significant impact on how deep intracerebral hemorrhages are treated.

Subsequent Neurological Critical Care of ICH

Similar to ischemic stroke patients, ICH patients are at risk for delayed neurological deterioration. Although delayed rebleeding may occur in TICH patients whose coagulopathy remains uncorrected, rebleeding in noncoagulopathic ICH patients beyond 24 hours post-presentation is rare, occurring in ≤1% of patients. Delayed hydrocephalus and seizures can, however, occur. The most common delayed neurological complication of ICH is the development of perihematomal edema.

Most patients have a thin (1 mm or less) low attenuation rim of perihematomal edema evident on the baseline or 24 hour follow-up head CT. This may represent serum proteins diffusing out to the periphery of the hematoma after the plasma, red cells, and platelets within the hematoma have clotted. Patients with TICH and those with actively bleeding ICH often lack this thin initial rim of perihematomal edema. It does not contribute to the mass effect of the hematoma and, in fact, as the hematoma clots and this initial hyperacute rim of edema forms, hematoma volume actually contracts approximately 6% on average over the first 24 hours. This type of edema does NOT result in neurological deterioration and does NOT result in reactive gliosis, blood–brain barrier breakdown, or inflammation.

Delayed perihematomal edema, by contrast, represents a substantial threat to neurological recovery and survival. It may occur as soon as 48 hours post-ICH onset or as late as 2 to 3 weeks after ICH onset, and may persist for days or weeks before subsiding. Its pathophysiological basis is complex and multifactorial. Experimental and human evidence indicate that perihematomal inflammation occurs due to microglia activation, direct injury to neurons, and direct injury to cerebral blood vessel tight junctions due to breakdown products of lysed red blood cells and hemoglobin byproducts (iron free radicals). This results in the development of both vasogenic and cytotoxic edema. Specific mediators of injury biochemically include matrix metalloprotease 9, iron free radicals, and direct microglial invasion. A pilot trial of desferoxamine (an iron chelater), has been completed and a larger trial is in progress examining the potential therapeutic effects of chelating away the iron free radicals and the oxidative injury they mediate.

Clinically, delayed perihematomal edema presents most often as a delayed and subacute onset of a declining LOC from a previously stable or even previously (transiently) improving focal neurological deficits that were observed upon presentation. It may also present as a new or worsening focal neurological deficit. Delayed herniation and death may occur as far out as 3 weeks post-presentation in rare instances, but the typical period of concern ranges from 2 to 14 days post-ICH onset.

Practitioners should prepare families for the possibility of a delayed and prolonged neurological decline and risk of death. Unexpected deterioration (especially when a patient is initially improving), if unexplained, is an ideal environment for the genesis of malpractice litigations. Ongoing communication of realistic expectations with the family members of critically ill ICH patients generally maximizes patient and family satisfaction. Establishing and periodically re- evaluating the goals of care and level of aggressiveness desired to achieve those goals, is advised.

Treatment of delayed perihematomal edema is often very challenging. Osmotic diuretics, hyperventilation, and hypertonic saline are options. While intuitively one might think that corticosteroids would play a potentially useful role in this setting, current guidelines recommend against their use. Two randomized clinical trials showed not only no benefit in outcome for using them, but also an increased risk of hyperglycemic and infectious complications. Furthermore, their mineralcorticoid effects lead to increased fluid retention in the intravascular space, which may exacerbate cerebral edema and hypertension.

There is a great need for drugs that will directly inhibit glial cell activation and perihematomal inflammation that are not corticosteroids. In cases where delayed perihematomal edema is intractable and refractory to medical therapy, hemicraniectomy is a reasonable consideration to prevent herniation and death. It may be particularly useful in young patients with more superficially located hematomas, though it could also be considered, in principal, for large deep hematomas.

Prophylactic treatment with anticonvulsants for patients with ICH is controversial. Seizures, both clinical and "subclinical" nonconvulsive status epilepticus, represent another common cause of delayed neurological deterioration. Up to 45% of patients with ICH in the NICU setting who undergo continuous bedside EEG monitoring have electrical evidence of seizure activity. However, no difference in the rate of such activity was noted in those receiving "prophylactic" anticonvulsants who had not had clinical seizure activity preceding such monitoring. If anticonvulsants are used (mostly for superficial cortical or temporal lobe hemorrhages), levateracitam may be a good choice based on its accessibility and safety profile. Valproic acid is generally avoided, especially during the first 24 hours post-ICH, and in those on antiplatelet medications, due to its thrombocytopathic effects. Oral anticonvulsants should initially be avoided and given only to those having passed a dysphagia evaluation. *Continous bedside EEG monitoring should be considered where available for any ICH patient with unexplained paroxysmal or a persistent decline in the LOC.*

☆ TIPS & TRICKS

For ICH patients with a persistent or paroxysmal unexplained decline in the LOC, consider a 24-hour, or more, duration of continuous bedside EEG monitoring to rule out nonconvulsive status epilepticus. Avoid narcotics (especially meperidine, tramodol, and morphine) and other commonly used NICU medications ("penem" antibiotics [imipenem/meropenem], dopamine agonists like bromocriptine, diphenhydramine) which may trigger seizures.

ICP monitoring with preservation of cerebral perfusion pressure of at least 50 mmHg (and ideally 70 mmHg) may be useful in patients with large hematomas with substantial mass effect. Its ability to improve the outcome is controversial.

Subsequent Medical Critical Care of ICH

The focus of medical care for the patient after ICH is to prevent subsequent medical complication. This can be accomplished through ongoing attention to DVT prevention and surveillance with bi-weekly lower extremity venous duplexes, skin breakdown assessment, prevention and treatment, aspiration prevention, regular changes of Foley catheters, central lines, and EVDs, which are all potentially effective strategies to minimize the risk of delayed medical complications. Monitoring and treating fever with acetaminophen may improve neurological status. Early discussion and consideration of tracheostomy and PEG in those ICH patients with larger or poorer prognosis ICH in whom prolonged respiratory failure and/or aspiration risk is anticipated, helps to minimize the risks of pulmonary complications.

Bibliography

Andersen CS, Huang Y, Wang JG, et al. Intensive blood pressure reduction in acute intracerebral haemorrhage trial (INTERACT): a randomized pilot trial. *Lancet Neurol* 2008; **7:**391–399.

Auer LM, Deinsbergerg W, Niederkorn K, et al. Endoscopic surgery versus medical treatment for spontaneous intracerebral hematoma: a randomized study. *J Neurosurg* 1989; **70:** 530–535.

Brott TG, Broderick JP, Kothari RU, et al. Early hemorrhage growth in patients with intracerebral hemorrhage. *Stroke* 1997; **28:**1–5.

Gebel J, Jauch E, Brott T, et al. Natural history of perihematomal edema in patients with hyperacute spontaneous intracerebral hemorrhage. *Stroke* 2002; **33:**2631–2635.

Gebel J, Jauch E, Brott T, et al. Relative edema volume is a predictor of outcome in patients with hyperacute spontaneous intracerebral hemorrhage. *Stroke* 2002; **33:**2636–2641.

Gebel J, Sila C, Sloan M, et al. Thrombolysis-related intracranial hemorrhage: a radiographic analysis of 244 cases from the GUSTO-1 trial with clinical correlation. *Stroke* 1998; **29:**563–569.

Manno EM, Atkinson JLD, Fulgham JR, Wijdicks EFM. Emerging medical and surgical management strategies in the evaluation and treatment of intracerebral hemorrhage. *Mayo Clin Proc* 2005; **80:**420–433.

Mendelow AD, Gregson BA, Fernandes HM, et al. (STICH investigators.) Early surgery versus initial conservative treatment in patients with spontaneous supratentorial intracerebral haematomas in the International Surgical Trial in Intracerebral Haemorrhage (STICH): a randomized trial. *Lancet* 2005; **365:**387–397.

Morganstern L, Hemphill JC, Anderson C, et al. Guidelines for the management of spontaneous intracerebral hemorrhage: a guideline for health care professionals from the American Heart Association/American Stroke Association. *Stroke* 2010; **41:**2018–2129.

Quereshi AI, Tuhrim S, Broderick JP, et al. Spontaneous intracerebral hemorrhage. *New Engl J Med* 2001; **344:**1450–1460.

Qureshi A. Antihypertensive treatment of acute cerebral hemorrhage (ATACH) trial. Presented at the International Stroke Conference, New Orleans, La, February 20–22, 2008.

Qureshi AI. Antihypertensive treatment of acute cerebral hemorrhage (ATACH): rationale and design. *Neurocrit Care* 2007; **6:**56–66.

Acute Management of Status Epilepticus

Jan Claassen

Division of Neurocritical Care and the Comprehensive Epilepsy Center, Department of Neurology, Columbia University, New York, NY, USA

Introduction and Definition

Status epilepticus (SE) is an acute life-threatening neurological emergency. Most recent literature agrees that any convulsions lasting for more than 5 minutes, or two or more convulsions in a 5-minute interval without return to preconvulsive neurological baseline, are sufficient to qualify for the diagnosis of SE. Since very few isolated seizures will last for 5 minutes or longer the traditional requirement for seizures to last for a minimum of 30 minutes has been abandoned by most authors. Patients with nonconvulsive SE (NCSE) do not exhibit overt signs of convulsions but have seizure activity documented on the EEG.

⚴ SCIENCE REVISITED

In animal models permanent damage and pharmacoresistance can be demonstrated earlier than 30 minutes after onset of seizures. The majority of clinical and electrographic seizures last less than 5 minutes and seizures that last longer often do not stop spontaneously.

Diagnosis and Clinical Presentation

Convulsive SE presents classically with generalized tonic–clonic movements or rhythmic jerking of the extremities, mental status is impaired, and additional neurological findings such as aphasia, amnesia, staring, automatisms, blinking, facial twitching, agitation, nystagmus, eye deviation, and perseveration may be seen. Transient benign post-ictal focal findings such as Todd's paralysis may persist. Typically, patients with generalized convulsive SE are expected to awaken gradually after the motor features of seizures disappear. Approximately half of all patients with generalized tonic–clonic seizures will have nonconvulsive seizures after convulsions have subsided and 14% will have NCSE. Classic findings of NCSE include ictal discharges on EEG, with or without subtle convulsive movements that may include twitching of the arms, legs, trunk, or facial muscles, tonic eye deviation, and nystagmoid eye jerking.

The differential diagnosis for convulsive and NCSE includes movement disorders (myoclonus, asterixis, tremor, chorea, tics, dystonia), herniation (decerebrate or decorticate posturing), limb-shaking transient ischemic attacks (TIAs) most commonly associated with perfusion failure due

Emergency Management in Neurocritical Care, First Edition. Edited by Edward M. Manno.
© 2012 John Wiley & Sons, Ltd. Published 2012 by John Wiley & Sons, Ltd.

to severe carotid stenosis, and psychiatric disorders also known as pseudostatus. Findings that suggest the presence of pseudostatus include poorly coordinated thrashing, back arching, eyes held shut, head rolling, pelvic thrusting, and preserved consciousness or purposeful movements. However, when in doubt, always assume that status is real and treat it adequately. Additionally, the differential diagnosis for NCSE is very broad and any condition that can lead to a decreased level of consciousness (e.g. toxic-metabolic encephalopathies, including hypoglycemia and delirium, anoxia, and CNS infections), transient global amnesia, sleep disorders (e.g. parasomnias), or syncope may be considered.

✶ TIPS & TRICKS

If the level of consciousness is not improving within 20 minutes of cessation of the movements, or if the patient's mental status remains abnormal 30 to 60 minutes after the convulsions cease, NCSE must be considered and urgent EEG is advised.

Epidemiology and Underlying Etiology

Convulsive SE occurs with an estimated incidence of 5 to 30 per 100,000 person years. The most common cause of SE is a prior history of epilepsy (22–26%). However, more than half of the episodes of SE occur in patients without prior seizures, often precipitated by an acute illness. In adults without a prior seizure history, stroke (19–20%) is the most frequent underlying etiology. In children, a major cause of SE is infection accompanied by fever, while alcohol intoxication or withdrawal is very common among young adults. No good data exists on the incidence of NCSE. Case series have reported that 10–30% of patients in neuro ICUs have nonconvulsive seizures or NCSE and found them to be particularly prevalent in patients with epilepsy, CNS infections, brain tumors, post-neurosurgery, and stroke. Interestingly, 10% of medical ICU patients without brain injury (particularly those with sepsis) will have nonconvulsive seizures and most

of these will be in NCSE. In one of the few prospective studies, 37% of 198 patients undergoing urgent EEG for altered MS were found to have nonconvulsive seizures. Electrographic seizures are more likely in those with coma, young age, a past medical history of epilepsy or remote risk factors for seizures, documented convulsive seizures prior to monitoring, periodic discharges (lateralized or generalized) or suppression-burst patterns on EEG, oculomotor abnormalities (i.e. nystagmus, hippus, or eye deviation), cardiac or respiratory arrest, and sepsis.

Acute Management
Prehospital Treatment

Several studies have shown that the most important variable predicting seizure control is the time that has elapsed prior to initiating antiepileptic drugs (AEDs). Following this principle, patients should receive benzodiazepine treatment as soon as they are diagnosed with SE. This may be in the form of the intravenous administration of lorazepam (4 mg IV given over 2 minutes) or diazepam, or diazepam (5 mg IV), but alternative routes of administration are also possible, including 20 mg of diazepam per rectum, and intranasal, buccal, or intramuscular 10 mg of midazolam – all of which were shown to be effective alternatives to IV administration (see Table 8.1).

Other important considerations for the prehospital phase of SE treatment include airway support, assuring stable circulation, if possible obtaining IV access, diagnosing hypoglycemia and administration of D50W 50 mL IV and thiamine 100 mg IV for those found to be hypoglycemic. As a side note, lorazepam needs to be refrigerated; for this reason it is usually impractical for emergency medical service (EMS) use and diazepam or midazolam are used as alternatives.

EVIDENCE AT A GLANCE

Alldredge et al. (2001) investigated if initiation of SE treatment in the prehospital setting could be safely done and lead to a better outcome. Patients treated with lorazepam by the EMS prior to reaching the hospital had better acute seizure control than those that received diazepam or a placebo. Importantly, these authors found that respiratory decompensation was more commonly seen in patients who got a placebo than those who were given benzodiazepine. Recently, Silbergleit et al (2012) demonstrated that intramuscular midazoalm is at least as effective and safe for prehopsital treatment of status epilepticus when compared to intravenous lorazepam.

Immediate Management Steps, Including First-Line Antiepileptic Medication

In the emergency room the following should be addressed immediately: secure the airway and breathing, support the blood pressure, obtain IV access, and administer first-line antiepileptic

Table 8.1. Simplified outline for management of SE

- Diagnose; ABCs, IV access, EKG monitoring; draw blood
- Thiamine 100 mg, D50W 50 mL IV
- Lorazepam 4 mg/2 min IV (or diazepam 5 mg IV) or 10 mg IM midazolam
↓
- Fosphenytoin load: 20 mg/kg IV at up to 150 mg/min (phenytoin is an alternative) (or valproate load: 40 mg/kg IV over 10 min)
- May skip this step and go straight to the next box if seizures continue after lorazepam
- If possible connect to EEG unless the patient wakes up or returns to preconvulsive baseline
- Consider intubation if the patient requires more sedative medications
↓
- Continuous IV midazolam or continuous IV propofol (dosing, see Table 8.2)
- Alternative IV valproate
- Continuous EEG needed
↓
- Continuous IV pentobarbital (dosing, see Table 8.2)
- Continuous EEG needed

Table 8.2. Initial diagnostic work-up

All patients
1. Fingerstick glucose
2. Pulse oximetry, supplement as needed
3. Monitor BP, HR, O_2 sat, support if needed
4. Obtain IV access
5. Head CT (for most cases)
6. Order labs: blood sugar, complete blood count, basic metabolic panel, calcium, magnesium, liver function tests, troponin, toxicology screen (urine and blood), anticonvulsant levels (at least for phenytoin, valproate, carbamazepine), type and hold, coagulation studies
7. continuous EEG monitoring – Notify EEG tech if available (as soon as available unless patient returns to prestatus epilepticus baseline)

Depending on clinical presentation
1. Brain MRI
2. Lumbar puncture
3. Toxins that are frequently associated with seizures (i.e. INH, tricyclics, theophylline, cocaine, sympathomimetics, alcohol, organophosphates, cyclosporine)
4. Labs: phosphorous, ABG, inborn errors of metabolism.

medication (see Table 8.2). It is crucial to diagnose hypoglycemia promptly and, if present, treat it with 50 mL of D50W IV together with thiamine (100 mg IV).

Lorazepam (4 mg IV over 2 min) should be given as the first-line antiepileptic medication or, if this is unavailable, diazepam 5 mg IV may serve as an alternative. In patients where IV access cannot be secured, benzodiazepine administration should not be delayed and diazepam 20 mg per rectum (given either as a diastat or as an IV solution of diazepam), or midazolam 10 mg intranasal, buccal, intramuscular, or IV are options. As mentioned above, the single most important factor in predicting seizure control is time elapsed prior to initiating AEDs. If unable to get intravenous access, benzodiazepines should be given promptly via an alternative route (i.e. rectal, buccal, or intramuscular).

EVIDENCE AT A GLANCE

Treiman et al. (1998) foud that lorazepam was superior to alternatives in this large randomized, double-blind, multicenter trial of four regimens: diazepam plus phenytoin, phenytoin alone, lorazepam alone, and phenobarbital alone. The best seizure control was seen with lorazepam.

✶ TIPS & TRICKS

A complete work-up of the underlying etiology needs to be initiated as soon as possible since seizures due to underlying uncorrected metabolic problems (i.e. hypoglycemia) are difficult to control with antiepileptic mediations.

✶ TIPS & TRICKS

Most physicians would not give first- and second-line antiepileptic medications in a sequential order, but together. Seizures may stop after the initial benzodiazepines but have a high chance of recurrence if longer-acting antiepileptics are not started.

☝ CAUTION

- Ongoing convulsions may be masked when using paralytics for intubation.
- Hypotension may be seen with loading phenytoin or fosphenytoin.
- Give a loading dose of phenytoin or fosphenytoin that is weight based, and not 1 g for everyone.
- Do not adjust loading doses for renal or hepatic insufficiency.

Second-Line Antiepileptic Medications

While most experts agree that benzodiazepines should be given as first-line therapy, a number of alternatives are recommended for additional treatment. Generally, most physicians would load any patient that has received first-line therapy with phenytoin/fosphenytoin (load: 20 mg/kg IV at up to 150 mg/min, while phenytoin needs to be given at a rate of up to 50 mg/min; more caution may be needed with elderly patients) or valproic acid (load: 40 mg/kg IV over 10 min; an additional 20 mg/kg may be given over 5 min if still seizing) and start maintenance therapy with either medication. Blood pressure and heart rate should be monitored closely since hypotension can be seen during the loading of phenytoin or fosphenytoin. In patients in whom convulsions persist after the administration of benzodiazepines, experts increasingly recommend skipping second-line antiepileptic medications and starting continuous antiepileptic medications, such as midazolam or propofol. This will be discussed in detail below. Levetiracetam (load: 2.5 g IV over 5 min at 1–4 g over 15 min) may be an attractive alternative as a second-line agent but data is limited so far. Phenobarbital may be an alternative choice if the above medications are contraindicated or not available (load: 20 mg/kg IV up to 60 mg/min; maintenance 1–3 mg/kg/day in 2–3 divided doses).

If logistics allow, all patients that do not return to a preconvulsive neurological baseline within 20 minutes after convulsions have ceased should be connected to EEG monitoring to diagnose nonconvulsive electrographic seizures. As mentioned above, a substantial number of patients will continue to have electrographic seizures after convulsions have stopped. Clinical expression of seizures may also be masked in patients that received paralytics for purposes of intubation. It is unclear how aggressive electrographic seizures and NCSE should be treated, but most evidence suggests that, in the acute brain injury setting, electrographic seizures should be treated aggressively.

Refractory Status Epilepticus

Patients are generally classified as refractory status epilepticus (RSE) if seizures persist after treatment with standard regimens. Most experts would call any ongoing SE refractory after receiving an initial benzodiazepine and a second acceptable anticonvulsant agent. Recommendation for treatment of RSE is primarily based on case series and expert opinion and, as a result, practices vary widely. Conceptually, therapeutic approaches should be stratified into an initial approach for those that have failed second-line AEDs and into those that require advanced treatment of RSE. Most experts would recommend treatment with a continuous IV AED such as midazolam or propofol (see Table 8.3 for dosing and administration information) as the initial step, but valproic acid may be a reasonable alternative, particularly in patients that have previously expressed a desire not to be intubated.

Table 8.3. Treatment of refractory status epilepticus

Continuous infusions of midazolam
- Load: 0.2 mg/kg IV over 2–5 min; repeat 0.2–0.4 mg/kg boluses every 5 min until seizures stop, up to a maximum loading dose of 2 mg/kg
- Initial rate: 0.1 mg/kg/h. Bolus and increase rate until seizure control
- Maintenance: 0.05–2.9 mg/kg/h

Continuous infusions of propofol
- Load: 1–2 mg/kg IV over 3–5 min; repeat boluses every 3–5 min until seizures stop, up to maximum total loading dose of 10 mg/kg
- Initial rate: 33 µg/kg/min (2 mg/kg/h). Bolus and increase rate until seizure control
- Maintenance: 17–250 µg/kg/min (1–15 mg/kg/h)

Valproic acid (if not chosen already as second-line agent)
- 40 mg/kg IV over 10 min (may give additional 20 mg/kg over 5 min if still seizing)

Phenobarbital
- Load: 20 mg/kg IV up to 60 mg/min
- Maintenance: 1–3 mg/kg/day in 2–3 divided doses

Pentobarbital
- Load: 5 mg/kg IV up to 50 mg/min; repeat 5 mg/kg boluses until seizures stop.
- Initial rate: 1 mg/kg/h
- Maintenance: 0.5–10 mg/kg/h traditionally titrated to suppression-burst on EEG but titrating to seizure suppression is reasonable as well

Table 8.4. Alternative therapies for refractory status epilepticus

Pharmacological
- Ketamine
- Corticosteroids
- Inhaled anesthetics
- Immunomodulation (IVIG or PE)

Nonpharmacological
- Vagus nerve stimulation
- Ketogenic diet
- Hypothermia
- Electroconvulsive therapy
- Transcranial magnetic stimulation
- Surgical management

Case reports and small case series
- Lidocaine
- Verapamil
- Paraldehyde
- Azetazolamide
- Deep brain stimulation

Most experts would not use phenobarbital in these circumstances. (See alternative therapies in Table 8.4.)

There is controversy regarding the target of continuous drips. Some advocate for seizure control or a burst suppression pattern on EEG monitoring, while others argue for complete background suppression. The best duration of maintaining continuous IV AEDs is similarly unclear. After seizures are controlled most physicians would continue IV therapy for at least 24 hours before starting to wean them. The speed of weaning is also controversial but should not be done too abruptly unless the agent is pentobarbital.

> **⚜ SCIENCE REVISITED**
>
> All patients should be connected to continuous EEG at this point if available since breakthrough and withdrawal seizures are frequent when treating with continuous IV AEDs. Initiate a consultation for a possible transfer if continuous EEG monitoring is not available at the institution (Claassen et al., 2002).

It is unclear how aggressive electrographic seizures and nonconvulsive status epilepticus should be treated, but most evidence suggests that, in the acute brain injury setting, electrographic seizures should be treated aggressively (Vespa et al., 2010). There is evidence from animal literature and in humans in a number of acute brain injury settings that electrographic seizures may cause additional brain injury.

Be sure to continue all second-line antiepileptic medications when starting treatment with continuous IV AEDs and follow serum levels when available (i.e. phenytoin or valproic acid). Serum levels may be obtained immediately post-infusion of valproic acid but should not be drawn before 2 hours after the infusions of fosphenytoin and phenytoin have passed.

Advanced Treatment of RSE

Many physicians will elect to use continuous infusions of pentobarbital (see Table 8.3 for dosing recommendations). All patients on pentobarbital for RSE will need continuous EEG monitoring. Often switching to pentobarbital will be performed in the ICU setting but at times, with patients that are highly refractory, pentobarbital infusions may need to be started while in the ER and within the first hour of SE onset. Similar controversies exist for treatment duration and titration goals for advanced therapy, as those mentioned above for the initial treatment of RSE. When comparing different treatment strategies of RSE, pentobarbital was less frequently associated with breakthrough and withdrawal seizures and more frequently associated with hypotension when compared with propofol or midazolam. Breakthrough seizures can be expected in 20–50% of patients and are usually treated with extra boluses of the current c.IV AED, together with optimization or addition of noncontinuous

IV AEDs. A long list of less-well-studied new approaches exists (see Table 8.4). Of particular interest are medications that target the refractoriness of SE to treatment (see Science Revisited 8.3) and therapies that may also be neuroprotective (i.e. therapeutic hypothermia). All of these are currently poorly studied and at this point should be considered investigational.

Hypotension is a frequent side effect of pentobarbital, and vasopressors should be readily available. Other side effects include gastric stasis, myocardial suppression, thrombocytopenia, metabolic acidosis.

Evidence from Chen and Wasterlain (2006) suggests that a number of mechanisms primarily related to the impairment of GABA-mediated inhibition might be involved in the development of refractoriness to treatment. These include internalization of GABA receptors, reduced sensitivity of GABA receptors, increased numbers of AMPA and NMDA receptors at the synaptic membrane, and drug efflux transporters. The development of drugs that specifically target these mechanisms may be most promising for the treatment of RSE.

Treatment Endpoints

As mentioned above, the duration of continuous IV AEDs is controversial but suppression should be sufficient to prevent a recurrence of seizures, with 24–72 hours of EEG suppression most frequently employed. When weaning is initiated this should be done under EEG monitoring. Withdrawal seizures may be seen in approximately half of the patients and should be treated adequately. One approach is to restart the continuous IV AED at the same rate that the patient was having prior to the taper, maximize or add noncontinuous IV AEDs and then repeat tapering after 24 hours without seizures. Alternatively patients may be switched to a different continuous IV AED.

Continuous EEG Monitoring

As outlined above all patients that do not return to their pre-SE baseline and those that have RSE should undergo continuous EEG monitoring since the majority of SE in the ICU is nonconvulsive. Intermittent EEGs will miss a large portion of seizures recorded in acutely brain-injured patients.

★ TIPS & TRICKS

Practically comatose patients should undergo a minimum of 48 hours of monitoring, while those that are noncomatose may only require 24 hours. In those patients where periodic epileptiform discharges are recorded, prolonged monitoring may be warranted since these patients may develop electrographic seizures. Limited montages are discouraged since focal seizures may be missed (minimum of 16–21 electrodes).

Effects of SE On Other Organ Systems

- *Cardiac.* Cardiac arrhythmias are frequent in the setting of ongoing SE. Interestingly, contraction band necrosis – presumably secondary to massive catecholamine release – has been associated with death during SE. Patients with SE and particularly RSE should have cardiovascular monitoring and cardiac enzymes checked.
- *Pulmonary.* Many patients with SE and most with RSE warrant intubation. Hypoxia, pulmonary edema, and aspiration are frequently seen after SE and a chest Xray should be obtained for most patients.
- *Infectious disease.* Infections may be the cause but also may be seen due to SE (i.e. pneumonia). Fever should prompt blood, urine, and CSF cultures as well as a chest X-ray. A mild elevation in the white blood cell count may be seen in the serum and CSF as a consequence of ongoing seizure activity.

- *Electrolytes.* Metabolic derangements (glucose, sodium, phosphate, calcium, pH) can be the underlying cause or the effect of SE. These should be corrected aggressively as outlined above since seizures may be very difficult to control with persistent metabolic abnormalities.
- *Renal.* Rhabdomyolysis and myoglobinuria leading to renal failure may be seen after prolonged convulsive SE and should be treated with adequate hydration.

Prognosis

In population-based studies, 10–20% of patients admitted with convulsive SE are dead at hospital discharge. Survivors have an increased risk of developing epilepsy and 10–23% of them are left with new or disabling neurological deficits such as cognitive decline. The in-hospital mortality of patients with NCSE is 18–52% and goes up to 65% at one month follow-up. Most studies found a worse outcome in older patients, those presenting with an acute symptomatic etiology (i.e. anoxic brain injury or stroke), and particularly those with a long duration of seizure. The presence of electrographic status, and ictal and periodic discharges, carries a worse prognosis. On the other hand, patients with SE due to withdrawal from antiepileptics or alcohol have a better prognosis. Approximately half of all patients with RSE are dead at hospital discharge in most studies and only a little more than half of survivors return to their premorbid functional baseline. Predictors of poor outcome are similar to those reported for convulsive and nonconvulsive SE.

Bibliography

Alldredge BK, Gelb AM, Isaacs SM, et al. A vcomparison of lorazepam, diazepam, and placebo for the treatment of out-of-hospital status epilepticus. *New Engl J Med* 2001; **345(9)**: 631–637.

Chen JW, Wasterlain CG. Status epilepticus: pathophysiology and management in adults. *Lancet Neurol* 2006 Mar; **5(3)**: 246–256.

Claassen J, Hirsch LJ, Emerson RG, Mayer SA. Treatment of refractory status epilepticus with pentobarbital, propofol, or midazolam: a systematic review. *Epilepsia* 2002; **43(2)**:146–153.

DeLorenzo RJ, Waterhouse EJ, Towne AR, et al. Persistent nonconvulsive status epilepticus after the control of convulsive status epilepticus. *Epilepsia* 1998; **39(8)**: 833–840.

Hesdorffer DC, Logroscino G, Cascino G, Annegers JF, Hauser WA. Incidence of status epilepticus in Rochester, Minnesota, 1965–1984. *Neurology* 1998; **50**: 735–741.

Lowenstein DH, Alldredge BK. Status epilepticus. *New Engl J Med* 1998; **338(14)**: 970–976.

Manno EM, Pfeifer EA, Cascino GD. Cardiac pathology in status epilepticus. *Ann Neurol* 2005; **58(6)**: 954–957.

Rossetti AO, Oddo M, Logroscino G, Kaplan PW. Prognostication after cardiac arrest and hypothermia: a prospective study. *Ann Neurol* 2010; **67**: 301–307.

Silbergleit R, Durkalski V, Lowenstein D, Conwit R, Pancioli A, Palesch Y, Barsan W; NETT Investigators. Intramuscular versus intravenous therapy for prehospital status epilepticus. New Engl *J Med.* 2012 Feb 16; **366(7)**: 591–600.

Towne AR, Waterhouse EJ, Boggs JG, et al. Prevalence of nonconvulsive status epilepticus in comatose patients. *Neurology* 2000; **55(9)**: 1421–1423.

Treiman DM, Meyers PD, Walton NY, et al. (Veterans Affairs Status Epilepticus Cooperative Study Group). A comparison of four treatments for generalized convulsive status epilepticus. *New Engl J Med* 1998; **339**(12):792–798.

Vespa PM, McArthur DL, Xu Y, et al. Nonconvulsive seizures after traumatic brain injury are associated with hippocampal atrophy. *Neurology* 2010 Aug; **75(9)**: 792–798.

Young GB, Jordan KG, Doig GS. An assessment of nonconvulsive seizures in the intensive care unit using continuous EEG monitoring: an investigation of variables associated with mortality. *Neurology* 1996; **47(1)**: 83–89.

Part II

Cerebrovascular Critical Care

Post-procedural Management of Patients with Aneurysmal Subarachnoid Hemorrhage

Tomoko Rie Sampson and Michael N. Diringer

Neurology/Neurosurgery Intensive Care Unit, Department of Neurology and Neurological Surgery, Washington University School of Medicine, Saint Louis, MO, USA

Introduction

Morbidity and mortality related to aneurysmal subarachnoid hemorrhage (aSAH) has improved greatly over the last 20 years. This is, in part, due to the improved management of complications in patients who survive the initial ictus. The complications associated with aSAH can be some of the most difficult to manage in a critical care setting.

In this chapter, we will discuss the management of neurologic and medical complications of subarachnoid hemorrhage (SAH) after an aneurysm has been secured.

Vasospasm and Delayed Cerebral Ischemia

Once the offending aneurysm is repaired surgically or endovascularly, the risk for rebleeding of the aneurysm is markedly reduced, thus emphasizing the need for early intervention. After the ruptured aneurysm is "secured," the main concern then becomes the prevention and management of delayed cerebral ischemia (DCI), as well as other medical complications associated with SAH. Therefore, a major focus of care in the

ensuing days and weeks involve minimizing the impact of DCI and complications.

Survival after aSAH is most affected by the impact of DCI in the days after the initial bleed, accounting for approximately half of deaths of those who survive to treatment. DCI is closely linked to the narrowing of large cerebral arteries (cerebral vasospasm) that can occur as early as 3 days after hemorrhage, with maximal narrowing occurring between 5 and 10 days after the bleed. Patients with an increased risk of developing DCI include those with poor clinical grade, thick subarachnoid clot or intraventricular hemorrhage, evidence of early angiographic vasospasm, younger age, hypertension, or a history of smoking.

> ## ⚙ SCIENCE REVISITED
>
> - *Vasospasm in aneurysmal subarachnoid hemorrhage:* In subarachnoid hemorrhage (SAH), the development of vasospasm reflects a very complex cascade of cellular dysfunction in addition to pathologic changes in the arterial walls of affected

Emergency Management in Neurocritical Care, First Edition. Edited by Edward M. Manno.
© 2012 John Wiley & Sons, Ltd. Published 2012 by John Wiley & Sons, Ltd.

vessels. Though the actual mechanism of post-SAH vasospasm remains unclear, it has been linked to the release of free hemoglobin from red blood cell lysis in the subarachnoid space. This may result in numerous mechanisms leading to vasospasm that include, decreased nitric oxide (NO) production, changes in endothelin levels, differential gene up-regulation, and increased oxidative stresses on the cells.

- *Anatomic changes in vessels:* In addition to changes in vascular reactivity and enhanced vasoconstriction structural changes occur in cerebral vessels following SAH. Vessel wall thickness is increased due to the remodeling of smooth muscle cells narrowing the lumen. In addition, collagen fiber reorganization impairs vessel dilation.
- *Impaired vascular reactivity:* In addition to luminal narrowing and impaired relaxation of large vessels, the function of small penetrating arterioles is impaired following SAH. Autoregulation of CBF in response to changes in perfusion pressure is frequently impaired, as well as reactivity to changes in carbon dioxide tension. This impaired reactivity is more common in poor grade patients and confers an increased risk of DCI.
- *Other potential factors:* Several other factors have been implicated in the development of DCI following SAH that are not related to vessel constriction. Microthrombi may develop in regions with low flow. Spreading cortical depression, slow-moving waves of neuronal depolarization, have been associated with DCI, even in the absence of large vessel vasospasm.

★ TIPS & TRICKS

Clinical grading of subarachnoid hemorrhage: Some of the scales that are used to gauge the severity of subarachnoid hemorrhage (SAH) can help to predict the development of DCI in these patients. Traditionally the Hunt and Hess score and the Fisher scales have been used. More recently they have been

supplanted by the World Federation of Neurologic Surgeons (WFNS) scale and the Modified Fisher scale. The Modified Fisher scale uses radiologic appearance to grade severity, while the Hunt & Hess score and the WFNS scale grade the clinical condition. Both scales provide best predictive value with evaluation at the initial clinical presentation. Higher scores represent a worse grade and prognosis.

WFNS scale

Grade	GCS score	Motor deficit
I	15	Absent
II	14–13	Absent
III	14–13	Present
IV	12–7	Present or absent
V	6–3	Present or absent

Modified Fisher scale

Score	Radiologic appearance
0	No SAH or IVH
1	Minimal or thin SAH, no IVH in lateral ventricles
2	Minimal or thin SAH, with IVH in lateral ventricles
3	Thick SAH (completely filling one or more cistern or fissure), no IVH in lateral ventricles
4	Thick SAH, with IVH in lateral ventricles

Angiographic vasospasm is seen in up to 70% of patients with aSAH (see Figure 9.1). Only about half of patients with angiographic vasospasm will actually develop clinical vasospasm, which emphasizes that arterial narrowing and DCI are not synonymous. Clinically, DCI manifests as an acute or subacute change in neurologic status, including an altered level of consciousness, agitation, focal neurologic deficits, or a new-onset aphasia or abulia. Signs and symptoms may wax and wane. These deficits may be reversible with treatment, but permanent ischemic damage is possible.

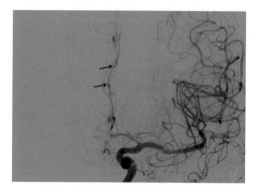

Figure 9.1. Angiographic evidence of vasospasm. This is from an angiogram performed on day 7 after aneurysm rupture and shows severe vasospasm of the left anterior cerebral artery (arrows).

Monitoring for DCI typically consists of serial neurologic examinations, transcranial Doppler examination, and cerebral angiography. Angiography remains the gold standard for the detection of vasospasm. Newer, potentially useful monitoring tools include computed tomography (CT) and magnetic resonance (MR) perfusion, and focal probes that perform microdialysis and measure brain oxygen tension. In addition to its diagnostic power, angiography also allows for the intraprocedure treatment of vasospasm.

Monitoring for DCI

Patients who have undergone the repair of an aneurysm are typically monitored in an intensive care unit setting. This allows for frequent serial neurologic examination and prompt recognition and initiation of treatment for clinical vasospasm. A change in neurologic status should always be investigated quickly and thoroughly. Alternative causes for neurologic changes must be considered prior to making the diagnosis of clinical vasospasm (see Figure 9.2).

Transcranial doppler (TCD) examination involves the serial measurement of blood flow velocities in cerebral vessels. The velocity rises either as a vessel diameter decreases or cerebral blood flow (CBF) increases. This modality is best suited for the assessment of vasospasm in the larger caliber vessels, such as the middle cerebral artery or the intracranial portion of the internal carotid artery. While TCD is a noninvasive and safe method, it is not without its disadvantages. About 10% of patients lack adequate "bone windows" making it impossible to detect blood flow velocities. As with other ultrasound modalities, it is a user-dependent technology. It also can be misleading when used to monitor the impact of interventions. In patients who are treated for vasospasm with hemodynamic augmentation, flow velocity can rise as blood pressure is elevated and CBF rises, leading to a conclusion of worsening vasospasm when, in fact, the rising velocities reflect the desired response to induced hypertension.

There are other methods for the detection of DCI that are under investigation. Cerebral microdialysis may offer some insight in the understanding and detection of DCI. This method can measure the level of substances in the extracellular fluid in a very small region of the brain. Increases in lactate, the lactate/pyruvate ratio, and glycerol have been observed in patients with symptomatic vasospasm. Other focal probes are available that measure brain tissue oxygen tension and local CBF. It remains to be determined if DCI can be detected prior to the onset of symptoms. Additionally, a major limitation to these methods is that they sample a single very small region of the brain that may or may not include the areas susceptible for developing DCI.

Imaging methods for the detection of vasospasm include perfusion CT, Xenon CT, diffusion–perfusion MRI, and SPECT. These methods offer the advantage of sampling a significant volume of brain tissue but only provide a snapshot of the physiologic state rather than the continuous data provided by focal probes. Current studies are investigating the clinical utility of these imaging techniques. They may be complementary to established modalities and focal probes rather than sole methods for the diagnosis of DCI.

Treatment for clinical vasospasm is aimed at minimizing permanent ischemic damage to the brain parenchyma and is accomplished by attempts to improve oxygen delivery to tissue at risk. Vasospasm treatment involves a combination of prophylactic treatment and intensive interventions that are instituted as vasospasm manifests. Prophylactic interventions include

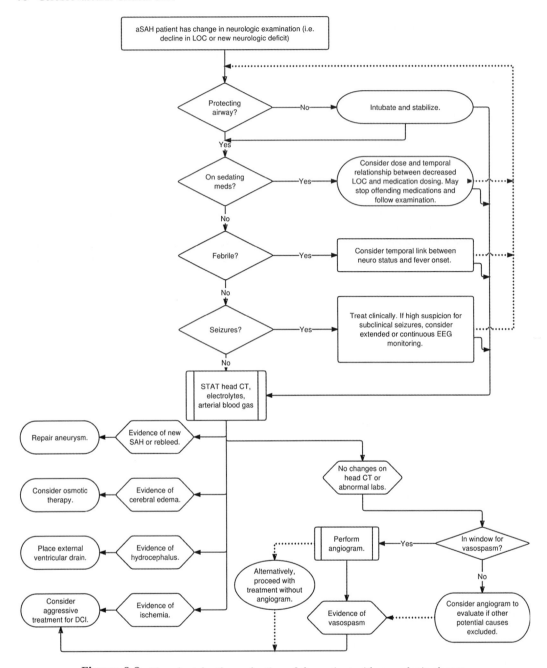

Figure 9.2. Flowchart for the evaluation of the patient with neurologic change.

nimodipine administration and the prevention of hypovolemia.

Nimodipine, a calcium channel blocker, reduces the impact of cerebral ischemia and improves the functional outcome. It does not, however, affect the presence of angiographic vasospasm. It can be given orally or via nasogastric tube, dosed at 60 mg every 4 hours. Hypotension is infrequent if the patient is well hydrated. Treatment with nimodipine begins at the time of admission and should continue to 21 days out from the ictus.

⚠ CAUTION

IV administration of nimodipine:
Nimodipine has no intravenous formulation; however, the FDA had received several reports on the IV administration of nimodipine, inducing the maker to put a black box warning on the drug. There were several reports of adverse cardiovascular events, including death. The drug comes in a capsule and requires aspiration of the contents with a standard needle. Careful labeling of syringes containing nimodipine with "NOT FOR IV USE" can be helpful in preventing inadvertent IV administration.

★ TIPS & TRICKS

Adjusting nimodipine dosing: Nimodipine administration can be adjusted to minimize precipitous decreases in blood pressure by giving it in smaller, more frequent doses (30 mg every 2 h).

Hemodynamic Interventions

Several decades ago it was recognized that SAH patients tend to develop hypovolemia which was associated with, symptomatic DCI and cerebral infarcts. While the mechanisms responsible for this continue to be debated, the administration of large volumes of fluids has been widely accepted as a means of ameliorating hypovolemia. This led to the concept that inducing hypervolemia may be useful in the prevention and treatment of DCI.

Prospective studies indicate that prophylactic hypervolemia does not improve CBF and is associated with increased risk of medical complications, including pulmonary and cerebral edema. Current guidelines recommend *maintenance of euvolemia* in the prevention of symptomatic vasospasm, and frequent assessments of volume status should be made to determine the normal

circulating blood volume. This may be accomplished by following volume balance, and body weight. The use of arbitrary central venous pressure (CVP) or pulmonary capillary wedge pressure (PCWP) targets does not appear to add additional benefit. Though no studies have addressed the use of continuous hemodynamic monitoring using either arterial pulse pressure waveform analysis systems, these monitors can provide valuable information regarding cardiac function. They can be useful in titrating hemodynamic intervention, particularly in patients with comorbidities, such as congestive heart failure or cardiomyopathy.

The trigger for more aggressive therapy for DCI varies across centers. In some the decision is guided by rising TCD velocities, angiographic vasospasm or clinical symptoms. These treatments include "triple-H" therapy, also referred to as hemodynamic augmentation with various degrees of volume expansion, augmentation of cardiac output, and elevation of blood pressure. Additionally, endovascular manipulation, including angioplasty and infusion of intra-arterial vasodilators, is often employed.

In most institutions implementation of hemodynamic augmentation is reserved for patients who have had the ruptured aneurysm repaired to minimize the risk of inducing rebleeding. Uncertainty exists as to how safe the therapy is in patients with multiple aneurysms when only the ruptured aneurysm has been repaired. The goal of this approach is to improve CBF and oxygen delivery. The relative contribution of each component of hemodynamic augmentation has been debated however, as the benefit of each approach has never been subjected to a controlled trial.

Of the three treatment modalities, induced hypertension probably provides the greatest contribution in improving both the CBF and oxygen delivery. Agent selection will be dependent on the patient's cardiovascular function and comorbidities. Phenylephrine and norepinephrine are the most commonly used vasopressors, and the inotropes commonly employed are dobutamine and milrinone.

The use of prophylactic hypervolemia does not improve the CBF or outcome and has been associated with cardiovascular complications related to fluid overload. Acute volume expansion at the time of symptomatic DCI may result in a modest improvement in the CBF in regions with low baseline flow. However, the verdict on its utility is mixed. In patients who are well hydrated prior to developing DCI, the administration of large volumes of fluid may result in increased medical complications, notably pulmonary edema. The individuals most likely to benefit from the administration of large volumes of fluid are likely to be those patients who are hypovolemic.

Hemodilution has been the least understood of the interventions considered in hemodynamic augmentation. Reduction in the viscosity of blood by hemodilution results in improved CBF. Unfortunately, this also results in a reduction of the oxygen-carrying capacity of the blood, ultimately reducing oxygen delivery. One study found that hemodilution resulted in a net fall in oxygen delivery, and it has largely fallen out of favor in the treatment of patients with aSAH.

Induced hypertension with vasopressors has been more consistently associated with an improvement in CBF, although this effect seems to be limited to patients with impaired autoregulation. There are differing approaches to the choice of blood pressure targets. Some target a particular systolic blood pressure, others target mean blood pressures. A more rational approach widely used is to raise blood pressure by 15–20% from the patient's baseline pressures. Further adjustments are guided by the patient's clinical response and ability to tolerate the use of vasopressors and/or inotropes.

★ TIPS & TRICKS

Inducing hypertension with pressors: The choice of vasopressors in hemodynamic augmentation should take into account the goal of induced hypertension balanced with the patient's underlying cardiovascular function and the risk of concomitant organ damage (heart failure, etc.) by these agents. The adrenergic vasopressors, phenylephrine, and norepinephrine act on alpha-adrenergic receptors to produce vasoconstriction Norepinephrine also has powerful beta-adrenergic properties so that it improves cardiac output. Vasopressin acts on vasopressin receptors; while dopamine acts on both adrenergic and dopaminergic receptors. These may be used in conjunction with inotropic agents to optimize cardiac output (CO) in the hypertensive state.

- Phenylephrine is an alpha-1 agonist, which increases blood pressure by increasing the systemic vascular resistance (SVR). It is well tolerated in patients without heart disease, and CO is not affected. In patients with poor CO, increased afterload can precipitate congestive heart failure. In addition, in the presence of pre-existing coronary artery disease, phenylephrine can precipitate myocardial ischemia. Usual dosing: 10–1500 µg/min.
- Norepinephrine is an alpha-1 and beta-1 agonist with dose-based receptor preference. At low doses it affects CO because of its preference for beta-1 receptors; while at high doses it is associated with increased systemic vascular resistance and to greater affinity for alpha-1 receptors. It is preferred over phenylephrine in patients with impaired cardiac function. Usual dosing: 2–80 µg/min.
- Vasopressin acts on V1 receptors to cause vasoconstriction, leading to increased vascular resistance. Because it also acts at V2 receptors as an ADH receptor, it must be used with caution due to the potential risk for hyponatremia. Usual dosing: 0.04 units/min.
- Dopamine acts on the dopamine receptor DA1, as well as adrenergic receptors alpha-1 and beta-1. Similar to norepinephrine, dopamine also has a dose-dependent profile. At moderate doses it can result in increased SVR and CO, and at high doses it primarily results in increased SVR only. However, the use of dopamine is limited because dysrhythmias are often seen even at moderate doses. Usual dosing: 1–20 µg/kg/min.

Although, under normal conditions, changes in cardiac output have no effect on the CBF, there is evidence to suggest that the use of inotropic agents can be helpful in treating DCI. In patients with symptomatic vasospasm, improved cardiac output has been reported to improve the CBF.

Both dobutamine and milrinone have been used in this way. There are no recommended guidelines for cardiac indices when intropic therapy is used, but it is largely based on individual response to therapy. In these cases, patients may benefit from the use of continuous hemodynamic monitoring to prevent complications such as congestive heart failure. In the past, Swan–Ganz catheters were used for this purpose, but more recently devices that calculate cardiac output using arterial pulse contour analysis, such as the PiCCO or LiDCO, have become popular.

Endovascular Interventions for DCI

Endovascular manipulation is often undertaken after patients fail to improve with optimal medical management, or whose poor cardiac function makes the administration of vasopressors or inotropes too risky. Both transluminal balloon angioplasty and intra-arterial infusion of vasodilators have been used to treat vasospasm. The timing of treatment is uncertain, as is the definition for failure of medical management.

Transluminal balloon angioplasty of the affected vessels can return the vessel caliber to normal and improve the CBF; however, *correction of angiographic vasospasm does not always lead to clinical improvement*. The use of prophylactic angioplasty among affected intracranial vessels in high-grade patients has been studied, and while it appears to benefit some patients, this was more than offset by complications of the therapy, including vessel rupture and death. It continues, however, to be used in symptomatic patients. As its application is limited by the ability to pass the balloons into smaller diameter vessels, it has no role in treating distal vasoconstriction.

Intra-arterial infusion of vasodilators has been used to treat distal vasospasm. Although initially very popular, most centers have abandoned the use of papaverine because of its short duration of action and increased risks of complications, including intracranial hypertension. Calcium-channel blockers (nicardipine and verapamil) are now used because of their lower risk of complications. Others have proposed the use of intra-arterial milrione because of its robust vasodilatory properties.

Emerging Therapies

Several emerging therapies for the treatment of vasospasm are on the horizon. In addition to the injection of vasodilators, which have a limited duration of action, there has been an investigation into the implantation of drug-eluting nimodipine wafers at the time of surgery to allow for the extended release of vasodilators. Preliminary studies suggest that this sustained release of nimodipine reduces arterial narrowing and may improve the outcome.

There has been considerable excitement about the use of statins in the prevention and treatment of DCI. Smaller studies have suggested some benefit, but larger studies are needed. Completed studies to date have been limited in terms of sample size, heterogeneous outcome definitions, and methodology. Larger trials are underway, and the routine use of statins remains controversial in the care of patients with aSAH.

Hypomagnesemia is seen in about half of patients with SAH and is associated with DCI and worsened long-term outcomes. There may be a theoretical benefit from a magnesium supplementation in patients with SAH, due to magnesium's effect on calcium voltage-gated channels, resulting in vasodilation. Pilot studies have shown feasibility and potential effectiveness in prevention and treatment of DCI, but subsequent larger studies failed to demonstrate any impact on outcome. Supplementation is fairly well tolerated, but it can induce bradycardia, hypotension, or hypocalcemia. Currently, there are two ongoing randomized clinical trials in magnesium supplementation which may help to define the utility of this treatment.

Endothelin is an extremely potent vasoconstrictor and receptor antagonist that has been shown to reduce the incidence of angiographic vasospasm in animal models.

⚗ SCIENCE REVISITED

Endothelin in vasospasm: While much of the pathophysiology of vasospasm remains unclear, endothelin is thought to play a significant role in the development of vasospasm. Endothelin is a potent, long-acting, endogenous vasoconstrictor. In SAH, vasospasm may be promoted by the elevation of endothelin in the CSF, coupled with up-regulation of endothelin receptors in the cerebral vessels.

Clazosentan, one such receptor antagonist, was shown to reduce angiographic vasospasm in acute SAH patients in a Phase II study, although its use was associated with increased pulmonary complications, possibly related to fluid retention induced by the study drug. Unfortunately a phase 3 trial of the endothelium antagonist Clazosentan failed to show a benefit.

Hydrocephalus and Edema

Hydrocephalus (defined by the presence of ventricular enlargement) often occurs early (within 72 hours) in the course of hospitalization for approximately 20–30% of patients with SAH. Early hydrocephalus may be associated with intraventricular blood or have a higher burden of subarachnoid blood. The significance of asymptomatic hydrocephalus in the acute period is unclear, as many of these patients do not deteriorate. Many patients who have a decreased level of consciousness and undergo extraventricular drain placement display improvement in their symptoms (improvement is seen in about 40–80% of patients). Late or chronic hydrocephalus can occur after 72 hours, and several risk factors have been identified for the development of chronic hydrocephalus, including older age, early ventriculomegaly, intraventricular hemorrhage, high-grade SAH, and female gender. Rates of chronic hydrocephalus do not differ by aneurysm treatment. Up to a quarter of these patients may require permanent shunting. There are no established protocols examining the time with which external ventricular drains (EVDs) are weaned in patients with hydrocephalus. The time required to discontinue an EVD does not appear to affect the need for permanent shunting.

Cerebral Edema

Poor grade patients commonly develop diffuse cerebral edema. Cerebral edema may develop as a result of intra-operative brain retraction, ischemia and/or infarction. Unfortunately, there are limited options for its treatment. Hyperosmotic therapy such as the use of mannitol can be useful. Care must be taken to balance the risk of hypovolemia potentially worsening of DCI with the risk of intracranial hypertension. Hypertonic saline (23.4%) provides volume expansion with less osmotic diuresis than that seen in mannitol. Additionally, hypertonic saline may exert a beneficial effect on aquaporin-4 channels, which may play a role in the development of cerebral edema. If intracranial hypertension is recalcitrant to medical management, decompressive craniectomy can be considered. The utility of this procedure, however, is not yet known.

> ### ☆ TIPS & TRICKS
>
> *Dosing of hypertonic saline for cerebral edema:* Dosing for hypertonic saline (23.4%) is weight-based. One gram of mannitol is equiosmolar to 0.686 mL of 23.4% saline. For a 70-kg individual, mannitol would be given as an initial dose of 70–105 g (0.5–1 g/kg). An equivalent dose of 23.4% saline would be approximately 25–50 mL. Remember that 23.4% saline must be given via central line.

Cardiopulmonary Complications

Patients with aSAH can show signs of early cardiac dysfunction with arrhythmias and electrocardiogram (EKG) changes that often differ from those of acute myocardial infarction. These should be treated expectantly with serial EKGs and cardiac biomarkers, as well as echocardiogram.

A more severe form of cardiac dysfunction following SAH is neurogenic stunned myocardium. This, is likely related to excessive catecholamine release at the ictus and is characterized by cardiogenic shock, severe heart failure, pulmonary edema, and hypotension. Older age patients (>50 years) with a poor clinical grade have a higher risk of developing this complication. The management of neurogenic stunned myocardium may require the use of pressors and inotropic agents, as well as strict control of fluids.

The most common pulmonary complications include pulmonary edema (both cardiogenic and neurogenic) and ventilator-associated pneumonia. Neurogenic pulmonary edema is seen in about 30–70% of patients with aSAH. This occurs soon after the ictus, and can resolve over several days. Ventilator-associated pneumonia is a well-known complication of mechanical ventilation and typically develops several days after intubation.

Occasionally aSAH patients may develop acute respiratory distress syndrome with marked impairment of oxygenation. This complication is associated with an increased length of stay and a worse short-term outcome. It does not, however, affect long-term outcome.

Anemia and Transfusion

Anemia in aSAH has been a subject of considerable interest. When defined as a hematocrit < 30% or hemoglobin concentration <9 g/dL, anemia is seen in a substantial proportion of patients. It has been associated with more DCI and worse outcome. There are several reasons why these patients develop anemia, including extracorporeal blood loss, hemodilution from volume expansion, and female gender. The threshold and systemic effects of transfusion after aSAH are ill defined; thus transfusion to correct anemia remains controversial.

In critically ill medical patients, a randomized clinical trial indicated improved outcomes if a conservative threshold were used to trigger transfusion (<7.0 g/dL). This study, however, did not include patients with cardiac or cerebral ischemia. It is argued that a more liberal transfusion threshold (∼10 g/dL) would result in an improve oxygen delivery to ischemic brain regions. This must be balanced with concerns that the rise in blood viscosity with transfusion and nitrous oxide (NO) depletion in stored blood might lead to a reduced CBF and actually reduce oxygen delivery. Retrospective reviews have suggested that this might be the case, but PET studies indicate that transfusion improves oxygen delivery, though a definitive target hematocrit level has not been determined. Additionally, the systemic consequences of transfusion, such as increased risk for infection and their impact on outcome, must be considered; a large prospective trial of liberal and conservation transfusion thresholds is planned.

☆ TIPS & TRICKS

Considering transfusion in the aSAH patient: Many questions remain with regard to the threshold hemoglobin or hematocrit for transfusion. Raising hemoglobin improves arterial oxygen content and, if cerebral blood flow (CBF) is unchanged, it will improve cerebral oxygen delivery. As hemoglobin increases, however, viscosity rises which can lower the CBF. It is the net balance of these two factors that ultimately determines if transfusion will improve oxygen delivery. Preliminary studies with PET suggest that raising hemoglobin to 10 or 11 g/dL improves oxygen delivery in SAH patients at risk for DCI; however, raising hemoglobin to higher levels does not appear to confer additional benefit. The age of transfused blood is also important. When blood is stored, 2–3 DPG and NO levels fall over time, which favor vasoconstriction and potentially offset any beneficial effect on arterial oxygen content. Finally, transfused blood has been associated with an increased risk of infection and worse outcome in medical patients.

Erythropoietin has been investigated as a potential treatment for anemia after aSAH. A limitation of this treatment is its delayed effect on blood hemoglobin (usually seen more than 1 week after administration). Data has been limited, though somewhat promising. Its benefit may potentially be derived from the secondary mechanisms of erythropoietin, rather than the correction of anemia. This approach must be considered in the light of a recent randomized trial in ischemic stroke where high-dose erythropoietin resulted in a worse outcome.

Thermoregulation

Fever (defined as temperature > 38.3 °C) is seen in up to 70% of patients during the first week after

SAH. Up to 50% of these patients do not appear to have an infection as the cause of fever. There is considerable evidence from animal studies that an elevated temperature worsens the impact of cerebral ischemia and that hypothermia is protective. There has been some research examining fever control in SAH patients, but the results have not been definitive.

Fever, however, likely improves the ability to fight infection and treating fever due to an infection is associated with longer courses of illness. Therefore, hyperthermic SAH patients should be evaluated for potential infectious sources prior to treating for hyperthermia. The decision to treat fever must balance the risk for ongoing cerebral ischemia with that of the beneficial effects of fever in treating infections.

There are a variety of interventions used to lower temperature. Many units have protocols for fever management for those with no identified source of infection. These protocols involve an escalation of interventions, which typically start with scheduled antipyretics (acetaminophen, ibuprofen, or both), with or without a water-circulating cooling blanket. If the patient continues to have prolonged hyperthermia despite these measures, cold intravenous fluids may be infused prior to employing surface or intravascular cooling devices.

Glucose Management

Hyperglycemia is a common medical complication of SAH. It occurs in about one-third of patients, though, dependent on the definition used, it may include all patients with aSAH. It is associated with increased risk of DCI and worse long-term outcome. Despite the potential for altered cerebral metabolism of glucose after SAH, there is no known optimal glycemic range. For many, moderate control of hyperglycemia is the goal in the care of these patients, but this must be balanced with the concern for cerebral hypoglycemia in the setting of serum euglycemia.

Hypoglycemia should be avoided. Studies in head injury suggest that tight glucose control (80–100 g/dL) may impair cerebral metabolism and less strict control has been recommended. The use of intensive insulin therapy should be

considered carefully, as hypoglycemia is also associated with worse long-term outcomes in patients with brain injury, including SAH.

Hyponatremia

Hyponatremia is a common complication seen in about one-third of patients after aSAH. Mild hyponatremia is often asymptomatic, but acute decrements in sodium concentrations can lead to cerebral edema, decreased mental status, and potential seizures. Hyponatremia in aSAH is most commonly attributed to cerebral salt wasting (CSW) syndrome, though it appears that the Syndrome of Inappropriate Secretion of AntiDiuretic Hormone (SIADH) may play a role.

Cerebral salt wasting is a syndrome characterized by inappropriate natriuresis, leading to volume contraction and hyponatremia. The mechanism responsible for this syndrome is unknown, although elevated levels of natriuretic factor and the effects of sympathetic activation on renal function have been implicated. The SIADH occurs when the central osmotic regulation of the release of antidiuretic hormone is impaired, resulting in ADH release in hypo-osmolar states.

These entities have different effects on intravascular volume; CSW can lead to marked hypovolemia whereas in SIADH intravascular volume is normal or elevated. Given the strong association between hypovolemia and delayed cerebral ischemia, the appropriate management of hyponatremia is crucial. SIADH is often treated with fluid restriction – a strategy that has been linked to more infarcts in SAH patients with DCI.

The aggressive administration of isotonic fluids (2–3 mL/kg/h), and the restriction of free water intake in oral fluid and tube feeding, can help to prevent hypovolemia and ameliorate hyponatremia. More severe or symptomatic hyponatremia can often be treated with mild hypertonic saline solutions (1.5%, 3%). Fludrocortisone and hydrocortisone have been utilized to reduce fluid requirements and natriuresis, but while they reduce the sodium and volume administered they have no impact on hyponatremia. Conivaptan blocks the effect of ADH on the kidneys and is effective in correcting hyponatremia via aquaresis, but must be used with caution to avoid hypovolemia.

⚠ CAUTION

Conivaptan and volume status: Use conivaptan with extreme caution when in the window for vasospasm, as it can cause a significant rise in urine output and lead to hypovolemia.

⚠ CAUTION

Hypotonic saline in SAH: Do not use hypotonic fluids for volume expansion in patients with SAH. While hypervolemia may be helpful in CSWS, the use of hypotonic fluids may worsen hyponatremia.

Seizures and Prophylaxis

Patients with aSAH may present with reports of seizure-like activity at the ictus. The true nature of these events, epileptic or posturing due to a sudden rise in intracranial pressure, is debated. The risks for and implications of subsequent seizures are not well understood. Antiepileptic drugs (AEDs) are commonly used in the acute period following SAH for seizure prophylaxis, although its benefit has recently been questioned. The presence of cortical hematomas and DCI-related infarcts may increase the risk of delayed seizures. Of note, early and delayed seizures do not appear to confer an increased risk for long-term epilepsy. Recent studies suggest that the use of AEDs may actually worsen the cognitive outcome, possibly by impairing brain recovery. Their routine use is being re-evaluated.

Questions remain with regard to the specific anticonvulsant and the duration of treatment. Phenytoin was commonly used for prophylaxis, partly because it can be given intravenously, but its use is not without consequences. A few observational studies have shown that the short-term use of phenytoin (3 days) does not significantly differ from longer courses of treatment in the development of seizures. Levetiracetam has become popular of late due to its more favorable side effect profile, but its efficacy in SAH and its effect on long-term impairments in SAH are unknown. Current practice is to administrator prophylactic AEDs from several days to 1 week after SAH. Routine long-term prophylaxis for seizures after SAH is no longer recommended.

⚠ CAUTION

Induced hypertension with only one of multiple aneurysms repaired: About 20% of patients presenting with aSAH have more than one aneurysm detected on evaluation. While some centers consider more conservative blood pressure goals when inducing hypertension for the treatment of DCI to minimize the risk of bleeding from the unprotected aneurysms, others consider the risk low and focus on the treatment of symptomatic DCI.

Bibliography

Bederson JE, Connolly ES Jr, Batjer HH, et al. Guidelines for the Management of Aneurysmal Subarachnoid Hemorrhage: A Statement for Healthcare Professionals from a Special Writing Group of the Stroke Council, American Heart Association. *Stroke* 2009; **40;**994–1025.

Diringer MN. Management of aneurysmal subarachnoid hemorrhage. *Crit Care Med* 2009; **37:**432–440.

Macdonald RL, Higashida RT, Keller E, et al. Clazosentan, an endothelin receptor antagonist, in patients with aneurysmal subarachnoid haemorrhage undergoing surgical clipping: a randomised, double-blind, placebo-controlled phase 3 trial (CONSCIOUS-2). *Lancet Neurol* 2011; **10:** 618–25.

Piuta RM, Hansen-Schwartz J, Dreier J, et al. Cerebral vasospasm following subarachnoid hemorrhage: time for a new world of thought. *Neurol Res* 2009; **31:**151–158.

Rabenstein AA, Lanzino G, Wijdicks EFM. Multidisciplinary management and emerging therapeutic strategies in aneurysmal subarachnoid hemorrhage. *Lancet Neurol* 2010; **9:**504–519.

Care of the Neurointerventional Patient in the Neurointensive Care Unit

Rishi Gupta

Department of Neurology, Neurosurgery and Radiology, Emory University School of Medicine, Marcus Stroke and Neuroscience Center, Grady Memorial Hospital, Atlanta, GA, USA

Introduction

Patients are admitted to the neurointensive care unit for emergent and elective endovascular and neurosurgical procedures. This chapter will review the patients frequently admitted after procedures and the potential complications that may occur during their stay in the intensive care unit. Many of the key principles will overlap the medical management of the disease states described in earlier chapters. The first section will review medications employed during endovascular procedures and the potential complications relevant to the management from a critical care perspective. Individual procedure types will be reviewed for more specific details on potential issues that may occur with each type of intervention.

Medications Used

Heparin

Intravenous heparin is commonly used during endovascular interventional procedures to prevent thromboembolic complications from catheter manipulations along the arterial vessels. The target for achieving adequate anticoagulation is an activated clotting time 1.5 to 2 times that of normal value. Heparin is typically administered

as a bolus intravenously in addition to flush lines that are connected to each catheter. Although weight-based approaches are used to determine dosing, there is inconsistency in achieving target anticoagulation levels leading to either under- or over-treatment. The half-life for unfractionated heparin is roughly 1 to 2 hours and thus patients will return to the intensive care unit fully anticoagulated after many types of endovascular procedures. More recently, there has been consideration for the use of direct thrombin inhibitors such as Bivalirudin to replace unfractionated heparin as they have the advantage of a shorter half-life and may avoid the phenomenon of heparin-induced thrombocytopenia. The coronary literature has shown that, compared to unfractionated heparin, the use of Bivalirudin was associated with less bleeding complications without any differences in thromboembolic complications.

Clopidogrel

Clopidogrel is commonly used in patients undergoing stenting or angioplasty. Stents may be used for wide-necked cerebral aneurysms that require a bridge to maintain the coil mass in the aneurysm. Additionally stents are used for intracranial and extracranial atherosclerosis. Bleeding risks

Emergency Management in Neurocritical Care, First Edition. Edited by Edward M. Manno.
© 2012 John Wiley & Sons, Ltd. Published 2012 by John Wiley & Sons, Ltd.

associated with antiplatelets are well established, with rare complications such as neutropenia and thrombotic thrombocytopenic purpura also being reported. More recently, there have been reports of patients who are poor metabolizers of clopidogrel due to variants in CYP2C19 and its association with ischemic events. Point of care testing such as the Verify Now may aid clinicians in determining if patients are biochemical nonresponders to clopidogrel. Similarly, genotyping kits are available to assess for the gene mutation. Many interventionalists adjust dosing of clopidogrel based on point of care testing in order to reduce thromboembolic complications after the placement of the stent. Unfortunately, there is no prospective data correlating biochemical nonresponders to clinical events with neurovascular stent procedures. There is also variability in response of critically ill patients with infections that may alter the efficacy of the drug. Additionally the use of proton-pump inhibitors concomitantly has been shown to reduce the efficacy of platelet inhibition. Patients who develop bleeding complications due to clopidogrel are typically transfused with platelets although the efficacy of such an approach has not been proven to improve outcomes in intracranial hemorrhagic complications from the drug.

Glycoprotein IIb/IIIa Antagonists

Glycoprotein IIb/IIIa antagonists are used in patients who are biochemical nonresponders to clopidogrel or in patients that have an in situ thrombus discovered at the time of angiography. Abciximab is a large compound with a strong receptor affinity and a long half-life. This makes it difficult to reverse bleeding complications that may occur as a result of infusion of this drug. Platelet transfusions can be given, but with a biological half-life of 12–24 hours, the additional platelets will potentially be inactivated with abciximab. Eptifibatide is a smaller molecule with a lower receptor affinity and shorter half-life. The biological half-life is 2 to 4 hours and the use of cryoprecipitate, fresh frozen plasma, and platelet transfusions may aid in reversing the bleeding issues that may arise from the medication. One of the rare complications associated with eptifibatide is the development of thrombocytopenia.

There have been case series describing the use of both agents intraprocedurally that report the safety of using these drugs either through direct infusion into the thrombus or via intravenous approaches without significant hemorrhagic complications. Given the limitation of the small single center case series it is difficult to ascertain the true incidence of complications arising from the utilization of these agents.

✮ TIPS & TRICKS

Anticoagulants and antiplatelet medications are commonly utilized during endovascular procedures. Understanding which drugs are used during the procedure can help better tailor the care of the critical care patient particularly with regards to monitoring for bleeding complications.

Carotid Revascularization Procedures

Carotid artery stenting (CAS) and carotid endarterectomy (CEA) are utilized in patients with symptoms of ischemic stroke or TIA that is referable to the ipsilateral vessel or in patients with severe luminal narrowing in asymptomatic patients. The procedure selected depends upon the anatomy, medical comorbidities, and presence of a contralateral carotid occlusion. There have been several randomized-controlled studies assessing the efficacy of either approach for patients with high risk (medical comorbidities) and conventional risk patients. Due to differences in trial designs and operator experience there has been variable complication rates reported in patients treated with CAS.

During CAS, patients are fully heparinized to help to reduce the risk of thromboembolic events. Additionally patients are placed on dual antiplatelet agents in anticipation of stent deployment. Such procedures are typically performed with conscious sedation to reduce the potential increased risk of myocardial infarction when general anesthesia is used. Neurological exams are performed at each step of the procedure. If any focal neurologic deficit is detected,

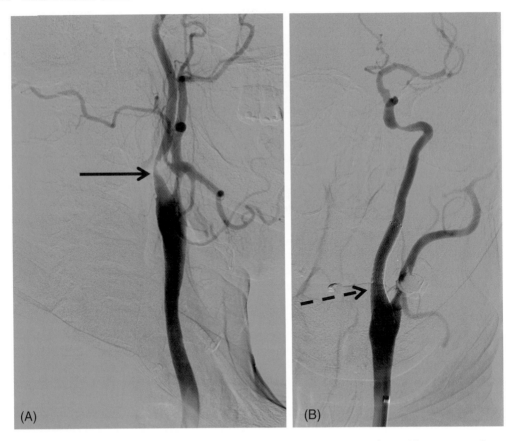

Figure 10.1. A 75-year-old man with a history of a symptomatic left internal carotid artery stenosis deemed high risk for CEA due to need for coronary revascularization. (A) Angiography of the left common carotid artery showing the stenosis prior to treatment (black solid arrow). (B) Angiography of the left common carotid artery showing the stent implanted with reduction of the stenosis (black dashed arrow).

angiography is performed to assess for an embolus. After placement of a guide catheter in the target carotid artery, a distal protection device is placed distal to the stenosis. The stent is deployed and typically angioplasty is performed to post-dilate the stent. Figure 10.1 shows an example of a patient who underwent successful placement of a carotid stent.

The most common complication from either procedure is hemodynamic instability due to manipulation of the carotid bulb during balloon angioplasty. Patients treated with CAS may experience hypotension or bradycardia at the time of balloon inflation or stent implantation. This is the result of compression of the carotid baroreceptors that lead to inhibition of adrenergic output

and increased parasympathetic tone. The phenomenon is common during CAS procedures, and requires vasopressor support in roughly 20% of procedures. Patients with calcified plaques located at the carotid bulb appear to be most vulnerable, while diabetic patients who have had prior CEA appear to have a lower frequency of hemodynamic perturbations. When patients require vasopressor support post-operatively they appear to be at a higher risk for periprocedural stroke and myocardial infarction. Careful hemodynamic monitoring is required post-CAS. Care should be taken to monitor for hypertension to avoid reperfusion injury particularly in patients with severe contralateral carotid stenosis. Such patients appear to have the highest risk for reperfusion hemorrhage when blood pressure is poorly controlled after the procedure.

Patients typically present with bradycardia after CAS. This can be treated with robinal or atropine, particularly if symptomatic. Pseudophedrine 30 to 60 mg every 8 hours can be given orally to help with vasoconstriction and reduce the vasodilatation that occurs after CAS. In rare instances, persistent bradycardia may arise due to the development of an AV block. Such patients may require a pacemaker to prevent further hemodynamic instability.

Intracranial Stenting and Angioplasty

Intracranial atherosclerosis is the etiology of ischemic stroke in 5 to 10% of cases. There appears to be a higher prevalence of the disease in China and Japan where reported rates are as high as 30%. Patients with a stroke due to a severe (>70%) intracranial stenosis have a risk of subsequent stroke of 23% at one year. There are two types of stents currently utilized. The Wingspan stent (Boston Scientific, Natick, MA) is a self-expanding stent that is FDA approved. The balloon expandable coronary stent is also commonly used but is difficult to deliver in tortuous intracranial vessels.

Given the risk of subsequent stroke, some patients are considered for endovascular stenting and angioplasty. Currently there are two randomized-controlled studies assessing the effectiveness of stenting compared to medical therapy for symptomatic lesions. Patients who may not meet criterion for these trials may be offered endovascular therapy outside of the trials.

The procedure is typically performed under general anesthesia. Care must be taken to maintain mean arterial pressure during the induction of anesthesia. Patients are given aspirin and clopidogrel prior to the procedure and receive systemic heparinization intraprocedurally. After deployment of the stent, the blood pressure is typically reduced to achieve lower mean arterial pressures in order to avoid reperfusion hemorrhage (Figure 10.2). The incidence of this entity is rare; however patients with more severe lesions may be more prone to develop this phenomenon.

The clinical syndrome of reperfusion injury typically manifests with seizures and cerebral edema in the ipsilateral hemisphere. Additionally, hemorrhage may occur in the region of the infarct or remote from the infarct (Figure 10.2). It is vital to keep the blood pressure close to a mean arterial pressure of 65 to 70 mmHg when this occurs.

If clinical fluctuations occur post-procedure, monitoring for subconvulsive seizures with continuous EEG monitoring may be helpful. There have been reports of utilizing hypothermia for patients with reperfusion syndromes even in the setting of a hemorrhage. Further data is required to determine if this approach is efficacious.

Acute Endovascular Stroke Reperfusion

There are currently roughly 750,000 ischemic strokes in the United States each year. Intravenous tPA is utilized for patients who present under 3 hours from symptom onset that meet inclusion and exclusion criteria. Recently, there is evidence that IV tPA has a modest benefit when administered within 4.5 hours of symptom onset. Unfortunately due to time delays in patients presenting to the emergency room, poor recognition of stroke symptoms, the utilization of intravenous tPA remains under 3% for all stroke patients. Moreover, tPA does not seem to have a tremendous impact on reperfusion for large vessel occlusion. Patients with carotid terminus occlusions who are treated with IV tPA have a 4% chance of successful recanalization. In recent years, there has been rapid advancement of the development of endovascular techniques to treat acute ischemic stroke. Roughly 75% of all ischemic strokes are due to the occlusion of a large to medium-sized cerebral vessel. In 1999, the PROACT II study was performed to determine if intra-arterial pro-urokinase was superior to placebo in patients with MCA occlusion. The study revealed an absolute benefit of 15% in achieving a modified Rankin Score less than or equal to 2. Based on this, the use of intra-arterial thrombolysis is now a level of evidence IB in the American Stroke Association guidelines for MCA occlusion under 6 hours.

Patients who are candidates for endovascular therapy are rapidly triaged to the angiography suite (Figure 10.3). At this point, there has been debate in the recent literature regarding whether

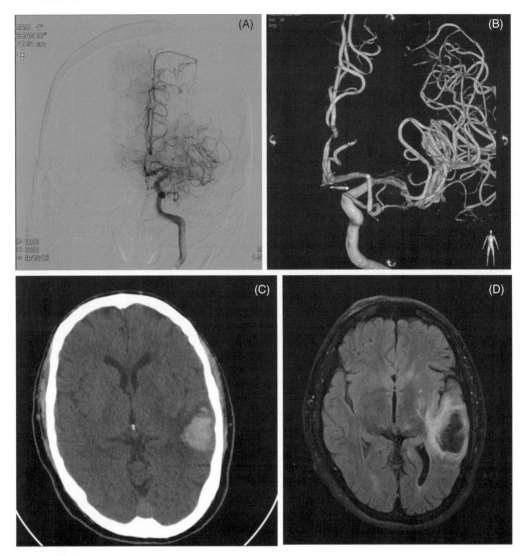

Figure 10.2. A 48-year-old man with recurrent strokes and transient ischemic events within 2 months who was noted to have a left middle cerebral artery occlusion. (A) Angiography in the AP projection confirms the subtotal left MCA occlusion (circle). (B) 3D rotational angiography post-stenting shows marked improvement in antegrade flow with reduction of the stenosis. The patient returned post op day 6 with aphasia and seizures. (C) CT scan of the brain showing a left posterior temporal lobe intraparenchymal hemorrhage due to reperfusion injury. (D) MRI of the brain showing extensive edema around the hemorrhage. The patient was placed on antiseizure medication and the blood pressure was further reduced. His examination markedly improved but he remained with a partial receptive aphasia.

to utilize a general anesthesia to limit the movement of the patient and perhaps improve the safety of the procedure versus conscious sedation that may be associated with better clinical out-come. Patients who undergo acute interventional stroke procedures with conscious sedation have a low rate of conversion to general anesthesia. The concern with anesthesia is that during induction

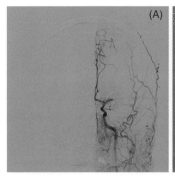 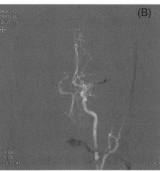 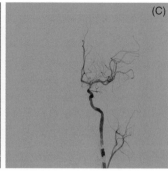

Figure 10.3. A 71-year-old man with atrial fibrillation who presented with acute onset of aphasia and right-sided hemiplegia. The patient was 4 hours and 30 minutes from symptom onset and brought to angiography after a CT of the brain was negative. (A) An AP projection angiogram reveals the presence of a left mid M1 middle cerebral artery occlusion (black arrow). (B) The Merci device was deployed (circle) distal to the thrombus and the clot was removed via an embolectomy. (C) Post-embolectomy angiography reveals successful removal of the thrombus.

there is significant hemodynamic variability that may impact the ischemic penumbra. Additionally, the patients who are intubated tend to remain intubated for a longer period of time thereby impacting rates of pneumonia and perhaps the family's perception of the severity of the condition. After an endovascular stroke intervention, a CT of the brain immediately after the procedure can help to determine the presence of a hemorrhage. Intra-arterial tPA is often administered. If hemorrhage does occur, assessing a fibrinogen level can help to determine if patients may benefit from cryoprecipitate to help with hemostasis. Some centers also administer glycoprotein IIb/IIIa antagonists during the procedure. If successful reperfusion has been achieved, the blood pressure can be lowered to a mean arterial pressure of 65 to 75 mmHg in order to reduce the risk of reperfusion bleeding. Patients are typically placed in the intensive care unit for careful neurological and blood pressure monitoring. Many of these patients require antihypertensives after reperfusion. Continuous infusions of these medications is typically required.

Post-reperfusion edema has also been reported and may lead to rapid development of swelling with significant midline shift and possible herniation. Hemicraniectomy can be utilized in patients with large ischemic strokes at risk for herniation or patients with extensive reperfusion injury.

> ☆ **TIPS & TRICKS**
>
> The need for intubation should be assessed for each individual patient prior to initiating the endovascular procedure as there may be an association of poor clinical outcomes with the use of general anesthesia during these procedures.

Coil Embolization of Cerebral Aneurysms

Patients harboring ruptured or nonruptured cerebral aneurysms are frequently treated with coil embolization. The decision of the surgical approach should be performed by an open vascular surgeon and endovascular specialist to determine the best and safest treatment strategy for the patient. Patients with subarachnoid hemorrhage have been studied as part of the ISAT study which randomized patients to microsurgical clipping and coil embolization. Patients treated with coil embolization were noted to have a 6.9% absolute reduction in mortality compared to clipping. Figure 10.4 shows an example of a patient who has undergone successful embolization of a ruptured anterior communicating artery aneurysm.

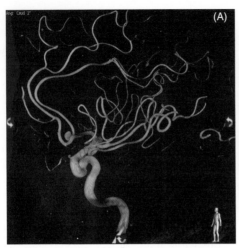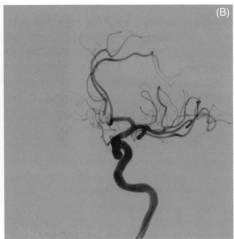

Figure 10.4. A 66-year-old man presented with a Hunt–Hess grade I subarachnoid hemorrhage and was found to have a narrow-necked anterior communicating artery aneurysm. (A) A 3D rotational angiogram showing the 5.5 mm aneurysm. (B) After coil embolization of the aneurysm.

Patients undergoing coil embolization in the setting of a ruptured aneurysm can be challenging to manage in the endovascular suite. Patients with subarachnoid hemorrhage tend to have a hypercoagulable state and thus care must be taken during the procedure to avoid thromboembolic events. This is particularly concerning if the patient is placed on amicar (epsilon caproic acid) prior to the procedure. Additionally, endovascular procedures are performed with the patient lying flat, and this may make the treatment of intracranial hypertension more difficult. During the procedure, protocols should be implemented with the anesthesiologist regarding the external ventricular drainage catheter.

> ⋆ **TIPS & TRICKS**
>
> The table position is frequently manipulated to identify the optimal working projection to treat an aneurysm. Intracranial pressure readings may not be accurate unless the drainage system is adjusted to the height of the table.

The most concerning complications from the procedure include intraprocedural rupture of the aneurysm or thromboembolic events. Patients are typically given intravenous heparin during the procedure to prevent thromboembolic events and thus protamine must be readily available in the case of intraprocedural rupture. After the aneurysm has been secured, many operators prefer the use of an antiplatelet agent to prevent platelet aggregation at the site of the coil mass and neck interface. The risk of platelet aggregation is likely linked to wider-necked aneurysms with larger amounts of coil mass. Blood pressure can be liberalized particularly in patients who may be at risk for vasospasm after the aneurysm has been secured.

Arteriovenous Malformations

Arteriovenous malformations (AVMs) have been associated with the development of seizures or intraparenchymal hemorrhage. Treatment of such lesions requires a multidisciplinary approach with specialists in radiosurgery, open neurovascular surgery, and endovascular surgery. Embolization of an AVM is performed for cure if the lesion is small or for treatment of intranidal aneurysms. More commonly, however, embolization is used to reduce the volume of the lesion for surgical resection or targeted radiosurgery.

The biggest challenge in the treatment of these lesions is blood pressure control. Arteriovenous malformations have surrounding areas of brain that have disturbed cerebral autoregulation. Patient's presenting with intracerebral hemorrhage have an ischemic penumbra surrounding the hematoma. Preservation of this penumbra by avoiding steep reductions of blood pressure may improve clinical outcomes. Patients being considered for embolization procedures may have challenging hemodynamics.

There are two theories of how intracerebral hemorrhage and edema occur during embolization. The first is normal perfusion pressure breakthrough. This theory stipulates that the tissue around the AVM is under-perfused and thus there is maximal vasodilatation of the arterioles. After embolization these vessels are unable to constrict, thereby leading to impaired autoregulation and increased flow causing hemorrhage. The second theory is that partial embolization of the venous side of the AVM prior to complete cure leads to outflow obstruction. In this condition, a reduction in blood pressure may theoretically exacerbate the condition and lead to hemorrhage.

In clinical practice it is important to communicate with the endovascular specialist post-procedure to understand the details of the procedure. Aggressive embolizations of larger AVMs with poorly controlled blood pressure can lead to catastrophic hemorrhages. In scenarios where the vein may have been partially occluded consideration can be given for emergent open surgical evacuation of the AVM in order to prevent rupture. Additionally, in planning AVM resections, minimizing the time from embolization to surgical resection may be the safest approach.

Conclusions

Endovascular therapies are rapidly evolving with technological advancements. Optimizing clinical outcomes requires a team approach with the intensivist having a thorough understanding of the details of the procedure and how best to manage the hemodynamics and anticoagulants.

Bibliography

Abou-Chebl A, Lin R, Hussain MS, et al. Conscious sedation versus general anesthesia during endovascular therapy for acute anterior circulation stroke: preliminary results from a retrospective, multicenter study. *Stroke* 2010; 31:1175–1179.

Combescure C, Fonana P, Mallouk N, et al. Clopidogrel and vascular ischemic events meta-analysis study group. *J Thromb Haemost* 2010; 8(5):923–933.

Fiorella D, Albuquerque FC, Han P, McDougall CG. Strategies for the management of intraprocedural thromboembolic complications with abciximab (Reopro). *Neurosurgery* 2004; 54(5):1089–1097.

Gupta R, Abou-Chebl A, Bajzer CT, et al. Rate, predictors and consequences of hemodynamic depression after carotid artery stenting. *J Am Coll Cardiol* 2006; 47(8):1538–1543.

Hassan AE, Memon MZ, Georgiadis AL, et al. Safety and tolerability of high-intensity anticoagulation with bivalirudin during Neuroendovascular procedures. *Neurocrit Care* 2010; Aug 19 (EPub ahead of print).

Kasner SE, Chimowitz MI, Lynn MJ, et al. Predictors of ischemic stroke in the territory of symptomatic intracranial stenosis. *Circulation* 2006; 113:555–563.

Kollmar R, Staykov D, Dörfler A, et al. Hypothermia reduces perihemorrhagic edema after intracerebral hemorrhage. *Stroke* 2010; 41:1684–1689.

Leslie-Mazwi TM, Sims JR, Hirsch JA, Nogueira RG. Periprocedural blood pressure management in neurointerventional procedures. *J Neurointerv Surg* 2011; 3:66–73.

Molyneaux A, Kerr R, Stratton I, Sandercock P, Clarke M, Shrimpton J, Holman R. International subarachnoid aneurysm trial (ISAT) of neurosurgical clipping versus endovascular coiling in 2143 patient with ruptured intracranial aneurysms: a randomized trial. *Lancet.* 2002; 360:1267–1274.

Yi HJ, Gupta R, Jovin TG, et al. Initial experience with the use of intravenous eptifibatide bolus during endovascular treatment of intracranial aneurysms. *Am J Neuroradiol* 2006; 27:1856–1860.

New Treatment Strategies in the Management of Large Hemispheric Strokes and Intracerebral Hemorrhages

Edward M. Manno

Neurocritical Critical Care, Cleveland Clinic, Cleveland, OH, USA

Introduction

Large hemispheric strokes and intracerebral hemorrhage is a mainstay of patients treated in neurological intensive care units and continue to have significant morbidity and mortality. Recent changes in our understanding of the underlying physiological mechanisms involved with the development of post-ischemic stroke cerebral edema and intracerebral hemorrhage have altered our approach to the management of these diseases. This chapter will review our historical understanding of these processes, discuss how our understanding has changed, and examine the recent strategies designed to implement this new understanding.

Large Hemispheric Strokes

Large hemispheric strokes refer to ischemic strokes that involve greater than 50% of the middle cerebral artery (MCA) territory. They primarily occur due to occlusions of the MCA stem or through occlusion of the internal carotid artery (ICA). The most common mechanisms include direct carotid thrombosis of a severely stenotic carotid lesion or are secondary to cardiogenic emboli.

The term "malignant cerebral edema" was utilized to denote the development of cerebral edema of significant magnitude to lead to the displacement of brain tissue shifts associated with neurological deterioration.

Mortality rates vary among studies but all are greater than 50%. Mortality approaches 80% with medical management alone for patients that develop malignant cerebral edema. Morbidity in survivors has been significant and has only recently been better documented.

History and Background

The initial studies and clinical observations of patients with large strokes were documented in the late 1950s and early 1960s. Through serial neurological assessments performed rigorously and continually over several days, the progression of neurological deterioration was documented. This documentation was recorded in McNealy and Plum's monograph on brainstem dysfunction and supratentorial lesions and served as the basis for Plum and Posner's textbook the diagnosis of stupor and coma. The conclusion from these observational studies was that clinically patients displayed evidence of increased intracranial pressure. Neurological deterioration was attributed to transtentorial herniation due to central or downward tissue shifts caused by increased intracranial hypertension. Treatment strategies were subsequently designed to lower the intracranial pressure.

Pathological studies, however, began to document horizontal (not vertical) tissue shifts with large hemispheric infarctions. Ropper's seminal radiographic study on horizontal tissue shifts (Ropper, 1986) documented neurological deterioration associated with horizontal displacement of the pineal. Finally, direct measurements of intracranial pressure found increased intracranial pressure in only a minority of patients with large hemispheric infarctions. Thus, it was presumed that neurological deterioration after large hemispheric infarctions occurred secondary to horizontal displacement of the rostral diencephalon (the pineal serves as a marker for this). These tissue shifts did not occur secondary to global increases in intracranial pressure, but were due to hemispheric pressure differentials established by a focal expanding mass lesion.

SCIENCE REVISITED

The Monroe–Kellie doctrine states that the cerebral contents inside of the skull represent a fixed volume. Any increase in contents (i.e. hemorrhage, edema, tumor) must be met with an equal displacement of some brain contents. Intracranial pressure in this hypothesis represents the pressure needed to displace certain fluids (i.e. CSF, blood, or brain). A corollary of this hypothesis is that intracranial pressure is equal in all areas of the brain. This has been proven not to be true. Cushing first described intracranial pressure gradients that could lead to intracranial tissue shifts. Subsequent studies with bihemispheric ICP monitoring with expanding mass lesions have documented these pressure gradients.

In addition to the documentation of horizontal tissue shifts as the source for neurological deterioration, concerns were raised that treatments designed to lower intracranial pressure may worsen neurological deterioration by preferentially shrinking normal tissue to a greater degree

than edematous tissue (Figure 11.1). Manno et al. (1999) directly measured horizontal and vertical tissue shifts radiographically in patients with large hemispheric infarctions after large doses of mannitol. Significant tissue shifts could not be documented but subsequent volumetric analysis did report an 8% decrease in the noninvolved hemisphere.

SCIENCE REVISITED

Much concern has been raised about the effects of mannitol or hypertonic solutions on damaged brain tissue: the theory being that mannitol can leak into brain tissue and become trapped inside this tissue thus worsening focal brain edema. Radiographic labeling of mannitol used in a stroke patient undergoing dialysis, however, suggested that damaged blood–brain barriers allow for both the influx and efflux of mannitol depending upon the local osmotic gradient.

Medical Management

The results of medical management for patients with large hemispheric infarcts have been disappointing. Supportive management, including mechanical ventilation, has not improved results. In fact the mortality for stroke patients undergoing mechanical ventilation for any reason is 66–75%.

Also, measures designed to lower the intracranial pressure have not proved to be effective in decreasing mortality. Mannitol has not been shown to improve mortality after large strokes. Schwab et al. (1997) utilized barbiturates titrated to burst suppression on EEG monitoring to treat malignant cerebral edema. Intracranial pressure did not respond in 20% of patients and all patients returned to similar intracranial pressure within 3 hours of treatment. Induced hypothermia was also used in a series of 25 patients. Mortality improved to 53% compared to historical controls, with most deaths occurring after passive rewarming. Steiner (2001) has suggested that more controlled rewarming protocols may improve outcomes.

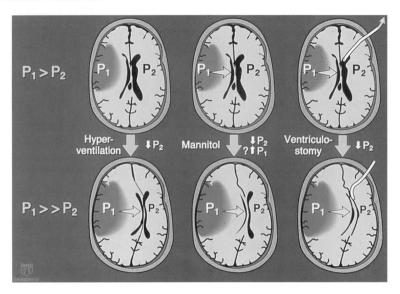

Figure 11.1. Methods to decrease intracranial pressure (i.e. use of hyperventilation, placement of an external ventricular drain, use of osmotic agents) may preferentially shrink tissue with an intact blood–brain barrier. This will decrease the pressure in nondamaged tissue and may potentially increase the pressure gradients that can worsen midline tissue shifts associated with neurological deterioration. (Reproduced from Frank (1995) with permission from LWW.)

Hemicraniectomy

The discovery of intracranial pressure differentials and the significant limitations of medical management mandated a new approach to the management of malignant cerebral edema post large hemispheric infarction. The concept of performing a hemicraniectomy to allow the expansion of edematous tissue outside of the skull was actually proposed and initiated in a series of case studies in the 1970s and 1980s. Rodent studies suggested that hemicraniectomy performed early post-infarct may actually preserve cerebral tissue through increased collateral circulation.

The first randomized study evaluating hemicraniectomy was the hemicraniectomy and durotomy upon deterioration from infarction-related swelling trial (HEADFIRST). This study randomized 26 patients with large hemispheric infarctions and neurological deterioration to standard medical management versus hemicraniectomy. The surgery involved a large hemicraniectomy with durotomy to allow for brain expansion outside of the skull (Figure 11.2). The

results revealed a trend toward improved outcome with surgery.

> ### ☆ TIPS & TRICKS
>
> The key to performing a hemicraniectomy is to ensure that the craniectomy is large enough to allow complete expansion of edematous tissue outside of the skull. Some early studies did not perform a large enough craniectomy. The result was incarcerated tissue coming out of the skull leading to worse edema and tissue shifts.

This trend for improvement encouraged several European studies evaluating the effectiveness of hemicraniectomy after large hemispheric infarcts. The hemicraniectomy after MCA infarction and life-threatening edema trial (HAMLET), decompressive craniectomy in malignant middle cerebral artery trial (DECIMAL), and decompressive surgery for the treatment of malignant

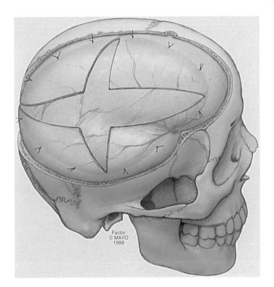

Figure 11.2. Schematic representation of a hemicraniectomy with the bone flap removed, incision of the dura, and placement of a dural sac to accommodate for expanding brain tissue outside of the cranial cavity. (Reproduced from Wijdicksl (2000) with permission from Dowden Health Media.)

infarction of the middle cerebral artery trial (DESTINY) were all initiated soon after. Individually, each of these studies did not reach completion due to limited enrollment or a predetermined or pooled analysis suggesting a significant benefit to surgery. A meta-analysis of these studies enrolling 93 patients aged 18–60 years of age undergoing randomization within 48 hours of infarction revealed a significant impact on both morbidity and mortality. Mortality was reduced from 71 to 21% in these studies. Modified Rankin Scores (MRS) analyzed for scores of 0–3 and 0–4 revealed an absolute risk reduction of 51% with surgery. The numbers needed to treat for survival were 2 and for a MRS of 0–3 were 4.

The success of the hemicraniectomy trials led to considerable interest in defining the timing and indication for surgery. Also, long-term outcomes for survivors became scrutinized. Gupta et al. (2004) reviewed a series of 15 studies enrolling 138 patients: 7% were independent, 35% were mild or moderately disabled, and 58% were severely impaired or died. Age appears to be a significant factor on defining the outcome. 80% of patients older than 50 were dead or disabled compared to only 32% of patients younger than 50. The clinical trials suggest that the utility of hemicraniectomy may be limited to patients under 60. DESTINY II is currently enrolling patients to evaluate this. Interestingly, hemispheric side and the timing of surgery have not been shown to affect quality outcome years. Post-hoc surveys have found that 83% of survivors at one year found life "satisfying" and that 80% of survivors would have surgery again if faced with the same circumstances.

Identifying those patients who are going to deteriorate and require surgery has also proved problematic. A review of the thrombolytic stroke trials involving tPA and streptokinase revealed several possible radiographic predictors, including > 50% MCA involvement, hyperdense MCA sign, decreased perfusion or increased diffusion on MRI diffusion/perfusion imaging, early midline shift, and effacement of the basilar cisterns. Manno et al. (2003), in a retrospective analysis of CT data from the Mayo clinic, identified a positive predictive value of 0.93 for the hyperdense MCA sign found anytime post-infarction. Involvement of > 50% of the MCA territory was only predictive of neurological deterioration if found within 12 hours of the initial infarct. The Heidelberg group has been developing computerized anatomic models to predict tissue shifts and subsequent deterioration.

Intracerebral Hemorrhage

Introduction

Our recent understanding of the dynamic changes that occur after intracerebral hemorrhage (ICH) has altered both our study and approach to this disease. Several demographic changes have occurred in the last few decades: improved control of hypertension in some populations has decreased the number of ICH attributed to this disease; the aging of the population and increased use of anticoagulation has increased the number of hemorrhages attributed to amyloid angiopathy and/or use of anticoagulation. Clearly studies designed to limit or control hemorrhages secondary to anticoagulation will be paramount in the future.

ICH was originally believed to be a monophasic event, but recent radiographic evidence has clearly documented that ICH is a dynamic process often evolving over several hours. Hematoma expansion is common and mortality is directly correlated with the size of the hemorrhage. Thus, new treatment strategies have been explored to prevent or decrease this expansion.

The long-term functional deficit after ICH is disproportionately larger than the actual cellular loss discovered at pathology, suggesting that there is some post-ICH secondary damage that must occur to account for these differences. Pathologically, iron (Fe) has been suggested as a possible source of this secondary damage acting as both a metabolic poison and increasing focal cerebral edema through the breakdown of the blood–brain barrier. Recent treatment strategies have thus focused on preventing expansion of the initial hematoma and subsequent secondary damage.

Prevention of Hematoma Expansion

Treatments designed to decrease hematoma expansion have included the trials using recombinant factor VII and more recently trials to decrease post-hemorrhage hypertension. A phase II block trial randomized 399 patients to placebo or escalating doses of recombinant factor VII within 4 hours of ICH. The initial results were promising, revealing an overall decrease in hematoma size by 14%, improved stroke scale and modified Rankin scores, and a 38% decrease in mortality. However, concerns with increased thromboembolic complications in the treatment group mandated a phase III study. A phase II study randomized 841 patients to a placebo or 20 or 80 µg of recombinant factor VII. The 80 µg dose reduced hematoma size by 11%; however, there was no difference in outcomes between groups. In addition, there were increased arterial thromboembolic complications in the 80 µg group. The discrepancy between studies may have represented either randomization imbalances or improvement in overall treatment since the placebo groups did much better in the phase III trial.

There has been interest in attempts to identify specific groups that could benefit from the use of recombinant factor VII. Patients receiving warfarin may benefit from rapid reversal of the anticoagulation effect. More recently a radiographic "spot sign" has been identified on early CT imaging, suggesting active bleeding of the hemorrhage. Treatment focused on these patients may prove beneficial. Subgroup analysis of the phase III study suggested that patients younger than 70 had an improved outcome with recombinant factor VII.

The management of hypertension after ICH has been debatable. Patients after ICH have multiple reasons to be hypertensive. These include the population being hypertensive at the baseline, a large sympathetic response with the hemorrhage, pain, etc. Historically, there had been some concerns that over-aggressive treatment of hypertension post-ICH could lead to an extension of the hemorrhage. This was based on PET data, suggesting that a ring of dysautoregulated brain surrounded the initial hemorrhage. Subsequent studies, however, identified the perilesional area as having matched perfusion to metabolism. Similar studies revealed that a modest control of hypertension post-ICH did not extend the size of the hemorrhage.

A systemic review of hypertension after ICH suggested that hypertension was correlated with hematoma expansion and poorer outcomes. The intensive blood pressure reduction in acute cerebral hemorrhage (INTERACT) trial was a radiographic study that evaluated the role of acute blood pressure reduction in hematoma expansion and the subsequent development of cerebral edema. The study randomized patients post-ICH to blood pressure management of less than 180 mmHg (considered standard management) versus less than 140 mmHg (considered aggressive management). Baseline 24 hour and 72 hour CAT scans were obtained. The results revealed 2.8 mL less hematoma expansion and 10 mL less perihematomal edema. The antihypertensive control of acute cerebral hemorrhage (ATACH) trial randomized patients to aggressive blood pressure reduction post-ICH, defined as greater than a 60 mmHg reduction in systolic blood pressure compared to a less aggressive group. Hematoma expansion and perihematoma edema was reduced and modified Rankin scores were similarly improved. These promising preliminary results have led to the development of ATACH II, a phase II trial currently enrolling patients.

Prevention of Secondary Injury

Medical and surgical strategies have been designed to decrease secondary injury after ICH. Deferoxamine, an iron chelator, has shown promising results in a rodent model, decreasing perihematomal edema and improving post-ICH performance. Clinical trials are currently underway evaluating the effectiveness of this medication after ICH.

One rational for surgery after ICH is to remove blood prior to the formation of toxic byproducts. Unfortunately almost all randomized surgical trials have shown no benefit to surgery post-ICH. The most recent trial for the surgical treatment of intracerebral hemorrhage (STICH) similarly did not find a benefit to surgery post-ICH. Subgroup analysis, however, did suggest that lobar ICH within 1 cm of the surface of the brain did better with surgery. This study, however, was not powered to evaluate this possibility and STICH II is currently underway to study this population.

The failure of surgical trials to show a benefit after ICH has renewed interest in minimally invasive efforts to remove intracerebral blood while preserving normal neurological tissue. The minimally invasive surgery plus tPA (MISTIE) trial is currently being evaluated. In this study deep basal ganglia hemorrhages greater than 30 cc in volume will be treated with CT-guided insertion and initial aspiration of the clot. Subsequently, 2 mg of tPA will be instilled into the catheter (clamped for 1 hour) and drained every 12 hours while the patient is in the ICU. The intra-operative CT-guided endoscopic surgery for ICH (ICES) trial has recently joined with MISTIE investigators to compare the safety of endoscopic clot removal with sterotactic thrombolysis.

Other surgical possibilities include hemicraniectomy for large basal ganglia hemorrhages.

Treatment of Intraventricular Hemorrhage

Intraventricular hemorrhage (IVH), whether primary or secondary to parenchymal ICH, portends a worse outcome for patients. Treatment has been largely supportive and may include external ventricular drainage if obstructive hydrocephalus develops. The amount of IVH correlates directly with outcome and may be responsible for some of the previous negative trials in ICH. Secondary tissue injury due to the release of inflammatory mediators can be mediated through the removal of the clot.

The initial study on this topic used urokinase for clot lysis but had to be abandoned after discontinuation of this drug in the United States. Follow-up studies substituting tPA were thus initiated. The CLEAR IVH trial enrolled patients within 48 hours of IVH. Patients were randomized to placebo or 1–3 mg of tPA every 12 hours for eight doses. Dosing was developed after a dose escalation scale and safety study. IVH resolution is followed with CT-guided measurements. Preliminary results on the first 36 patients have revealed adequate safety and improved lysis rates. Clear IVH is currently a phase III trial enrolling 48 active sites.

> ### ⚛ SCIENCE REVISITED
>
> Recombinant tPA must be given early to the patient with intraventricular hemorrhage (IVH). Clot resolution within the first 72 hours follows first-order kinetics suggesting that the clot resolution is dependent upon the amount of drug administered. Some time after this period, clot resolution follows zero-order kinetics which is independent of drug concentration.

Conclusions

Our understanding of the cerebral hemodynamics involved with expanding supratentorial mass lesions and ICH have increased significantly over the last few decades. Hemicraniectomy, allowing for the expansion of edematous cerebral contents outside of the skull, appears crucial for decreasing the secondary compressive injury to vital neurological structures. Patients must be selected on an individual basis. Identifying patients prior to neurological deterioration and the timing of surgery remain under study.

The treatment for ICH has focused on preventing or limiting hematoma expansion or decreasing secondary neurological injury. Initial promising results of recombinant factor

VII could not be validated on the phase III analysis. Blood pressure management is currently being investigated.

Surgical treatment designed to prevent secondary damage has similarly not proved beneficial. The concerns over structural damage during open surgery has led to renewed interest in minimally invasive surgical methods to decrease or eliminate ICH. The instillation and aspiration of thrombolytics both for ICH and IVH are currently being investigated.

Bibliography

Anderson CS, Huang Y, Arima H, et al. (INTERACT study investigators). Effects of early intensive blood pressure lowering treatment on the growth of hematoma and perihematoma edema in intracerebral hemorrhage: the intensive blood pressure reduction trial after cerebral hemorrhage trial (INTERACT). *Stroke* 2010; **41**:307–312.

Delgado, Almandoz JE, Yoo AJ, Stone MJ, et al. Systemic characterization of the computed tomography angiography spot sign in primary intracerebral hemorrhage identifies patients at highest risk for hematoma expansion: the spot sign score. *Stroke* 2009; **40**:2994–3000.

Frank JI. Large hemispheric infarction, clinical deterioration, and intracranial pressure. *Neurology* 1995; **45**:1286–1290.

Gupta R, Connolly ES, Mayer S, Elkind MSV. Hemicraniectomy for massive middle cerebral artery territory infarction. A systematic review. *Stroke* 2004; **35**:539–543.

Hanley DF. Intraventricular hemorrhage. Severity factor and treatment target in spontaneous intracerebral hemorrhage. *Stroke* 2009; **40**:1533–1538.

Manno EM, Adams RE, Derdeyn CP, et al. The effects of mannitol on cerebral edema after large hemispheric cerebral infarct. *Neurology* 1999; **52**:583–587.

Manno EM, Nichols DA, Fulgham JR, Wijdicks EFM. Computed tomographic determinants of neurological deterioration in patients with large middle cerebral artery infarctions. *Mayo Clin Proc* 2003; **78**:156–160.

Mayer SA, Brun NC, Begtrup K, et al. Efficacy and safety of recombinant activated factor VII for acute intracerebral hemorrhage. *New Engl J Med* 2008; **358**:2127–2137.

Plum F. Brain swelling and edema in cerebral vascular disease. *Res Publ Assoc Res Nerv Mental Dis* 1966; **41**:318–348.

Plum F, Posner JB. *The Diagnosis of Stupor and Coma* (3rd edition). F.A. Davis Company: Philadelphia, 1980.

Qureshi AI, Palesch YY, Martin R, et al. (ATACH study investigators). Effect of systolic blood pressure reduction on hematoma expansion, perihematomal edema, and 3-month outcome among patients with intracerebral hemorrhage: results from the antihypertensive treatment of acute cerebral hemorrhage study. *Arch Neurol* 2010; **67**:570–576.

Ropper AH. Lateral displacement of the brain and level of consciousness in patients with acute hemispheric mass. *New Engl J Med* 1986; **31**:953–958.

Schwab S, Schwartz S, Spranger M, et al. Moderate hypothermia in the treatment of patients with severe middle cerebral artery infarctions. *Stroke* 1998; **29**:2461–2466.

Schwab S, Spranger M, Schwarz S, Hacke W. Barbiturate coma in severe hemispheric stroke: useful or obsolete? *Neurology* 1997; **28**:1608–1613.

Steiner T, Friede T, Aschoff A, et al. Effect and feasibility of controlled rewarming after moderate hypothermia in stroke patients with malignant infarction of the middle cerebral artery. *Stroke* 2001; **32**:2833–2835.

Vahedi K, Hofmeijer J, Juettler E, et al. Early decompressive surgery in malignant infarction of the middle cerebral artery: a pooled analysis of three randomized controlled trials. *Lancet Neurol* 2007; **6**:215–222.

Videen TO, Zazulia AR, Manno EM, et al. Mannitol bolus preferentially shrinks non-infarcted brain in patients with ischemic stroke. *Neurology* 2001; **57**:2120–2122.

Wijdicksl EF. Management of massive hemispheric cerebral infarct: is there a ray of hope? *Mayo Clinic Proc* 2000; **75**:945–952.

Presentation and Management of Acute Cerebral Venous Thrombosis

Patrícia Canhão and José M. Ferro

Department of Neurosciences, Serviço de Neurologia, Hospital de Santa Maria, University of Lisbon, Lisboa, Portugal

Introduction

Thrombosis of the dural sinuses and cerebral veins is a distinct cerebral vascular disease, less common than other types of stroke (0.5–1% of all strokes). It can occur at any age, but is more frequent in children and young adults. Among adults, it predominates in females (3:1) Cerebral venous thrombosis (CVT) has a wide spectrum of clinical presentation and a multiplicity of causes or predisposing risk factors. The increasing clinician's awareness for the diversity of symptoms and signs that CVT can present, and the widespread use of neuroimaging, now allows for early recognition and treatment of patients. Although the overall prognosis is good, a few patients that have poor neurological condition at admission, or those who worsen during hospitalization, may require more intensive care.

Clinical Presentation

CVT can have an acute, subacute, or less often chronic presentation. The most frequent symptoms are headaches, seizures, focal deficits, altered mental status, decreased consciousness, diplopia, and visual loss. Symptoms and signs of CVT can be grouped in three major syndromes:

- Isolated intracranial hypertension syndrome (headache with or without vomiting, papilledema, and visual problems)
- Focal syndrome (focal deficits, seizures, or both)
- Encephalopathy (multifocal signs, mental status changes, stupor or coma)

Less common syndromes include cavernous sinus syndrome (cavernous sinus thrombosis), thunderclap headache, pulsating tinnitus, and multiple lower cranial nerve palsies (lateral sinus thrombosis).

Clinical presentation may be influenced by the site and number of occluded sinuses and veins, the presence and type of parenchymal lesions, the age and gender of the patient, and the underlying disease.

Headache is usually the first symptom of CVT. It can be the only symptom or precede other symptoms and signs by days or weeks. It is more frequent in females and young patients than in males or older patients. It can be localized or diffuse, usually increasing over several days. Typically, headache caused by intracranial hypertension from CVT is severe, dull, generalized, and worsens with Valsalva maneuvers and with recumbence. Occasionally, headache may

Emergency Management in Neurocritical Care, First Edition. Edited by Edward M. Manno.
© 2012 John Wiley & Sons, Ltd. Published 2012 by John Wiley & Sons, Ltd.

resemble migraine with aura. Some patients with CVT describe sudden explosive onset of severe head pain (i.e. thunderclap headache) mimicking subarachnoid hemorrhage.

Motor weakness with monoparesis or hemiparesis, sometimes bilateral, is the most frequent focal deficit associated with CVT, affecting more than one-third of the patients. Aphasia is particularly frequent in thrombosis of the left lateral sinus.

Focal or generalized seizures, including status epilepticus, are more frequent in CVT than in other types of stroke. In the International Study on Cerebral Vein and Dural Sinus Thrombosis (ISCVT) cohort of 624 patients, seizures at presentation occurred in 39%, and seizures after the diagnosis of CVT occurred in 7%. Supratentorial parenchymal brain lesions, superior sagittal sinus (SSS), cortical vein thrombosis, and motor deficits are associated with the occurrence of seizures. Seizures are also frequent in children (including neonates) with CVT.

A small percentage of patients (less than 6%) are comatose at the time of the diagnosis. In the ISCVT cohort, patients with a Glasgow Coma Scale score <9 were more likely to have an acute onset, seizures, motor deficits, occlusion of the SSS and of the deep venous system, and parenchymal lesions (in particular bilateral brain lesions).

In children, signs of diffuse brain injury, coma, and seizures are the main clinical manifestations, especially in neonates. In older children, the manifestations of CVT resemble those in adults, with headache and hemiparesis. Elderly patients have more vigilance and mental status disturbances.

★ TIPS & TRICKS

The clinical spectrum and presentation of cerebral venous disease is broad. Given the nonspecificity of the signs and symptoms of CVT, the key for a prompt diagnosis is having a high clinical suspicion for high-risk patients. These include women taking oral contraceptives, pregnant or puerperal females, patients with ear or sinus infection, known acquired or genetic prothrombotic condition, malignancies, or other systemic diseases with prothrombotic potential.

Diagnosis

The diagnosis of CVT requires the demonstration of an occluded dural sinus or vein by neuroimaging.

In clinical practice, computed tomography (CT) is usually the first investigation to be performed. It is useful to rule out cerebral disorders which have similar clinical presentations, such as brain tumors, subdural hematoma, subarachnoid hemorrhage, or encephalitis. It may be normal in up to 30% of cases, and most of the findings are nonspecific. CT may show: (1) direct signs of thrombosis, such as the cord sign and the dense triangle sign due to the hyperdensity of a thrombosed cortical vein or dural sinus; (2) indirect signs, such as parenchymal abnormalities, small ventricles and dilated transcerebral veins. After contrast injection the occluded sinus appears as the empty delta sign and there may be intense contrast enhancement of the falx and tentorium or areas of gyral enhancement (Figure 12.1).

Parenchymal abnormalities may occur in 60–80% of cases. This may include intracerebral hematomas, hemorrhagic infarcts, areas of hypodensity due to focal edema or venous infarction, and diffuse brain edema. Rarely, subarachnoid hemorrhage along the convexity or subdural hematoma may be observed. In repeated scans, new lesions may appear, some may undergo hemorrhagic transformation and some may vanish or disappear.

★ TIPS & TRICKS

Some brain locations are suggestive to CVT. These include frontal or parietal paramedian lesions in SSS thrombosis, posterior temporal lesions in the case of lateral sinus thrombosis, or bilateral thalamic lesions in cases of deep venous system thrombosis.

CT venography is useful to demonstrate filling defects in an occluded sinus or veins, sinus wall enhancement, and increased collateral venous drainage. Drawbacks to CT venography include radiation exposure, contrast allergy and the possibility of worsening of renal function.

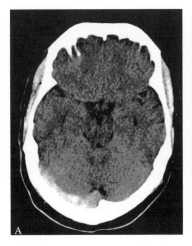 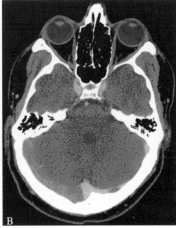

Figure 12.1. Direct signs of thrombosis of right lateral in CT scan: (A) CT scan without contrast shows a hyperdense signal in the right lateral sinus; (B) after contrast injection, there is poor visualization of the same sinus, consistent with the diagnosis of thrombosis.

Magnetic resonance imaging (MRI), combined with MR venography (MRV), is the most sensitive technique for the diagnosis of CVT.

> ★ **TIPS & TRICKS**
>
> The diagnosis of CVT requires the demonstration of an occluded dural sinus or vein. MRI with T1, T2, fluid-attenuated inversion recovery, and T2* sequences combined with magnetic resonance venography are the most sensitive examination techniques for the diagnosis.

The combination of an abnormal signal in a sinus and a corresponding absence of flow on MRV support the diagnosis of CVT (Figure 12.2). The thrombus may be difficult to be visualized in the first days, because it may be isointense on T1-weighted images and hypointense on T2-weighted images. In these circumstances, the MR venography is essential to confirm the absence of flow. After 5 days, the diagnosis becomes easier due to an increased signal on both T1- and T2-weighted images. The diagnosis again becomes difficult after the first month, while the thrombus may become isointense. A chronically thrombosed sinus may still demonstrate a low signal on gradient echo (GRE) and susceptibility weighted imaging (SWI). After contrast (Gadolinium) injection the thrombus appears as a central isointense lesion in a dural sinus with surrounding enhancement.

Specific MRI sequences should be used for improving the differential diagnosis of two tricky conditions: (1) isolated cortical venous thrombosis, where gradient echo T_2*-weighted images enable the diagnosis of CVT by the identification of the occluded vein as a hypointense linear area; (2) nonthrombosed hypoplastic sinus, where GRE and/or SWI will show a normal signal in the sinus.

MRI is also useful in showing the parenchymal lesions secondary to dural or venous occlusion. It is useful in differentiating vasogenic edema from venous infarct, where there is an increased signal in diffusion-weighted imaging (DWI).

Intra-arterial angiography is now rarely performed. It is reserved for cases with inconclusive or contradictory findings in other imaging modalities, or when endovascular treatment is planned.

Independent of the modality (CT, MR, or IA), venography has limitations related to anatomical venous variations, such as hypoplasia of the anterior part of the superior sagittal sinus (SSS),

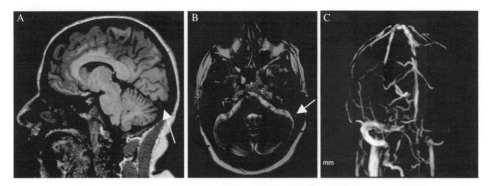

Figure 12.2. Acute thrombosis of the torculae and left lateral sinus diagnosed by MRI: (A) T1 sagittal MRI shows an isointense signal in the torculae (arrow); (B) in T2 axial MRI the thrombus has an isointense/hypointense signal (arrow); and (C) MR venography confirms the absence of flow in the corresponding dural sinus.

duplication of the SSS, intrasinus septa, giant arachnoid granulations and hypo- or aplasia of the transverse sinuses, which may be misdiagnosed as thrombosis.

A screening laboratorial test with a high sensitivity for CVT would be of clinical importance in emergency settings where MR is not readily available. Unfortunately, this test does not exist. Measurement of D-Dimers, a product of fibrin degradation, could be helpful to identify patients with a low probability of CVT. However, CVT patients presenting with isolated headache, those with a subacute or chronic presentations, and those with lesser clot burden may have normal D-Dimers levels. For that reason, D-Dimers cannot be used in clinical practice to rule out CVT.

Evaluation of CVT

The search for risk factors of CVT should be part of the evaluation of these patients. The more frequent risk factors are prothrombotic conditions, either genetic or acquired, oral contraceptives, puerperium or pregnancy, malignancy and infection.

Multiple risk factors may be found in about half of patients. Some of the risk factors are persistent and deserve life-long therapy, but others are transient predisposing the occurrence of CVT (Table 12.1).

Testing for the antiphospholipid syndrome (APL) and for genetic prothrombotic conditions is recommended in all CVT patients, even when another associated condition had already been identified. The diagnosis of APL requires abnormally high titters of lupus anticoagulant, anticardiolipin IgG or anti-β2-glycoprotein IgG antibodies on 2 or more samples at least 12 weeks apart. Testing for deficiencies of protein C, S, and antithrombin must be performed at least 6 weeks after the thrombotic event, and should be confirmed with repeat testing and genetic studies. Heparin reduces antithrombin levels, and protein C and S levels are lowered by oral anticoagulants. High levels of Factor VIII are also found in some CVT series, but high Factor VIII levels may be secondary to acute CVT or to systemic disease underlying CVT.

ENT consultation may be required if otitis or sinusitis is suspected, and cerebrospinal fluid examination through lumbar puncture is indicated if there is a clinical suspicion of meningitis.

The risk factors associated with CVT vary throughout life. In neonates, acute systemic illness, such as perinatal complications and dehydration, occurred in 84% of patients in the Canadian Pediatric Ischemic Stroke Registry. In infants older than 4 weeks of age and in children, head and neck disorders, mostly infections and chronic systemic diseases (e.g. connective tissue disease, hematological disorder, and cancer) are common. A prothrombotic state was found in 41% of these patients, most often in infants older than 4 weeks of age, and children.

The most frequent risk factor in young women is the use of oral contraceptives. The risk for CVT

Table 12.1. Risk factors for cerebral venous thrombosis

Persistent risk factors
Genetic prothrombotic conditions (protein C, protein S and antithrombin deficits; Factor V Leiden and prothrombin G20210A polymorphism
Malignancies
Hematological diseases (polycythemia, thrombocythemia)
Antiphospholipid syndrome
Behçet's disease
Systemic lupus erythematous, and other connective tissue disease or vasculitis
Other inflammatory systemic conditions (e.g. inflammatory bowel disease)
Nephrotic syndrome
Homocystinuria
Intracranial causes (meningeoma, brain vascular malformations)
Transient risk factors
Pregnancy and puerperium (or post-abortion)
Oral contraceptives and post-menopausal hormonal therapy
Other drugs with prothrombotic effect
Intracranial infection, including meningitis
Infection of neighboring structure (eye, sinus, ear, tooth, skin of face, scalp)
Other infections
Mechanical causes (head trauma, lumbar puncture, jugular catheter, neurosurgery)
Hyperhomocysteinemia
Severe dehydration
Severe anemia

in women using oral contraceptives is increased if they have a prothrombotic defect. In the elderly patients of the ISCVT, the proportion of patients with malignancies and hematological disorders, such as polycythemia, was higher than in younger patients. Therefore in the elderly patient and in cryptogenic CVT, a search for an occult neoplasm is recommended.

In almost 15% of adult CVT patients an extensive search is unable to identify an underlying cause. Sometimes the cause (e.g. vasculitis, antiphospholipid syndrome, malignancy, polycytemia, thrombocytemia) is revealed weeks or months after the acute phase or after repeated testing.

Clinical Course and Prognosis

CVT usually has a favorable prognosis compared with other types of stroke. However, the clinical course should be monitored because about one-fourth of patients suffer neurological deterioration after admission, and 5% of patients die during hospitalization. Neurological worsening can occur several days after diagnosis and the initiation of treatment. Symptoms can consist of depressed consciousness, and mental status disturbance while new signs may include seizures, Worsening of prior deficit or onset of new focal sign, increase in headache intensity, or visual loss. Some features that are associated with higher risk of early death include depressed consciousness at admission, altered mental status, thrombosis of the deep venous system, right hemisphere hemorrhage and posterior fossa lesions. The main cause of acute death is transtentorial herniation secondary to a large hemorrhagic lesion followed by herniation due to multiple lesions or to diffuse brain edema. Status epilepticus, medical complications, and pulmonary embolism are among other causes of early death. The acute mortality in children with CVT is similar to that in adults. In a European cohort of 396 children with CVT (median age 5.2 years), 3% of the patients died in the first 2 weeks after presentation.

The large majority of patients achieve complete neurological recovery on long-term follow-up (80% in the ISCVT). In a systematic review of prospective cohort studies the overall long-term death and dependency rate was 15%. Factors associated with the risk of poor long-term prognosis in the ISCVT cohort were: central nervous system infection, any malignancy, thrombosis of the deep venous system, intracranial hemorrhage on the admission CT/MR, Glasgow Coma Scale (GCS) score <9, mental status disturbance, age >37 years, and male gender. Isolated intracranial hypertension at the time of CVT diagnosis is usually associated with good outcome. After discharge, some patients may have long-term complications such as seizures, headaches, visual loss, dural arteriovenous fistulae, and recurrent thrombotic events.

Comatose patients have a poor prognosis. In the ISCVT cohort, among 31 patients with a GCS score <9 at admission, 16 (52%) worsened after diagnosis. More than half of patients who had repeated CT/MR had new cerebral hemorrhages or new venous infarcts. Mortality was high (35%, 9 acutely and 2 during the follow-up), but among the survivors the outcome was good: all but one patient acquired full independence, and none was left severely disabled. Patients without thrombosis of the deep venous system had a better prognosis.

Treatment

Treatment of CVT includes: (1) treatment of the associated risk factors; (2) specific antithrombotic treatment; and (3) symptomatic treatment and management of CVT complications.

Treatment of the Associated Risk Factors

Although the treatment of the multiple possible risk factors or diseases associated with CVT is out of the scope of this chapter, we would stress the importance of appropriate antibiotic treatment, whenever there is meningitis or other intracranial infection or an infection of a neighboring structure (e.g. otitis, mastoiditis).

Specific CVT Treatment
Heparin

There is a general consensus that anticoagulation with unfractionated or low molecular weight heparin (LMWH) is the main treatment for acute CVT. The use of heparin in acute CVT is supported by four clinical trials and a meta-analysis of two of these trials. These trials showed a nonsignificant relative risk of 0.33 (95% CI 0.08–1.21) for death and 0.46 (95% CI 0.16–1.31) of death or dependency after anticoagulant therapy as compared to placebo.

A nonmatched case control study of cases treated with IV heparin and LMWH in the ISCVT cohort showed that LMWH is at least equally as effective as IV heparin for the treatment of CVT. In this large cohort, death or dependency was more frequent in patients treated with IV heparin than with LMWH (16% vs. 9%, $p = 0.05$).

Several observational series showed that heparin is also safe and can be used in acute CVT patients with intracranial hemorrhagic lesions. Similarly, observational data from single and multicenter case series suggest that anticoagulant therapy is safe in children with CVT.

Endovascular Thrombolysis

Direct endovascular thrombolysis is an alternative treatment in severe cases or in patients who fail to improve despite anticoagulation. The aim is to dissolve the clot and reopen the occluded sinus or vein. The goal is to restore the venous outflow and decrease intracranial pressure. Catheterization of the sigmoid, transverse, straight and superior sagittal sinuses via the femoral venous, or jugular approach is followed by local injection of tPA or urokinase. Mechanical thrombolysis by disruption, removal or suction may be additionally performed or utilized alone.

No randomized trials of endovascular treatment for sinus thrombosis have been performed to assess its efficacy and safety. Data from the literature, including a systematic review (169 CVT patients treated with thrombolysis) and several other series suggest that thrombolytics may reduce case fatality in critically ill patients. These data, however, may reflect publication bias. A recent Dutch series (20 patients) could not confirm these findings. Patients that are good candidates for endovascular therapy are those patients with thrombosis of the deep venous system that progress to coma despite anticoagulation.

A randomized trial (TO-ACT) to compare endovascular treatment vs. heparin in acute CVT is in its final preparation stages and will randomize patients with severe forms of CVT, as defined by the presence of one or more intracranial hemorrhage, mental status disturbance, coma, or thrombosis of the deep cerebral venous system. Pending the results of this trial, endovascular thrombolysis should be considered a treatment option for CVT patients who worsen despite anticoagulant therapy. Those with thrombosis of the cerebral deep venous system, and without large hemispheric lesions with mass effect, should be considered.

Oral Anticoagulation

Prolonged oral anticoagulation with warfarin should be started after the acute phase of CVT to prevent further venous thrombotic events. Optimal duration of anticoagulation has not been addressed. Oral anticoagulation aims at an international normalized ratio (INR) of 2 to 3. The EFNS Guidelines recommend that anticoagulants should be given for 3 months if CVT is related to a transient risk factor. In patients with cryptogenic CVT or in those with mild thrombophilia, the period of anticoagulation must be extended for 6 to 12 months. Patients with "severe" thrombophilia or recurrent venous thrombosis, should be given anticoagulants for life.

Symptomatic Treatment and Management of CVT Complications
Treatment of Intracranial Hypertension

In patients presenting with increased intracranial pressure, headache, and papilloedema, intracranial hypertension can be reduced and symptoms relieved through a therapeutic lumbar puncture. This must be performed after CT, or MR excludes large parenchymal lesions or hydrocephalus.

Corticosteroids do not improve the outcome of CVT patients and should not be prescribed unless they are indicated to treat the cause of CVT. Acetazolamide may be used, despite lack of supporting evidence. Patients may need to be admitted to an intensive care unit. Measures to control acutely increased ICP include elevating the head of the bed, osmotic diuretics with mannitol, and initiating hyperventilation to a target $PaCO_2$ of 30 to 35 mmHg.

Decompressive Surgery

Herniation due to unilateral mass effect is the major cause of death in CVT. Decompressive surgery can be life saving in these patients (Figure 12.3). A recent case-control study, retrospective registry, and a systematic review of 68 cases treated by decompressive surgery (hemicraniectomy or hematoma drainage) showed that in patients with large parenchymal lesions causing herniation, decompressive surgery was life-saving and often resulted in good functional outcome. This was irrespective of age, coma, aphasia, bilateral lesions, or bilateral fixed pupils. A prospective registry is under way to confirm these encouraging results.

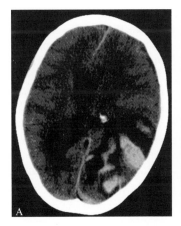 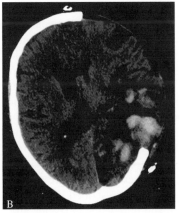

Figure 12.3. Large parieto-occipito-temporal venous infarct, with mass effect secondary to thrombosis of the left lateral sinus. CT (A) before and (B) after decompressive hemicraniectomy.

✷ TIPS & TRICKS

Heparin is the first-line treatment, but in a few cases more aggressive treatment may be attempted, such as local intravenous thrombolysis for patients with deep cerebral venous thrombosis progressing to coma, or decompressive hemicraniectomy for large hemispheric lesions with impending herniation.

Shunting

Ventriculostomy or ventriculoperitoneal shunts are usually not indicated in acute CVT. Exceptions can be made for the patients that develop hydrocephalus in response to CVT of the posterior fossa. In patients with increased intracranial pressure, a lumboperitoneal shunt may be indicated if severe headaches or visual loss develop or do not improve with measures to reduce intracranial pressure.

Visual Loss

Visual loss due to CVT rarely occurs (2–4%). Patients with papilledema or visual complaints should have a complete neuro-ophthalmological study, including visual acuity and visual field testing. The rapid diagnosis of CVT and treatment of intracranial hypertension are the main measures to prevent visual loss. Surgical fenestration of the optic nerve may be performed in specialized centers, but is rarely required.

Treatment and Prevention of Seizures

Prophylactic administration of antiepileptic drugs is not indicated. Anticonvulsants should be reserved for high-risk patients. These include patients with seizures prior to, or at, admission and those with supratentorial lesions. In these patients, anticonvulsants reduce the risk of subsequent seizures and should be prescribed during the acute phase. Anticonvulsants may also be considered in the patient with a single seizure even in the absence of parenchymal lesions. Prophylactic antiepileptics for a defined duration (usually 1 year) should be prescribed in patients with early seizure and parenchymal lesions and in those with post-CVT epilepsy.

Bibliography

Bousser MG, Russell RR. Cerebral venous thrombosis. In: *Major Problems in Neurology*, Vol **33** (Warlow CP, Van Gijn J, eds.). London, WB Saunders, 1997.

Bousser MG, Ferro JM. Cerebral venous thrombosis: an update. *Lancet Neurol* 2007; **6**:162–170.

Canhão P, Falcão F, Ferro JM. Thrombolytics for cerebral sinus thrombosis: a systematic review. *Cerebrovasc Dis* 2003; **15**:159–166.

Canhão P, Ferro JM, Lindgren AG, et al. ISCVT Investigators. Causes and predictors of death in cerebral venous thrombosis. *Stroke* 2005; **36**:1720–1725.

Dentali F, Gianni M, Crowther MA, Ageno W. Natural history of cerebral vein thrombosis: a systematic review. *Blood* 2006; **108**:1129–1134.

deVeber G, Andrew M, Adams C, et al. Cerebral sinovenous thrombosis in children. *New Engl J Med*. 2001 Aug; **345(6)**:417–423.

Einhäupl K, Stam J, Bousser MG, et al. EFNS guideline on the treatment of cerebral venous and sinus thrombosis in adult patients. *Eur J Neurol*. 2010 Oct; **17(10)**:1229–1235.

Ferro JM, Canhão P, Stam J, et al. ISCVT Investigators: Prognosis of cerebral vein and dural sinus thrombosis: results of the International Study on Cerebral Vein and Dural Sinus Thrombosis (ISCVT). *Stroke* 2004; **35**:664–670.

Idbaih A, Boukobza M, Crassard I, et al. MRI of clot in cerebral venous thrombosis: high diagnostic value of susceptibility-weighted images. *Stroke* 2006; **37**:991–995.

Kenet G, Kirkham F, Niederstadt T, et al. Risk factors for recurrent venous thromboembolism in the European collaborative paediatric database on cerebral venous thrombosis: a multicentre cohort study. *Lancet Neurol* 2007 Jul; **6(7)**:595–603.

Moharir MD, Shroff M, Stephens D, et al. Anticoagulants in pediatric cerebral sinovenous thrombosis: a safety and outcome study. *Ann Neurol* 2010 May; **67(5)**:590–599.

Pfefferkorn T, Crassard I, Linn J, et al. Clinical features, course and outcome in deep cerebral venous system thrombosis: an analysis of 32 cases. 2009 Nov; **256(11)**:1839–1845.

Stam J, de Bruijn SF, deVeber G. Anticoagulation for cerebral sinus thrombosis. *Cochrane Database Syst Rev* 2002; **4**:CD002005.

Stam J. Thrombosis of the cerebral veins and sinuses. *New Engl J Med* 2005; **352:**1791–1798.

Stam J, Majoie BLM, van Delden OM, et al. Endovascular thrombectomy and thrombolysis for severe cerebral sinus thrombosis: a prospective study. *Stroke* 2008; **39:** 1487–1490.

Part III

Infections of the Nervous System

Infections in the Neurocritical Care Unit

Denise H. Rhoney[1], Karen J. McAllen[2] and Dennis Parker[3]

[1]UNC Eshelman School of Pharmacy, University of North Carolina at Chapel Hill,
Chapel Hill, NC
[2]Department of Pharmacy Services, Spectrum Health Hospitals, Grand Rapids,
MI, USA
[3]Eugene Applebaum College of Pharmacy & Health Sciences, Wayne State
University, Detroit, MI, USA

Introduction

Patients in the NCCU can present with community-acquired infections (CAIs), but most commonly will develop nosocomial or hospital-acquired infections (HAIs) as a result of endogenous colonized flora that become virulent from the hospital environment. Recent statistics have shown that the four most common nosocomial infections (bloodstream, urinary tract, surgical site, and ventilator-associated pneumonia) account for up to 800,000 preventable infections, 60,000 preventable deaths, and $27 billion in excess costs annually in the United States. These patients have many risk factors for developing infections, including the exposure to invasive devices, mechanical ventilation, severity of the injury, surgical intervention, impaired protective oropharyngeal reflexes, co-administration of corticosteroids, stress hyperglycemia, presence of coma, and altered cellular immunity as a result of the neurologic injury. While there are numerous studies addressing nosocomial infections in medical and surgical intensive care units, there is limited information specifically for the NCCU. The limited studies available in the NCCU have reported a moderate to high incidence of nosocomial infections (20–30%) with pneumonia and urinary tract infections being the most common.

Fever and the NCCU

Fever is a common complication in NCCU patients. The presence of fever has recently been shown to increase intensive care unit (ICU) length of stay by 5.7 days. The definition of fever is variable. Recent recommendations define "febrile" in critically ill patients as a temperature equal to or greater than 38.3 °C. However, it is important to consider that the definition of fever in patients with brain injury has not been clearly defined and the threshold to treat is often lower since brain temperature is higher than body temperature.

Noninfectious causes account for half of the fevers in the general critical care units. Common noninfectious causes that are commonly present in NCCU patients include: central fever, posterior fossa syndrome, intracranial bleeding, seizures, thyroid storm, stroke, venous thromboembolism, drug fever, post-operative fever, fever from transfusions, alcohol/drug withdrawal, and adrenal insufficiency.

Emergency Management in Neurocritical Care, First Edition. Edited by Edward M. Manno.
© 2012 John Wiley & Sons, Ltd. Published 2012 by John Wiley & Sons, Ltd.

The most common classes of drugs that are associated with drug fever include β-lactam antibiotics, antiseizure agents (especially phenytoin), and antiarrhythmics. The time of onset of drug fever is not immediate, and may arise 3 weeks after initiating therapy and can take over 1 week to abate after discontinuing the offending agent.

Fever is believed to provide immunologic protection from infection, but in patients with neurologic injury it has been shown to be associated with a worse outcome. Fever is aggressively managed in the NCCU although there is currently no evidence to demonstrate that this is associated with improved outcomes.

Respiratory Tract Infections

Lower respiratory infections are associated with substantial morbidity and mortality in patients in the ICU. Hospital-acquired pneumonia (HAP), particularly ventilator-associated pneumonia (VAP), occurs in approximately 20% of all ventilated patients and is associated with twice the mortality rate of patients without VAP. Healthcare-associated pneumonia (HCAP) is the largest group of patients affected by pneumonia, and includes patients with recent exposure to the healthcare environment that may be at risk for multidrug-resistant pathogens. A joint consortium of the American Thoracic Society and the Infectious Diseases Society of America has published recommendations for the diagnosis, prevention, and treatment of pneumonia.

Diagnosis

The diagnosis of pneumonia is based largely upon symptoms such as fever, increased sputum production, and poor oxygenation, as well as the presence of leukocytosis or leukopenia and infiltrate on Chest X-ray. If clinical signs are present in the absence of a pulmonary infiltrate, then a diagnosis of tracheobronchitis can be made. Once a diagnosis of pneumonia is made, sputum and blood cultures should be obtained to aid in the identification of the infecting pathogen. Sputum may be obtained via endotracheal aspirates

(nonquantitative) or by bronchoalveolar lavage (BAL) with protected brush samples (quantitative) methods. Early and aggressive treatment with appropriate intravenous antibiotics is indicated in all patients requiring ICU admission. A study in patients with VAP had higher mortality when appropriate antibiotics were delayed by more than 24 hours.

There is conflicting data regarding the use of invasive quantitative sputum culture sampling methods such as PSB and/or BAL as opposed to obtaining nonquantitative cultures via endotracheal aspirates. To date, there is no definitive benefit of invasive methods over tracheal aspirates. Although either approach is acceptable, tracheal aspirates are much easier and cheaper to obtain. Furthermore, a negative bacterial culture result using tracheal aspirates carries a strong negative predictive value (>90%), which can be helpful in guiding appropriate antimicrobial therapy.

Appropriate Empiric and Treatment Recommendations

The most common organisms associated with community-acquired pneumonia (CAP), HCAP, and VAP, along with empiric antibiotic selections, are listed in Table 13.1. Risk factors for infections with multidrug-resistant organisms (MDRO) include prior antibiotic exposure, prolonged hospitalization (>5 days) and the presence of a MDRO within the hospital unit.

For patients with CAP, empiric antibiotic therapy must provide coverage against penicillin-resistant *Streptococcus pneumoniae*, along with enteric gram negatives and atypical pathogens such as *Legionella*, and *Chlamydia pneumoniae*. If patients have CAP requiring ICU admission, it is reasonable to suspect a MDRO. Furthermore, community-acquired methicillin-resistant *Staphylococcus aureus* (MRSA) infection has been reported, particularly in patients with recent influenza infection. Patients with HCAP,

Table 13.1. Treatment strategies for pneumonia

Diagnosis	Most Common Pathogen	Empiric Regimen
Community-acquired Outpatient	*Streptococcus pneumoniae, Haemophilus influenzae, Mycoplasma, Chlamydia, viruses*	1. Azithromycin 500 mg daily OR 2. Doxycycline 200 mg daily OR 3. Moxifloxacin 400 mg daily OR 4. Levofloxacin 750 mg daily
Inpatient (non-ICU)	Same as Outpatient PLUS *Legionella* and *Chlamydia pneumoniae*	1. Moxifloxacin 400 mg daily OR 2. Levofloxacin 750 mg daily OR 3. Ceftriaxone 1–2 g daily OR ampicillin-subbactam 1.5–3 g q6h PLUS azithromycin 500 mg daily
Presence of CA-MRSA Risk Factors		1. Add vancomycin OR linezolid 600 mg q12h
Inpatient (ICU)	Same as Inpatient non-ICU PLUS *Pseudomonas aeruginosa* and other Gram-negative organisms	1. Piperacillin-tazobactam 4.5 g q6h OR cefepime 1–2 g q8h OR meropenem 500 mg q6h PLUS azithromycin OR moxifloxacin OR levofloxacin
Healthcare-Associated OR Hospital acquired/ Ventilator-associated	MSSA/MRSA, *Streptococcus pneumoniae, Haemophilus influenzae*, enteric Gram-negative bacilli, *Pseudomonas aeuroginosa, Acinetobacter baumanii, Klebsiella spp.*	1. Vancomycin or linezolid PLUS cefepime OR ceftazidime 1–2 g q8h OR piperacillin-tazobactam OR meropenem 2. May add gentamicin (dosed for trough <1 μg/mL) OR amikacin (dosed for trough <4 mcg/ml) OR tobramycin (dosed for trough <1 μg/mL) to broaden initial coverage

MSSA = methicillin sensitive *Staphylococcus aureus*; MRSA = methicillin resistant *Staphylococcus aureus*

HAP, or VAP are all at risk for a MDRO such as *Pseudomonas aeruginosa, Acinetobacter baumanii,* and MRSA. Vancomycin or linezolid plus piperacillin/tazobactam or cefepime or a carbapenem (meropenem or imipenem) are all appropriate empiric options in most of these circumstances.

★ **TIPS & TRICKS**

Double-coverage against pseudomonas has been historically advocated for synergy; however, there is little clinical data to support this practice. The most appropriate reason to use combination therapy is to broaden coverage against MDRO.

Many pathogens may be isolated from sputum cultures but differentiating the pathogens from colonizing organisms is often difficult. A negative sputum culture result is fairly reliable in ruling out infecting organisms. Appropriate antimicrobial therapy should result in signs of clinical improvement within 72 hours of initiation of therapy. If patients exhibit clinical improvement (absence of fever, reduction in WBC, improved oxygenation), antibiotics should continue for no longer than 8 days. If symptoms continue or worsen, re-evaluation should include additional sputum cultures and assessment for other potential diagnoses.

Prevention

Several strategies have been evaluated for the prevention of pneumonia in hospitalized patients. Endotracheal intubation increases the incidence of pneumonia more than any other risk factor, and reintubation further enhances this risk. Elevation of the head of the bed 30–45 degrees should be maintained in all eligible neurological patients to prevent aspiration. Neuromuscular blocking agents should be avoided as they can suppress protective coughing mechanisms. Prophylaxis for stress-related mucosal bleeding, using acid suppressive therapy with histamine receptor 2-blocking agents or proton-pump inhibitors, may increase the risk of pneumonia and should not be used in patients at low risk for this complication. The prophylactic use of chlorhexidine and oral antibiotics (selective gut decontamination) has shown benefit in reducing the occurrence of VAP in some studies, however the routine use of these agents remains controversial. The use of systemic antibiotics routinely is discouraged over concerns of subsequent infections with MDROs. Recently, the Brain Trauma Foundation recommended utilizing periprocedural antibiotic prophylaxis prior to intubation (Level II). Although the specific antibiotic to be used is not stated, it would be appropriate to choose an antibiotic that covers common pathogens that colonize the respiratory tract, such as a second- or third-generation cephalosporin.

Urinary Tract Infections

The annual incidence of urinary tract infection (UTI) has been reported to be as high as 20%. Urinary tract infections account for approximately 30% of all nosocomial infections diagnosed each year. Symptoms range from asymptomatic to urosepsis, resulting in significant morbidity and mortality in some patient populations. This section will focus primarily on the healthcare, catheter-associated symptomatic UTI.

Risk Factors

Numerous risk factors have been shown to be associated with developing UTI in hospitalized patients. These include the presence of an indwelling catheter, increased length of hospital stay (LOS), age, invasive procedures, diabetes, other urinary tract disorders, prior surgery, duration of surgery, reoperation, other sites of infection, malnutrition, need for mechanical ventilation, and serum creatinine greater than 2 mg/dL at time of catheterization. Spinal cord injury patients suffering from paralysis are at a very high risk of developing a UTI.

Diagnosis

Differentiating catheter-associated urinary tract infections from bacteriuria or contamination may be difficult. In addition, in neurologically impaired patients it is often challenging to determine whether the patient is exhibiting symptoms. The current recommendations indicate that patients with indwelling catheters should have signs and symptoms of urinary tract infection along with $\geq 10^5$ cfu/mL of at least one bacterial species in a single catheter urine specimen.

✋ CAUTION

A positive culture of a urinary catheter tip is not an acceptable laboratory test to diagnose a urinary tract infection. Urine cultures must be obtained using an appropriate technique, such as clean catch collection or catheterization.

Symptoms of urinary tract infection in patients with spinal cord injury may include increased spasticity, autonomic dysreflexia or a sense of unease.

Appropriate Empiric and Treatment Recommendations

Common empiric antibiotic choices include trimethoprim/sulfamethoxazole, second- and third-generation cephalosporins and quinolones. When candiduria is present, no therapy is indicated in asymptomatic patients, but patients with fever or symptoms should be treated with an appropriate antifungal agent. Fluconazole is recommended for candida species that are susceptible. Alternative antifungal agents should be chosen for organisms that are not susceptible to fluconazole. If the urinary catheter has been in place for longer than a week, the catheter should be removed and replaced. The duration of therapy will depend on the patient's response to treatment. A 7-day course of antibiotics is appropriate for patients who have prompt resolution of symptoms and a 10–14-day course may be required for patients who have a delayed response to therapy. For symptomatic candida UTI, a course of 14 days is recommended.

Prevention

The most important factor in the prevention of UTI is to promptly remove indwelling catheters when they are no longer needed.

✋ CAUTION

Prophylactic antibiotics are not a recommended strategy for the prevention of CA-UTI or CA-bacteriuria.

Bloodstream Infections

Bloodstream infections can arise from infection anywhere in the body or exogenously from intravenous lines or catheters. Nosocomial bloodstream infections are defined as clinically significant positive cultures for bacteria or fungus obtained more than 72 hours after admission, or positive blood cultures obtained within 72 hours with the use of invasive lines. Primary nosocomial bacteremia is from an intravenous device while secondary infections are from a distant site. Catheter-related bloodstream infection (CRBSI) is a common cause of HAI in the ICU with an incidence of 10 infections/1000 catheter days.

Risk Factors

Risk factors for bloodstream infections in the ICU include: anatomic catheter insertion site, type of catheter used, number of ports, number of manipulations, length of time inserted, and the patient population (age, severity of underlying illness, presence of neutropenia, loss of skin integrity).

Diagnosis

Clinical signs of the systemic inflammatory response associated with sepsis include fever or hypothermia, change in leukocyte counts, chills, tachypnea, and tachycardia. Clinical signs of a CRBSI include difficulty drawing or infusing through the catheter, presence of inflammation at the insertion site, and recovery of microorganisms in multiple blood cultures. A definitive diagnosis of a CRBSI requires the presence of intravascular access with at least one positive blood culture obtained from a peripheral vein, clinical manifestation of infection, no other apparent source of bloodstream infection and, additionally, one of the microbiological methods: a positive result of semiquantitative (≥ 15 colony forming units per catheter segment) or quantitative culture ($>10^3$ cfu per catheter segment) with the same organism, paired quantitative blood cultures with a ≥ 5:1 ratio device versus periph- eral, differential time to positivity (blood culture obtained from a central venous catheter is posi- tive at least 2 hours earlier than a peripheral blood culture). The catheter should be removed if purulence or erythema is present. The catheter tip can be sent for culture and confirmation of the diagnosis for the presence of the same organism on the tip and in the blood. These blood cultures should be sent prior to the initiation of empiric antibiotics. If the fever persists after 48 hours despite empiric antibiotics and without a specific cause having been isolated, the patient should be assessed for fungal infections.

Microbiology

The most common pathogens associated with secondary bloodstream infections include staph- ylococci and Gram-negative bacilli. The most common bacteria associated with a CRBSI in- clude *Staphylococcus epidermidis* (37%), *Staphylococcus aureus* (13%), *Enterococcus* (13%), *Klebsiella-Enterobacter* (11%), *Candida* spp. (8%), and *Serratia* (5%).

★ TIPS & TRICKS

Gram-negative bacteria and *Candida sp.* have been associated with a higher incidence of severe sepsis and septic shock while coagulase-negative staphylococci have a reduced risk of severe sepsis relative to these other organisms.

Appropriate Empiric and Treatment Recommendations

Bloodstream infections in the ICU represent se- rious infections that can cause septic shock. The mainstay of therapy includes antimicrobial agents in conjunction with supportive care (refer to Surviving Sepsis Campaign recommenda- tions). Sepsis bundles have been developed to improve patient outcomes by combining compo- nent therapies.[1] When initiated early (within 3

[1] http://www.survivingsepsis.org/Bundles/Pages/de- fault.aspx.

hours of emergency department admission or 1 hour for non-ED ICU admissions), appropriate empiric antimicrobial intervention can reduce mortality.

The current guideline for CRBSI recommends vancomycin for empiric therapy in healthcare settings with an elevated prevalence of MRSA, and for institutions in which the preponderance of MRSA isolates have vancomycin minimum inhibitory concentration (MIC) values of 2 mg/mL, alternative agents such as daptomycin should be used. Empirical coverage for Gram- negative bacilli should be based on local antimi- crobial susceptibility data and the severity of disease. Initial broad-spectrum antibiotic thera- py for bloodstream infections should be directed toward *Pseudomonas aeruginosa* and *Staphylo- coccus aureus*. For the empirical treatment of a suspected CRBSI candidemia, may be used an echinocandin or, in selected patients, flucona- zole. Fluconazole can be used for patients with- out azole exposure in the previous 3 months and in healthcare settings where the risk of *Candida krusei* or *Candida glabrata* infection is very low. Therapeutic recommendations for selected pathogens are contained in Table 13.2.

Systemic antibiotic prophylaxis does not sig- nificantly reduce the risk of CRBSI and may increase MDRO in the ICU. Guidelines for CRBSI advise against a course of antibiotics in patients with an infected catheter and negative blood cultures unless the patient appears to be septic. Generally the length of therapy for these CRBSIs is 7–14 days unless there is concurrent osteomy- elitis or endocarditis, where therapy is for 6–8 weeks. These guidelines recommend as few as 5–7 days of therapy for some coagulase-negative staphylococci.

Prevention

Numerous infection control procedures have been directed toward preventing CRBSI, includ- ing maximal sterile barrier precautions during insertion, structured educational programs on the use of sterile precautions, maintaining non- soiled dressing at the catheter insertion site, and the use of antibiotic or antiseptic-coated cathe- ters. A meta-analysis suggests that chlorhexidine gluconate solutions reduce the incidence of CRBSI by 50% when compared to aqueous

Table 13.2. Intravenous Antimicrobial Agent Selection for Selected Pathogens in Nosocomial Bloodstream Infections[*]

Pathogen	Preferred Antimicrobial Agent	Alternative Antimicrobial Agent
Staphylococcus aureus:		
Methicillin sensitive	Nafcillin or Oxacillin 2g q4h	Cefazolin 2 mg q8h
Methicillin resistant	Vancomycin	Daptomycin 6–9 mg/kg/day or Linezolid
Coagulase-negative staphylococci:		
Methicillin sensitive	Nafcillin or Oxacillin 2g q4h	Cefazolin 2 mg q8h Daptomycin
Methicillin resistant	Vancomycin	6–9 mg/kg/day or Linezolid
Enterococcus faecalis:		
Amp senstive	Amp 2 g q4h or 6h ± AG	Vancomycin
Amp resistant, Vanco sensitive	Vancomycin ± AG	Linezolid or Daptomycin
Amp resistant, Vanco resistant	Linezolid or Daptomycin	Quin/Dalf
Escherichia coli or *Klebsiella* spp.:		
ESBL negative	3rd or 4th generation Csp (Ceftriaxone 1–2 g q24h or Cefepime 2 g q8h)	Ciprofloxacin or Aztreonam
ESBL positive	Carbapenem (Imi 500 mg q6h; Mero 1 g q8h; Erta 1 g q24h; doripenem 500 mg q8h)	Ciprofloxacin or Aztreonam
Enterobacter spp. or *Serratia marcescens*	Carbapenem (Imi 500 mg q6h; Mero 1 gm q8h; Erta 1g q24h)	Cefepime or Ciprofloxacin
Acinetobacter spp.	Ampicillin/Sulbactam 3 g q6h or Carbapenem (Imi 500 mg q6h; Mero 1 g q8h)	—
Pseudomonas aeruginosa	Cefepime 2 g q8h or Carbapenem (Imi 500 mg q6h; Mero 1 g q8h) or Pipercillin/Tazobactam 4.5 g q6h ± AG (dose to desired conc)	—
Candida albicans	Echinocandin (Caspofungin 70 mg LD then 50 mg/day; micafungin 100 mg/day; anidulafungin 200 mg LD then 100 mg/day) or Fluconazole 400–600 mg/day	Lipid Amphotericin B

Amp = ampicillin; AG = aminoglycoside; Quin/Dalf = quinupristin/dalfopristin; ESBL = extended spectrum beta lactamase; CSP = cephalosporin; Imi = imipenem; Mero = meropenem; Erta = ertapenem; conc = concentration; LD = loading dose
[*]Use this in conjunction with local antibiograms, which assess local susceptibility and resistance patterns

providone-iodine. In regards to impregnated catheters, the use of chlorhexidine/silver sulfadiazine catheters significantly reduces the risk of CRBSI, with larger risk reductions with minocycline-rifampin-coated catheters. Current guidelines suggest using these impregnated catheters only in patients with limited venous access, history of recurrent CRBSI, and patients with a heightened risk for severe sequelae from CRBSI. The best prevention is limiting the duration of use of these catheters. The practice of converting central catheters to peripherally inserted central catheters (PICC) may not reduce infection rates.

> ★ **TIPS & TRICKS**
>
> Central catheters should be removed as soon as possible and should have the least amount of lumens required.

Gastrointestinal Infections

Diarrhea is common in hospitalized patients and may be due to either infectious or noninfectious causes. *Clostridium difficile*, a spore-forming anaerobic bacillus, is the most common cause of infectious diarrhea. Although it accounts for only 10–30% of antibiotic-associated diarrhea, up to 30% of hospitalized patients who receive antibiotics can become asymptomatic carriers. *Clostridium difficile* has been shown to increase ICU costs, and is associated with prolonged length of hospital stay, especially if the infection is acquired in the ICU. More recently, a newer strain called NAP1/BI/027 appears to result in a more severe disease and has an increased propensity for quinolone resistance.

Risk Factors

There are numerous factors that have been associated with the development of *Clostridium difficile* infection. Therapy-related risk factors include antibiotic treatment, chemotherapy treatment, proton pump inhibitors, stool softeners, enemas, gastrointestinal stimulants, and antiperistaltic medications. Patient risk factors include severity of the patient's underlying illness, age > 65, malnutrition, chronic renal failure,

and HIV infection. Other associated risk factors include gastrointestinal surgery, gastrostomy, nasogastric tube, and prolonged length of hospital stay.

Diagnosis

Clostridium difficile infection is defined as: (1) the presence of diarrhea (3 or more unformed stools in no longer than 24 hours); (2) stool test result for the presence of toxigenic *C. difficile* or its toxins; or (3) colonoscopic or histopathologic findings demonstrating pseudomembranous colitis. The clinical suspicion and evaluation of risk factors is important in the diagnosis of *C. difficile* infection. This infection is most often associated with antibiotic administration, but is not a requirement for diagnosis. Testing should be performed on diarrheal stool unless ileus due to the infection is suspected. Diagnostic testing can be completed in a number of methods, including stool culture, ELISA immune assay (EIA), and polymerase chain reaction (PCR). The stool culture is the most sensitive but is clinically impractical due to the time needed to receive results. The EIA has low sensitivity. PCR is gaining more popularity since it is rapid, sensitive, and specific.

Appropriate Empiric and Treatment Recommendations

Treatment for *Clostridium difficile* depends upon the severity of the infection as well as whether it is an initial infection, reinfection, or relapse (Table 13.3). Probiotics are not recommended to prevent *C. difficile* infection in critically ill or immunocompromised patients due to the risk of developing bloodstream infections from the probiotic. The use of antidiarrheal medications in the patient with *C. difficile* infection should be avoided.

Prevention

Methods to prevent *C. difficile* infection include minimizing the use of unnecessary antimicrobials, hand washing, and implementation and adherence to antimicrobial stewardship programs.

Central Nervous System (CNS) Infections

Infections complications encountered in the NCCU include meningitis, ventriculitis, enceph-

Table 13.3. Treatment of *Clostridium difficile* infection

Definition	Clinical Information	Treatment	Duration
Initial episode, mild or moderate	WBC ≤ 15,000 cells/μL, Serum creatinine < 1.5 × baseline	Metronidazole 500 mg PO TID*	10–14 days
Initial episode, severe	WBC ≥ 15,000 cells/μL, Serum creatinine ≥ 1.5 × baseline	Vancomycin 125 mg PO QID	10-14 days
Initial episode, severe, complicated	Hypotension or shock, ileus, megacolon	Vancomycin 500 mg PO QID and Metronidazole 500 mg IV q8h*,**	10–14 days
First recurrence		Same as initial episode	
Second recurrence		Vancomycin PO tapered or pulse regimen**	Prolonged regimen can be used

*If complete ileus, consider adding rectal instillation of vancomycin
**Metronidazole should not be used beyond the first recurrence

alitis, brain abscess, and subdural or epidural empyema. (Please refer to Horan et al. (2008) for the current Center for Disease Control diagnostic definitions of CNS infections.)

Risk Factors

The risk of infection is primarily due to the placement of invasive, intracranial monitoring devices. Risk factors include; prolonged duration, underlying diagnosis of brain injury, concurrent infection in other body systems, open skull fracture, hyperglycemia, neurosurgical intervention, CSF leakage, catheter exchange, and technique of catheter placement. Infection is generally related to skin flora along the catheter tract or from direct inoculation when the system is accessed. Thus, the majority of isolates related to intracranial infectious complications are consistent with skin flora: *Staphylococcus aureus* and *Staphylococcus epidermidis*. Gram-negative pathogens are generally a result of contamination from a poor aseptic technique on insertion or from a concurrent systemic infection. The diagnosis is made with clinical signs of infection or deterioration in the level of consciousness in conjunction with positive CSF cultures and increased CSF white blood count and reduced CSF glucose levels.

Appropriate Empiric and Treatment Recommendations

Empiric antimicrobial regimans for intracranial infectious complications consists of ceftazidime 2gm q8h or cefepime 2gm Q6–8h with vancomycin dosed to achieve a serum trough concentration of 15–20 μg/mL.

★ TIPS & TRICKS

While vancomycin is a preferred agent for common pathogens related to ventriculitis, it has very poor tissue penetration particularly into the central nervous system. Thus it is important to achieve and maintain higher trough concentrations.

For patients with basilar skull fractures, metronidazole can be added to this regimen. Therapy can be streamlined once culture and sensitivity results are obtained. The general length of therapy is 14 days. The infected catheter should be removed.

Prevention

Strategies for the prevention of ventriculitis in patients with EVD include inserting the catheter under sterile conditions and minimizing manipulation and flushing. Antibiotic-coated catheters may reduce the infection rate in patients with EVD placement.

Currently, the Brain Trauma Foundation does not advocate prophylactic ventricular catheter exchange at 5 days or antibiotic prophylaxis. Unfortunately, the lack of well-controlled trials continues to keep the issue of antibiotic prophylaxis controversial. If antibiotic prophylaxis is used, prolonged antibiotics (greater than 24 hours) should be avoided.

Antimicrobial Considerations in the NCCU

Use of antimicrobial agents in the NCCU requires a systemic approach, starting first with a thorough assessment of the suspected source of the infection. Next, the possible source of infection should be thoroughly investigated and appropriate specimens should be collected for testing prior to the initiation of antimicrobial agents. Optimizing initial empiric therapy with broad-spectrum coverage is critical followed by de-escalation of the regimen once a source and pathogen have been isolated. The final step is appropriate antimicrobial selection with corresponding monitoring of the drugs and response to the therapy selected. The key is to individualize therapy and select and monitor for not only the desired response but also for possible adverse effects.

Pharmacokinetic Alterations in NCCU Patients

There are many possibilities for alterations in pharmacokinetics of drugs administered to patients in the NCCU. Some of the key alterations that may occur include reduced oral absorption, changes in volume of distribution, reductions in plasma proteins, and reduced or increased renal or hepatic elimination of agents. The potential exists for the underdosing of antibiotics in patients with high volumes of distribution, such as trauma or septic patients. It is essential to individualize therapy and monitor frequently when there is a suspicion of alterations.

Induced hypothermia can result in a 7–22% reduction in clearance of drugs metabolized by the cytochrome P450 system for every 1 °C below

37 °C. Drugs that are metabolized via the cytochrome P450 include the macrolides, fluoroquinolones, rifampin, and tetracyclines. During hypothermia the volume of distribution also changes, which may lead to therapy failure or toxicity. Rewarming patients to normothermia can also result in toxicity or therapy failure. Unfortunately there is a paucity of information on the impact of hypothermia on these agents, but it is important that clinicians are aware of these possibilities.

Pharmacodynamic Considerations

Correct dosing of antimicrobial agents requires adherence to principles of pharmacodynamics. Time-dependent antimicrobial agents (e.g. beta-lactams, carbapenems, glycopeptides, oxazolidinones) need to maintain plasma concentrations higher than the minimum inhibitory concentration (MIC). The administration of concentration-dependent antimicrobial agents (e.g. aminoglycosides, fluorquinolone) should be based on either the ratio between the area under the curve and the MIC or the ratio between plasma peak concentrations and the MIC.

Risk of Seizures

Antibiotics may lower the seizure threshold making seizures more likely. Many antibiotics act by antagonizing the action of GABA by various mechanisms. The clinician can minimize this risk by identifying predisposing conditions such as renal insufficiency, age, pre-existing CNS disease, and the use of proconvulsant drugs which may alter the pharmacokinetic profile.

Beta-lactams, isoniazid, and carbapenems are antibiotic classes most commonly associated with adverse CNS events. Traditionally, carbapenem, imipenem/cilastatin, has been associated with seizures at lower concentrations than other antibiotic agents and has a reported incidence of 1.8–6%. The proconvulsant effects of quinolones have been attributed to direct pharmacodynamic effects and to pharmacokinetic and dynamic interactions with co-administered drugs. Direct pharmacodynamic proconvulsant mechanisms of quinolones may relate to gamma-aminobutyric acid (GABA)-like substituents, which act as GABA-receptor antagonists.

Antimicrobial Resistance

The utilization of broad spectrum antibiotics has led to the emergence of MDRO in all ICUs. Approaches to limiting drug resistance includes prompt de-escalation and a reduction in the duration of treatment.

⚗ SCIENCE REVISITED

Pathogens continually exposed to multiple classes of antibiotics will acquire multiple mechanisms of resistance including: (1) production of antibiotic degrading enzymes; (2) mutations that prevent antibiotic binding to bacterial targets; (3) efflux pumps that remove the antibiotic from the cell; and/or (4) down-regulation of outer membrane protein that prevent antibiotic penetration into periplasmic space.

✶ TIPS & TRICKS

The correct selection of empiric therapy is critical to ensure a favorable prognosis. The current approach is to initiate broad-spectrum therapy, which is then de-escalated or discontinued based on culture results.

The use of cultures or biomarkers, such as procalcitonin, may facilitate these strategies.

✶ TIPS & TRICKS

Procalcitonin is a biomarker that is elevated in the serum of patients who are exposed to bacterial pathogens or who currently have an active bacterial infection. Low serum levels of procalcitonin ($<0.5\,\mu g/L$) suggest that an initial use of antibiotics is not warranted. A decrease of $\geq 80\%$ from peak concentration suggests the need to discontinue antibiotics. Note: This should not be applied to serious infections such as sepsis and meningitis.

Every institution has different susceptibility patterns, therefore it is essential to assess local antibiotic profiles to assist in appropriate empiric antibiotic selection. Susceptibility patterns may also vary between ICUs within the same institution. Antimicrobial stewardship programs involve a multidisciplinary approach to optimize the safe and appropriate use of antibiotics. These are designed to enhance clinical outcome, while minimizing the unintended consequences of antimicrobial use (e.g. toxicity, resistance), and reduce healthcare costs without adversely affecting the quality of care.

Conclusion

Although infections are very commonly encountered in the NCCU, every effort should be directed toward the prevention of infections and the subsequent development of MDROs in order to improve patient outcome. The choice of empiric antibiotics is based upon the treatment of the most likely infecting pathogens based upon institutional data as well as pharmacokinetic, pharmacodynamic, and cost considerations pertaining to antibiotic utilization. The initiation of antibiotics should be timely and include broad-spectrum coverage that can be de-escalated once the source of infection is identified.

Bibliography

American Thoracic Society; Infectious Diseases Society of America. Guidelines for the Management of Adults with Hospital-acquired, Ventilator-associated, and Healthcare-associated Pneumonia. *Am J Respir Crit Care Med*. 2005 Feb 15; **171(4)**:388.

Bayston R, de Louvois J, Brown EM, et al. Infection in neurosurgery. Working Party of British Society for Anticmicrobial Chemotherapy. Use of antibiotics in penetrating craniocerebral injuries. *Lancet* 2000: **355**:1813–1817.

Beer R, Pfausler B, Schmutzhard E. Infectious intracranial complications in the neuro-ICU patient population. *Curr Opin Crit Care* 2010; **18**:117–122.

Bratton SL, Chestnut RM, Ghajar J, et al. Guidelines for the management of severe traumatic brain injury. IV. Antibiotic prophylaxis. *J Neurotrauma* 2007; **24(Suppl 1)**:S26–31.

Coffin SE, Klompas M, Claassen D, et al. Strategies to prevent ventilator-associated pneumonia in acute care hospitals. *Infect Control Hosp Epidemiol* 2008 Oct; **29**(Suppl 1): S31–40.

Cohen SH, Gerding DN, et al. Clinical practice guidelines for *Clostridium difficile* infection in adults: 2010 update by the Society for Healthcare Epidemiology of America and the Infectious Diseases Society of America. *Infect Control Hosp Epidemiol* 2010; **31(5)**.

Dellinger RP, Levy MM, Carlet JM, et al. Surviving sepsis campaign: international guidelines for management of severe sepsis and septic shock, *2008. Crit Care Med* 2008 Jan; **36(1)**:296–327.

Dellit TH, Owens RC, McGowan JE Jr, et al. Infectious Diseases Society of America and the Society for Healthcare Epidemiology of America guidelines for developing an institutional program to enhance antimicrobial stewardship. *Clin Infect Dis* 2007 Jan; **44(2)**:159–177.

Hooten TM, Bradley SF. Diagnosis, prevention and treatment of catheter-associated urinary tract infection in adults: 2009 international clinical practice guidelines from the infectious disease society of America. *Clin Infect Dis* 2010 Mar: **50**:625–663.

Horan TC, Andrus M, Dudeck MA. CDC/NHSN surveillance definition of health care-associated infection and criteria for specific types of infections in the acute care setting. *Am J Infect Control* 2008 Jun; **36(5)**:309–332.

Mandell LA, Wunderink RG, Anzueto A, et al. Infectious Diseases Society of America/American Thoracic Society consensus guidelines on the management of community-acquired pneumonia in adults. *Clin Infect Dis* 2007 Mar 1; **44**(Suppl 2): S27–72.

Mermel LA, Allon M, Bouza E, et al. Clinical practice guidelines for the diagnosis and management of intravascular catheter-related infection: 2009 update by the Infectious Diseases Society of America. *Clin Infect Dis* 2009; **49**:1–45.

Muscedere J, Dodek P, Keenan S, et al. VAP Guidelines Committee and the Canadian Critical Care Trials Group. Comprehensive evidence-based clinical practice guidelines for ventilator-associated pneumonia: diagnosis and treatment. *J Crit Care* 2008 Mar; **23**(1):138–147.

O'Grady NP, Alexander M, Dellinger EP, et al. *Guidelines for the prevention of intravascular catheter-related infections.* 2002 Dec; **30**(8):476–489.

O'Grady NP, Barie PS, Bartlett JG, et al. Guidelines for evaluation of new fever in critically ill adult patients: 2008 update from the American College of Critical Care Medicine and the Infectious Diseases Society of America. *Crit Care Med* 2008 Apr; **36**(4):1330–1349.

Diagnosis and Management of Bacterial and Viral Meningitis

Maxwell S. Damian

Department of Neurology and the Neurocritical Care Unit, Cambridge University Hospitals, Cambridge, UK

Introduction

Fever, headache and neck stiffness are the clinical hallmarks of inflammation of the meninges, of which bacterial meningitis is the most severe. Acute bacterial meningitis (ABM), which develops within hours to 1–3 days, most frequently presents with altered mental status. Viral meningitis in contrast is, in most cases, a self-limiting aseptic meningitis with good prognosis that requires supportive treatment only. Chronic meningitis is caused by many different organisms as well as noninfectious conditions, and has a highly variable course; it is only briefly summarized in the differential diagnostic discussions.

This chapter gives an overview of the background and clinical features of bacterial and viral meningitis and provides a guide to the appropriate prevention and management.

Acute Community-Acquired Bacterial Meningitis (ABM)

Epidemiology and Etiology

ABM is the prototype of an infectious neurological emergency and is a leading cause of infection-related death. Young children and the elderly are more frequently affected; in developing countries the incidence may be 10 times higher than the estimated 1.5–6 per 100,000 annually in Europe and the USA.

Streptococcus pneumoniae and *Neisseria meningitides* cause >75% of cases in immunocompetent patients; *S. pneumoniae* is the leading agent world wide (47% of cases in the western population), and its relative frequency is increasing. The frequency of particular bacterial agents varies over time and in different environments. Meningococcal outbreaks are associated with crowded populations (colleges, the military). Hemophilus influenzae type B has become rare due to widespread immunization programs, but less so in the developing world; other vaccination programs may have significant future impact, for example conjugate pneumococcal vaccines and serotype C meningococcal vaccine. Listeria monocytogenes occurs more frequently in the elderly; listeria, staphylococci and Gram-negative bacilli (*Escherichia coli*, Klebsiella, Enterobacter and Pseudomonas) are particularly common in immunocompromised patients.

Pathophysiology

Bacterial meningitis develops mainly through hematogenous spread, often from colonization in the nasopharynx or respiratory tract; *S. pneumoniae* is a common colonizer of the nasopharynx

Emergency Management in Neurocritical Care, First Edition. Edited by Edward M. Manno.
© 2012 John Wiley & Sons, Ltd. Published 2012 by John Wiley & Sons, Ltd.

(up to 10% of healthy adults and >20% of children). Less common sources are the gastrointestinal or genitourinary tract, or infections of the skin. Direct spread from parameningeal sites (sinusitis, traumatic defects to the meninges or base of skull) is a less common path of infection. Retrograde neuronal spread through the olfactory tract is particularly recognized in amebic meningoencephalitis due to *Naegleria fowleri* or Acanthameba. Limited defences within the blood–brain barrier facilitate the agents' survival.

Cytokines, especially TNF-alpha and interleukin-1, play a prominent role in the early inflammatory process and are activated by bacterial products. Secondary mediators potentiate this inflammatory cascade. The inflammation starts in the subarachnoid space, where it causes headache and meningismus, and progresses to the subpial brain, causing encephalopathy, and in 25% of cases, seizures. Complement-mediated blood–brain barrier breakdown, brain swelling, and impaired cerebrospinal fluid flow result in rising intracranial pressure, and decreased cerebral blood flow. As the brain becomes ischemic, anaerobic metabolism will develop with the formation of lactate and reactive oxygen species. Clinically, patients at this point will become obtunded and can progress to coma. Focal signs may indicate vasculitis or the development of a cerebral abscess.

Clinical Features

Two-thirds of patients will present with the full clinical triad of fever (in 95% of cases with bacterial meningitis), headache and photophobia, and signs of meningeal irritation (nuchal rigidity, Kernig and Brudzinski signs).

Patients with altered mental status, papilledema, and focal signs are highly likely to have intracranial hypertension and/or focal brain swelling. More subtle manifestations are common in the elderly, who frequently appear lethargic but have few meningeal signs. Children may present with vomiting and irritability but less often display nuchal rigidity. Also, many patients with bacterial meningitis are partially treated with antibiotics on admission and may present with an incomplete meningitis syndrome.

The systemic investigation of the patient with meningitis should include a careful search for a rash (petechiae or purpura in meningococcal disease; vesicular or morbilliform rashes in viral infections) and an examination for sinusitis, otitis, and pharyngeal infections. Evidence of embolism should prompt a search for endocarditis. Signs of a bleeding tendency or peripheral circulatory failure indicate a potential need for resuscitation.

The overall mortality averages around 20%, but rises to 50% or more with rapid onset and early severe neurological impairment. Patients under 5 or over 60 years are at increased risk of death and residual disability.

Differential Diagnosis

The differential diagnosis of ABM includes other infective meningoencephalitic diseases (tuberculous, fungal, leptospiral, parasitic, and viral), paramenigeal infections, or other forms of aseptic meningitis. Fungal and tuberculous meningitis often present with a protracted course, featuring intracerebral or meningeal granulomas and subacute cranial nerve involvement. Hydrocephalus is particularly common due to the preferential basal meningeal inflammation encountered in this meningitis. Patients with tuberculous meningitis often feature generalized tuberculous infection. Amebic meningoencephalitis can present with a fulminant meningoencephalitis syndrome. The key to early recognition of this meningitis is a history of potential exposure, i.e. swimming in warm freshwater lakes and rivers in *Naegleria fowleri*; contact with soil through gardening or leisure sports in *Balmuthia mandrillaris*. Viral meningitis normally presents with a less severe meningitic syndrome without systemic instability, but acute viral meningoencephalitis, most often due to *Herpes simplex* type 1 can have a fulminant course.

Parainfectious immunological diseases such as hemorrhagic leukoencephalitis, Weston Hurst, or the severest forms of noninfectious inflammatory disease such as acute disseminated encephalomyelitis (ADEM), should be included in the differential diagnoses, particularly where brain swelling prevents CSF samples. Similarly, severe immune reactions such as graft-versus-host disease in transplanted patients can cause acute brain swelling and meningeal signs.

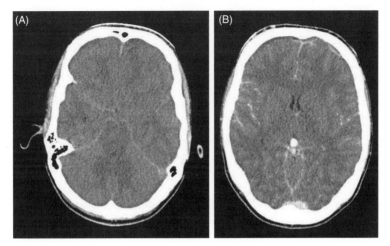

Figure 14.1. **(A).** Sulcal effacement and loss of basal cisterns in brain swelling due to acute bacterial meningitis in a noncontrast CT. (Courtesy of Dr. John Morlese, Department of Radiology, University Hospitals of Leicester, UK.) **Figure 14.1(B).** Post-contrast CT showing acute frontal empyema, sulcal effacement and cerebral edema together with generalized leptomeningeal enhancement. (Courtesy of Dr. John Morlese, Department of Radiology, University Hospitals of Leicester, UK.)

The past history can indicate potential entry ports (ventriculoperitoneal shunt; cochlear implants) or provide evidence for a relapsing disease such as the recurrent bouts of meningitis seen in Mollaret meningitis. Time of year (warmer months for arboviruses, colder for measles and varicella zoster), geographic location (especially for specific parasitic infections), exposure to affected individuals (meningococcal disease), sexual contacts (*Herpes simplex*, HIV), occupation, diet and animal contacts (leptospirosis, brucellosis) can all help to indicate potential infectious agents.

Emergency Management of ABM

Management starts with the immediate admission to a hospital with adequate facilities for assessment and treatment as soon as ABM is suspected. Prehospital antibiotics are recommended when the delay to hospital admission may exceed 90 minutes, or when an acute course and skin rash give suspicion for meningococcemia, in order to reduce the risk of acute adrenocortical necrosis with circulatory collapse (Waterhouse-Friderichsen syndrome). Recurrent seizures, status epilepticus, and cardiorespiratory compromise need to be stabilized according to standard guidelines. Signs of raised intracranial pressure such as coma and pupillary disturbances are ominous prognostic signs but cannot be adequately treated or monitored outside the hospital. Patients may need to be empirically hyperventilated as a bridging measure until some form of intracranial pressure monitoring can be arranged.

After hospital admission, baseline investigations include blood cultures, full blood count, and C-reactive protein. The diagnosis should be confirmed as soon as possible with a lumbar puncture, as long as it is considered safe. A CT scan of the head should be performed immediately if clinical features suggest potentially raised intracranial pressure (i.e. presence of focal neurological deficits, seizures, or reduced level of consciousness) (Figures 14.1a, 14.1b). Circulatory compromise and coagulation problems should be stabilized before lumbar puncture is performed; platelets levels below 50,000 per μL should be substituted. Absolute contraindications to lumbar puncture include infection at the puncture site, or clinical signs of raised intracranial pressure such as papilledema, or CT evidence of obstructive hydrocephalus, brain edema, or herniation.

Figure 14.2 provides an algorithm for the emergency management of bacterial meningitis,

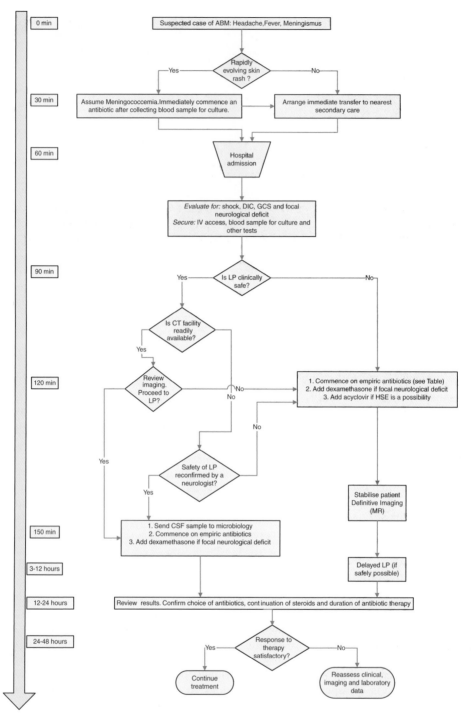

Figure 14.2. Flowchart of emergency management of patients with suspected bacterial meningitis. ABM, acute bacterial meningitis; DIC, disseminated intravascular coagulation; GCS, Glasgow Coma Scale; HSE, herpes simplex encephalitis; LP, lumbar puncture. (Courtesy of Dr. A. Chaudhuri; reproduced from Chaudhuri et al., 2008.)

included in the European Federation of Neurological Sciences (EFNS) guidelines.

The cerebrospinal fluid (CSF) is typically cloudy or purulent and opening pressure is often raised. The white cell pleocytosis in most cases exceeds 500 per μL (more often, several thousand) with a neutrophilic predominance. Patients may have a lower CSF leukocytosis if the patient has been partially treated with antibiotics. Bacterial infections, which may present with a "viral" type CSF profile in acute meningitis, include Mycoplasma, Listeria, and Leptospira. In these, meningitis CSF protein is elevated and CSF glucose is reduced below 2.5 mM with a CSF/serum glucose ratio under 0.4. CSF lactate is often increased. CSF cultures are also more likely to be negative if the patient has been pretreated with antibiotics. In children the CSF is sterilized of meningococci within 2 hours, and *S. pneumoniae* in 4 hours. Rapid methods for the detection of bacteria are available. Immune-based methods include antigen detection, ELISA, and latex agglutination which have a sensitivity of 60–90% and a specificity >90%. PCR methods are increasingly available and may have higher sensitivity.

Treatment of ABM

The time to antibiotic administration is crucial for prognosis, and delayed treatment is the most important cause of morbidity and mortality. Case-control studies have not confirmed a benefit for prehospital antibiotic treatment, possibly due to sample composition (i.e. earlier recognition in more severe cases), but a significant increase of mortality in ABM occurs if antibiotics are delayed for more than 3–6 hours after contact with medical professionals.

Third-generation cephalosporins are the current standard of care in the empiric management of ABM. The efficacy of cefotaxime (2 g tid) or ceftriaxone (2 g bid) is equivalent to newer and more expensive agents such as meropenem (2 g tid), which can be used if there is beta-lactam allergy. Variations in empiric therapy can include benzyl penicillin if a rash suggests meningococcal meningitis; amoxicillin 2 g q4h if Listeria is suspected or in an immunocompromised patient, or IV cotrimoxazole 20 mg/kg tid if there is penicillin allergy. Vancomycin 60 mg/kg/day may be added if penicillin or cephalosporin resistance is suspected. The results of cultures and sensitivity testing may indicate a change of the subsequent antibiotic regimen. The emergence of penicillin-resistant strains is a cause for concern; and patterns of resistance change over time and geographically.

Methodologic considerations may be important. In 1997 a CDC survey reviewed 3237 isolates of invasive pneumococcal disease in eight US states; 25% of isolates were nonsusceptible (11.4% intermediate susceptibility, 13.6% resistant), and resistance rates ranged from 15.3% in Maryland to 38.3% in Tennessee. This survey did not separate meningitis and nonmeningitis cases. In a more recent CDC report from 10 US states in 2006–2007 redefining susceptibility breakpoints, the overall susceptibility rate increased from 74.7% under former breakpoints to 93.2% using the new breakpoints for intravenous treatment. Resistance, however, was different among isolates associated with meningitis. Due to variations in CSF penetration of antibiotics, isolates previously categorized as having intermediate susceptibility to penicillin were recategorized as penicillin resistant. This increased the rate of resistant isolates from 10.7 to 27.5%.

The optimal duration of antibiotic treatment remains uncertain. The EFNS taskforce guidelines found highly variable durations of treatment in their data and recommended 10–14 days of antibiotic treatment for pneumococcal and unspecified bacterial meningitis; 5–7 days for meningococcal meningitis; 7–14 days for

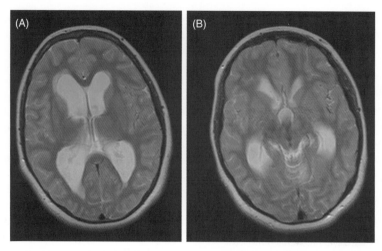

Figure 14.3. (A and B) Acute hydrocephalus causing secondary obtundation in a patient with acute meningitis. (Courtesy of Dr. John Morlese, Department of Radiology, University Hospitals of Leicester, UK.)

H. influenzae; 21 days for Listeria meningitis; and up to 28 days for Gram-negative bacilli and pseudomonal meningitis.

Dexamethasone has gained a role in the adjunctive treatment of pneumococcal ABM. There have been several randomized trials in different clinical settings in children and adults over the last 20 years, generally showing improved mortality and neurological residua. Current recommendations are to institute 10 mg dexamethasone qid for 4 days. Therapy is initiated with the first dose of antibiotics in immunocompetent patients with suspected *S. pneumoniae* or *H. influenzae* meningitis. Note that this may reduce CSF penetration of some antibiotics, e.g. vancomycin in penicillin-resistant meningitis.

Patients with severe ABM should be treated in a neurological intensive care unit (ICU). Early complications include septic shock and circulatory collapse. This can occur with or without adrenocortical necrosis (Waterhouse-Friderichsen syndrome in meningococcal meningitis). Brain swelling (Figures 14.1A and 14.1B) may cause progressive impairment of consciousness and is treated with standard measures including head elevation, osmotic substances, temperature control, and avoidance of hypercapnia; mild hypothermia may be useful for the control of raised intracranial pressure in meningitis and is currently the subject of further investigation (IHPOTOTAM: Induced HyPOthermia TO Treat Adult Meningitis trial). Neuroimaging is needed to exclude obstructive hydrocephalus requiring CSF drainage (Figure 14.3A and B). Seizures need to be treated with IV anticonvulsant drugs; phenytoin or fosphenytoin are the conventional choices, but levetiracetam is increasingly used due to its favorable side-effect profile. Nonconvulsive status epilepticus has been increasingly recognized as a cause of persistent coma in patients on ICU and can be identified by EEG monitoring.

Late complications can include stroke secondary to vasculitis or embolic complications from endocardial vegetations. CT or MR angiography is necessary to exclude vasoconstriction, vasculitic stenosis, or mycotic aneurysms, which are typically located in distal branches of the circle of Willis and may be the cause of secondary intracerebral or subarachnoid hemorrhage. A progressive focal deficit may be due to brain or subdural abscess and empyemas (Figure 14.4). Intraspinal abscesses may cause myelopathy and paraparesis. Meningitis may cause severe deficits of cranial nerves, most commonly deafness or visual impairment, as well as spinal radiculopathies. Long-term sequelae are reported in 30–50% of survivors.

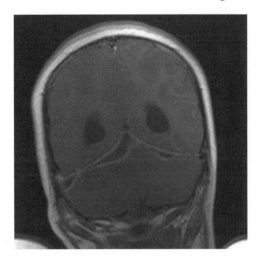

Figure 14.4. Post contrast T1-w MRI in bacterial meningitis showing subtentorial subdural empyema, sulcal effacement, obstructive hydrocephalus and cerebral edema, and generalized leptomeningeal enhancement.

☆ TIPS & TRICKS

- Acute bacterial meningitis (ABM) is a neurological emergency which must be correctly diagnosed and treated without delay.
- The most important cause of morbidity and mortality is late or inadequate administration of antibiotics.
- Antibiotic susceptibility can be highly variable according to local patterns.

Viral Meningitis

Viral meningitis shares the meningitic triad of fever, nuchal rigidity, and headache with bacterial meningeal infection, but in most cases is a relatively mild and self-limiting condition. Nevertheless, lumbar puncture is necessary to reliably differentiate the two, and to exclude other infectious agents and noninfectious etiologies.

Epidemiology and Etiology

The frequency of viral meningitis in the population varies significantly according to age and geographical location, and estimates are difficult through lack of reporting. In the USA, the overall annual incidence has been estimated at 5–10 per 100,000 and more recently the annual rate has been estimated at more than 36,000 cases per year. The condition is significantly more common in children, with an incidence in Finland of 209 per 100,000 infants and 27.8 per 100,000 in children aged under 14 years. Variation in immunization patterns lead to further differences, with prevalence of mumps, measles, and polio being much lower in western countries with robust vaccination practices than in the developing world. There are also differences in incidence according to gender, with mumps occurring 3 times more frequently in males.

Enteroviruses, spread by fecal–hand–oral contamination, are overall the most common cause of viral meningitis, and are responsible for over 80% of cases. This most likely accounts for the peak incidence in summer and autumn. Lymphocytic choriomeningitis virus was the first virus to be recognized to cause meningitis and is transmitted by mouse excreta; it is now rarely found but is associated with severe disease in immunocompromised patients. West Nile virus is an arthropod-born flavivirus which was first recognized in the USA in 1999; by 2008 it had caused over 28,961 cases, of which 11,822 were considered neuroinvasive, with 33% reported as meningitis (versus 63% encephalitis); its incidence is greatest from July through September. Toscanavirus is a further arbovirus that commonly causes viral meningitis in Europe.

Recognizing infection patterns is crucial for effective prevention strategies. These include vaccination programs (effective in mumps and measles, newly available for varicella zoster virus), personal and food hygiene (enteroviruses), and home hygiene (lymphocytic choriomeningitis), control of animal and insect vectors (arboviruses), and safe sexual practices (HIV).

Pathophysiology

After entering the body through the percutaneous, gastrointestinal, respiratory, or urogenital sources, replication and viremia develop prior to CNS penetration. Neural penetration and, more often, hematogenous spread through the choroid plexus or endothelium, are the two routes of viral access to the CNS. In meningitis, the endothelial and meningeal cells are the initial sites of damage and viral replication. This results in inflammation. Superficial cortical inflammation is common, but deeper brain structures are not affected in uncomplicated disease.

Clinical Features

The onset of viral meningitis may be sudden, or follow a flu-like viral prodrome of up to 48 hours with low grade fever, myalgia, and upper respiratory symptoms. Symptoms sometimes exhibit a biphasic course. Patients seldom appear as unwell or toxic as with bacterial meningitis, but extraneurological manifestations may indicate the causative virus. Rashes are common with enteroviruses. Other skin manifestations include zoster in varicella zoster infection, or herpangina in coxsackievirus A. Group B coxsackieviruses commonly cause cardiac manifestations (myocarditis/pericarditis). Pharyngitis as well as lymphadenopathy are common with Epstein–Barr virus infection.

The history must cover potential exposure and include the patient's travel history and outdoor activities, vaccination history, use of medication and drugs, and sexual history.

An acute retroviral syndrome can occur at seroconversion in up to 50% of HIV infections. This syndrome can include fever and nuchal rigidity and can manifest as an aseptic meningitis with CSF lymphocytic pleocytosis. Some cases with a normal CSF cell count have also been reported. Therefore, HIV testing should be included in the initial work-up.

Differential Diagnosis

The clinical triad is, in most cases, easily recognized. The clinical picture differs from bacterial meningitis mostly, through the absence of significant systemic illness. However, viral meningitis can be confused with an early evolving bacterial meningitis. In these circumstances procalcitonin levels may help differentiate viral from bacterial meningitis.

Patients who fail to improve within a few days require a more extensive work-up. Tuberculosis, fungal, and parasitic disease should be reconsidered. EEG and MRI may be indicated if encephalitis is suspected.

Partially treated bacterial meningitis due to antibiotic use must be excluded. Obtaining CSF is essential. The CSF profile typically reveals an asepticmeningitis with lymphocytic pleocytosis of up to 1000 cells/μL. A neutrophilic pleocytosis may be seen early in the course and cause confusion with bacterial infection. Protein is only moderately elevated. Glucose is normal in CSF in most cases of viral meningitis. This is in contrast to fungal meningitis, parasites, or tuberculosis that will generally lower the CSF glucose.

The Pediatric Emergency Medicine Collaborative has published a Bacterial Meningitis Score predicting the risk of bacterial meningitis. Risk is considered very low if pleocytosis does not exceed 1000 cells/μL, protein is less than 0.8 g/L, the cell count in blood does not exceed 10,000, and there is no Gram-positive stain. PCR testing is selected according to the likely viral infection suggested by history and clinical features. Other nonviral infections with a similar inflammatory CSF profile include Lyme disease, listeriosis, or rickettsial disease.

Noninfectious etiologies causing aseptic meningitis include connective tissue diseases (Lupus erythematosus, Sjogren syndrome, mixed connective tissue disease), drugs (nonsteroidal anti-inflammatories, antibiotics), and by chemicals secreted by dermoid or neuroepithelial cysts. Acute disseminated encephalomyelitis (ADEM) can initially present with a meningitis syndrome, although focal neurological deficits rapidly predominate. Meningeal infiltration secondary to malignancies can also present with aseptic meningitis. A prolonged course or cranial nerve involvement can be indications for more extensive investigation.

Management and Prognosis

Management is typically supportive, involving hydration, antipyretic, and analgesic medication. Antibiotics may be indicated initially if bacterial meningitis is under consideration, and acyclovir is advised if encephalitis is suspected. There should be a low threshold for using either of these if there is an initial clinical doubt.

Prognosis is mostly good with a self-limiting course and complete recovery in 1–2 weeks. Complications such as persistent lethargy, malaise, sleep disorders, and fatigue are seen in up to 5% of cases. There may be a link with learning difficulties and delayed language development in some affected children. However, the most severe complications are observed when meningeal inflammation extends to the brain.

Some forms of viral meningitis may develop a relapsing course and qualify as Mollaret relapsing aseptic meningitis. This is a syndrome of benign recurrent meningitis for which multiple viruses can be responsible, including Human herpesvirus 6, Herpes simplex viruses 1 and 2, and Epstein–Barr virus.

✋ CAUTION ⁃

- Viral meningitis may be the initial manifestation of serious chronic viral infection and work-up includes HIV testing.
- A prolonged clinical course is an indication for more extensive diagnostic assessment.

Acknowledgment

MRI and CT scans are courtesy of Dr. John Morlese, Department of Radiology, University Hospitals of Leicester, UK.

Bibliography

Anon, Centers for Disease Control and Prevention (CDC). Geographic variation in penicillin resistance in Streptococcus pneumoniae – selected sites, United States, 1997. *Morb Mortal Wkly Rep* 1999; **48(30)**:656–661.

Anon: Centers for Disease Control and Prevention (CDC). Effects of new penicillin susceptibility breakpoints for Streptococcus pneumoniae – United States, 2006–2007. *Morb Mortal Wkly Rep* 2008; **57(50)**:1353–1355.

Beghi A, Nicolosi A, Kurland LT, et al. Mulder DW, Hauser WA, Shuster L. Encephalitis and aseptic meningitis, Olmsted County, Minnesota, 1950–1981. *Ann Neurol* 1984; **16**:283–294.

Chaudhuri A, et al. EFNS guidelines on the management of community-acquire bacterial meningitis: report of an EFNS Task Force on acute bacterial meningitis in older children and adults. *Eur J Neurol* 2008; **15**:649–659.

Chaudhuri A. Adjuvant dexamethasone use in acute bacterial meningitis. *Lancet Neurol* 2004; **3**:54–61.

De Gans J, van de Beek D. Dexamethasone in adults with bacterial meningitis. *New Engl J Med* 2002; **347**:1549–1556.

Dubos F, Korczowski B, Aygun DA, et al. Serum procalcitonin level and other biological markers to distinguish between bacterial and aseptic meningitis in children: a European multicenter case cohort study. *Arch Pediat Adolesc Med* 2008; **162**:1157–1163.

Lepur D, Kutleša M, Baršić B. Hypothermia in adult community-acquired bacterial meningitis – more than a promise? *J Infect* 2010 Oct 13 (Epub).

Lindsey NP, Staples JE, Lehman JA, Fischer M. Centers for Disease Control and Prevention (CDC). Surveillance for human West Nile virus disease – United States, 1999–2008. *MMWR Surveill Summ* 2010 Apr; **59(2)**:1–17.

Nigrovic LE, Kuppermann N, Macias CG, et al. Clinical prediction rule for identifying children with cerebrospinal fluid pleocytosis at very low risk of bacterial meningitis. *J Am Med Assoc* 2007; **297**:52–60.

Rantakallio P, Leskinen M, von Wendt L. Incidence and prognosis of central nervous system infections in a birth cohort of 12, 000 children. *Scand J Infect Dis* 1986; **18**:287–294.

Scarborough M, Gordon SB, Whitty CJ, et al. Corticosteroids for bacterial meningitis in adults in sub-Saharan Africa. *New Engl J Med* 2007; **357(24)**:2441–2450.

Seupaul RA. Evidence-based emergency medicine/rational clinical examination abstract. How do I perform a lumbar puncture and analyze the results to diagnose bacterial meningitis? *Ann Emerg Med* 2007; **50(1)**:85–87.

Van de Beek D, de Gans J, Tunkel AR, Wijdicks EF. Community-acquired bacterial meningitis in adults. *New Engl J Med* 2006; **354(1)**:44–53.

Vardakas KZ, Matthaiou DK, Falagas ME. Adjunctive dexamethasone therapy for bacterial meningitis in adults: a meta-analysis of randomized controlled trials. *Eur J Neurol* 2009 Jun; **16(6)**: 662–673.

Encephalitis: Presentation and Management

Ali E. Elsayed[1] and Barnett R. Nathan[2]

[1]Mountainside Hospital, Montclaire, NJ, USA
[2]Departments of Neurology and Internal Medicine, NeuroCritical Care and NeuroInfectious Disease, University of Virginia, Charlottesville, VA, USA

Introduction

Encephalitis is defined by the presence of an inflammatory process of the brain in association with clinical evidence of neurologic dysfunction. The presence or absence of normal brain function is the important distinguishing feature between encephalitis and meningitis. Patients with meningitis may be uncomfortable, lethargic, or distracted by headache, but their cerebral function remains normal or close to normal. The diagnosis of encephalitis is suspected in the context of a febrile disease accompanied by headache, altered level of consciousness, and symptoms and signs of cerebral dysfunction which can be classified into four distinct categories:

1. Cognitive dysfunction (acute memory, speech, and orientation disturbances).
2. Behavioral changes (disorientation, hallucinations, psychosis, personality changes, agitation).
3. Focal neurological abnormalities (such as anomia, dysphasia, hemiparesis).
4. Seizures.

Note that many patients with a primary diagnosis of meningitis or encephalitis, frequently reflect signs and symptoms of meningoencephalitis – a combination of both meningitis and encephalitis.

Etiology

A wide variety of pathogens have been reported to cause encephalitis, most of which are viruses. The epidemiology of viral encephalitis in developed countries has changed significantly in the last few decades as a result of the initiation of vaccination protocols (such as measles and rubella vaccine).

Noninfectious encephalitis, such as acute disseminated encephalomyelitis (ADEM), is more commonly seen in children and adolescents. It is a type of encephalitis most likely mediated by an immunologic response to an antigenic stimulus after infection with viruses such as measles, mumps, rubella, herpes simplex, cytomegalovirus, influenza, and hepatitis A. It may also occur following immunization for measles, anthrax, Japanese encephalitis, yellow fever, influenza, smallpox, and rubella. In many cases of encephalitis, the etiology remains unknown (32–75%) despite extensive diagnostic evaluation.

Emergency Management in Neurocritical Care, First Edition. Edited by Edward M. Manno.

Diagnosis

History

Information will most likely need to be obtained from an accompanying person since most patients with encephalitis will be encephalopathic. Geographic location as well as travel history should be considered in identifying possible causative pathogens, such as malaria and avian H5N1 influenza virus, which are endemic to or prevalent in certain geographic regions. Seasonal occurrence is important for other pathogens such as West Nile viral infection and polio viral infection. Occupation or hobbies may be important (as in a case of a forestry worker or an outdoor enthusiast with Lyme disease). History of insect or animal bites can be relevant for arbovirus infection, as well as rabies. Other important historical features may include a history of contact with diseased individuals and the underlying immune system condition of the patient. An associated abnormality outside the nervous system (bleeding tendency in hemorrhagic fever) may also point to a specific pathogen.

☆ TIPS & TRICKS

Seasonal incidence of some viral CNS infections:

Summer/Fall: Enterovirus, West Nile virus, St. Louis encephalitis virus, Eastern equine encephalitis virus, California encephalitis viruses and Western equine encephalitis viruses.
Winter/Spring: Mumps and measles.
Any season: Herpes simplex virus (HSV) types 1 and 2, HIV virus.

General Examination

Viral infection of the nervous system is almost always part of a generalized systemic infectious disease. Other organs may be involved prior to or in association with CNS manifestations. A dermatomal pattern or a vesicular skin rash may be indicative of herpes zoster virus. Parotitis strongly suggests the diagnosis of mumps encephalitis in an unvaccinated patient with mental status change. Flaccid paralysis that evolves into an encephalitis strongly suggests the possibility of West Nile virus (WNV) infections, while gastrointestinal signs are associated with enteroviral disease, and upper respiratory findings may accompany influenza virus infection and HSV-1 encephalitis. Tremors of the eyelids, tongue, lips, and extremities may suggest damage to the basal ganglia or cerebellum and the possibility of St. Louis encephalitis or WNV encephalitis in the appropriate season, geographic location, or travel history. Hydrophobia, aerophobia, pharyngeal spasms, and hyperactivity are highly suggestive of encephalitic rabies.

Diagnostic Studies

General

Lymphocytosis is suggestive of a viral encephalitis and is helpful in differentiating viral from nonviral encephalitis.

A culture of body fluids other than cerebrospinal fluid (CSF) may be useful in establishing the etiology of encephalitis. All patients should have blood cultures sent for bacterial and fungal organisms. Positive cultures may be indicative of encephalopathy secondary to systemic infection rather than encephalitis. Specific clinical findings should direct other sites for culture (e.g. stool, nasopharynx).

Scraping and biopsy of skin rashes to identify viral antigens by direct fluorescent antibody in cases of varicella (herpes zoster encephalitis) may be useful.

Cerebrospinal Fluid Findings

Examination of the CSF, although not diagnostic, will usually confirm the presence of inflammatory disease of the CNS. Red cells are usually absent; their presence in the appropriate clinical setting suggests HSV-1 infection.

☆ TIPS & TRICKS

In a CSF analysis for viral infection, the peripheral white blood cell count is usually less than 250/mm^3, with a lymphocyte predominance. A very early infection may show a neutrophilic predominance. CSF protein is elevated but is usually less than 150 mg/dL. CSF glucose concentration (e.g. >50% of blood value) is typically normal, but moderately reduced values are occasionally seen with HSV, mumps, and some enteroviruses.

These findings are generally quite different from those associated with bacterial meningitis, which include a higher white blood cell count in the CSF (>2000/mm^3) with neutrophil predominance, a higher protein concentration (>200 mg/dL), and usually hypoglycorrhachia.

The exclusion of bacterial meningitis based only upon individual CSF parameters can be difficult, since the spectrum of CSF values in bacterial meningitis is so wide that the absence of one of more of these findings is of little value. This was illustrated in a review of 296 episodes of community-acquired bacterial meningitis; 50% had a CSF glucose above 40 mg/dL, 44% had a CSF protein below 200 mg/dL, and 13% had a CSF white cell count below 100/μL (see Duran et al., 1993).

Culture

Viral culture has been routinely ordered by most physicians after obtaining CSF samples. However, one review demonstrated that viruses were recovered from only 6% of 22,394 viral cultures of CSF samples. In subset analysis of the same study, 1290 CSF samples were evaluated for HSV by polymerase chain reaction (PCR) and culture. Of these, only nine samples were positive for HSV and all were identified only by PCR testing (see Polage and Petti, 2006). Therefore, in most circumstances, PCR testing of the CSF has replaced viral culture for the common viral encephalitides. Culture may still be important when rare causes of encephalitis are being considered (e.g. parainfluenza, measles, mumps) for which PCR testing is unavailable.

Polymerase Chain Reaction

With the advent of PCR technology, significant advances have been made in the ability to diagnose viral infections of the CNS. CSF PCR can be performed for HSV-1, HSV-2, and enteroviruses.

The identification of HSV-1 in the CSF is a rapid, sensitive, and specific diagnostic test for HSV-1 encephalitis. PCR testing for other viruses will depend on the clinical situation, epidemiology, and availability.

Serology

Serologic testing is most important for patients who are not improving and who do not have a diagnosis based upon CSF analysis, culture, and PCR. Most viral etiologies require paired sera for diagnosis; thus, in the setting of acute illness, it is prudent to save serum that can later be used if necessary. Convalescent serology should be obtained no sooner than 3 weeks after the onset of the clinical illness. As an example, the presence of IgM antibodies in a single serum sample provides presumptive evidence of St. Louis encephalitis; however, a significant rise or fall between appropriately timed acute-convalescent or early–late convalescent sera is diagnostic.

West Nile virus has emerged as the most common cause of viral encephalitis in the USA. A single specimen looking for IgM antibodies on the serum or CSF is sufficient for diagnosis. A single serum specimen can also be used to diagnose mumps. Serology may also be helpful in obtaining evidence for primary EBV infection, a rare cause of meningoencephalitis.

Brain Biopsy

A brain biopsy to establish the etiology of encephalitis is rarely used today and is not routinely recommended. A biopsy should only be considered in patients with encephalitis of unknown etiology, or patients who deteriorate clinically despite treatment.

Neuroimaging

CT and MRI are most frequently used to evaluate patients with encephalitis. MRI is more sensitive and specific, and CT with or without contrast should only be done if MRI is unavailable, impractical, or cannot be performed. Diffusion-weighted imaging is superior to conventional MRI for the detection of early signal abnormalities in viral encephalitis.

In certain patients with herpes encephalitis, some characteristic neuroimaging patterns have been observed. There may be significant edema and hemorrhage in the temporal lobes as well as hypodense areas on T1-weighted images. Many of these abnormalities can be found in 90% of patients with herpes simplex encephalitis documented by CSF PCR.

In cases of suspected ADEM, MRI is the diagnostic neuroimage of choice, often revealing multiple focal or confluent areas of signal abnormalities in the subcortical white matter and, sometimes, subcortical gray matter on T2 and flair sequences. MRI can be negative early in the clinical course of suspected ADEM. Repeat imaging should occur if clinically indicated.

Electroencephalogram (EEG)

An EEG is generally considered to be a nonspecific investigation. The main benefit of obtaining an EEG is to demonstrate cerebral involvement during the early stage of the disease. It can be used as an indicator of cerebral involvement and usually shows a background abnormality prior to evidence of parenchymal involvement on neuroimaging. Although an EEG is rarely useful in identifying the pathogen, it has a role in identifying patients with nonconvulsive seizures.

Specific Organisms

Herpes Simplex Viruses Types 1 and 2

HSV represents 5–10% of all cases of encephalitis. It is the most common cause of fatal sporadic encephalitis in the USA and affects all age groups (HSV-1 infection is more common in adult and HSV-2 infection is more common in neonates) and can occur in all seasons.

Herpes simplex encephalitis (HSE) arises via one of three routes: (1) direct CNS invasion via the trigeminal nerve or olfactory tract following an infection of oropharynx (most ot these patients are younger than 18 years of age); (2) CNS invasion after an episode of recurrent HSV-1 infection, which is believed to represent viral reactivation with subsequent spread; (3) CNS infection without primary or recurrent HSV-1 infection, which is felt to represent reactivation of latent HSV in situ within the CNS.

Patients usually present with headache, fever, personality changes, memory problems, and commonly seizures.

Diagnosis

Examination of the CSF is indicated. In patients with HSE, both CSF white cells (lymphocyte predominance) and CSF protein levels are elevated.

The gold standard for establishing the diagnosis is the detection of herpes simplex virus DNA in the CSF by polymerase chain reaction (PCR).

⋆ TIPS & TRICKS

PCR testing of CSF is the gold standard in the detection of HSV with 98% sensitivity and 94 to 100% specificity and is positive early in the disease.

CSF serologic testing for HSV antigen and antibody detection is not helpful in the early diagnosis of HSV encephalitis. The use of purified HSV glycoprotein B to detect CSF antibodies has a sensitivity of 97% and a specificity of 100%. However, viral antibody titers, which rise fourfold over the course of the illness, are first positive after 10 days to 2 weeks of illness and are thus only helpful retrospectively. HSV antigen can also be detected in the CSF, but as sensitivity and specificity of this test is lower than PCR assays, there are very few situations in which serology is preferred over PCR.

A viral culture of CSF is rarely positive in the early stages of infection and is only positive later in about 4 to 5% of patients with brain biopsy-proven HSV encephalitis.

Noninvasive neuroimaging studies support a presumptive diagnosis of HSE. Focal changes of the EEG are characterized by spike and slow wave activity and periodic lateralized epileptiform discharges (PLEDs) which arise from the temporal lobe.

⋆ TIPS & TRICKS

MRI usually detects changes earlier than a CT scan in temporal and/or inferior frontal lobe. Bilateral temporal lobe involvement is nearly pathognomonic.

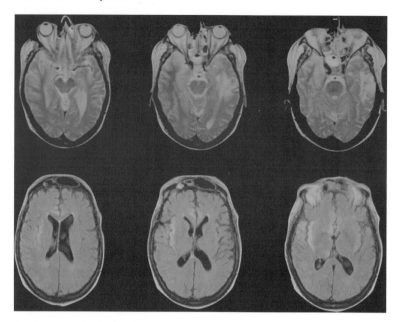

Figure 15.1. *Top row:* T2 MRI sequence demonstrating bilateral (R>L) temporal lobe increased signal intensity consistent with Herpes simplex encephalitis. *Bottom row:* Same patient with T1 post-contrast imaging demonstrating bilateral (R>L) enhancement of temporal lobes.

Treatment

Acyclovir is the treatment of choice for patients with HSE, but morbidity and mortality remain high. Predictors of an adverse outcome include age older than 30 years, a GCS level of consciousness <6, and duration of symptoms before starting acyclovir therapy >4 days. Dosage of acyclovir in normal renal function is 10 mg/kg intravenously every 8 hours for 14–21 days. Therapy may continue beyond that if patients have not had the appropriate clinical response and the repeated PCR for CSF is still positive.

West Nile Virus Infections

West Nile virus (WNV) was first isolated in 1937 from the blood of a woman with a febrile illness who lived in the West Nile region of Uganda. Until relatively recently, it was not considered to be a significant human pathogen. The virus historically was endemic throughout Africa, the Middle East, west and central Asia, and the Mediterranean. WNV infection first appeared in North America in 1999 when an outbreak in New York City resulted in encephalitis in 62 patients and 7 deaths. Since the beginning of the new millenni-

um, WNV has been epidemic in the USA with over 12,000 cases of meningoencephalitis. Nearly all human infections of WNV are due to mosquito bites. Peak transmission occurs between July and October, reflecting the seasonal activity cycle of the mosquito vectors. Persons of all ages are susceptible to WNV infection, though older and/or immunecompromised patients develop a more severe disease. Transmission has also been described via blood transfusion, organ transplant, and through transplacental transmission.

Most persons infected with WNV are asymptomatic, as symptoms are seen in only about 20 to 40% of infected patients. The illness is characterized by a flu-like illness with fever, headache, malaise, back pain, myalgias, and anorexia. About 35% of infected patients develop meningoencephalitis. Additionally, cranial nerve palsies and an acute flaccid paralysis, secondary to the infection of anterior horn cells, can complicate the disease.

The cerebrospinal fluid usually demonstrates a pleocytosis often with a predominance of lymphocytes as well as an elevated protein concentration. CSF for IgM is the preferred test with positive PCR in less than 60%.

Neuroimagings are usually nonspecific, but MRI may reveal hyperintense T2/FLAIR lesions in the thalamus, substantia nigra and basal ganglia, spinal cord, and cortical structures.

Treatment

Treatment is supportive.

St. Louis Encephalitis (SLE) Virus

SLE virus is widely distributed in the USA and is the second leading cause of epidemic viral encephalitis after West Nile virus. The original epidemic of the virus occurred in St. Louis, Missouri, in 1933 causing 1095 clinical cases. The disease is endemic in the western United States with occasional large periodic outbreaks in the eastern states, and Central and South America. Transmission is by *Culex* vector mosquitoes with birds as the intermediate host. SLE occurs during the summer months and peaks during August and September.

Infection with SLE virus only rarely results in clinical illness. Age is the most important risk factor for symptomatic encephalitis, with elderly persons at higher risk. The disease rarely affects children.

Prodromal symptoms of a flu-like illness usually precede the neurological symptoms. Patients always experience fever, malaise, myalgia, and typically a severe headache. Some patients develop a cough and a sore throat, while others develop dysuria and urgency. Neurological symptoms usually occur rapidly, with tremors of eyelids, tongue, lips, and extremities. These may persist for weeks after recovery from the acute illness. Cranial nerve dysfunction as unilateral facial motor weakness may be present. Motor and sensory deficits are rare.

The diagnosis of SLE is generally made by serology, particularly the IgM enzyme-linked immunosorbent assay (ELISA).

Treatment

Treatment is supportive.

Eastern Equine Encephalitis (EEE) Virus

EEE is widely distributed throughout North, Central, and South America and the Caribbean. Transmission is through mosquitoes with birds as the reservoir. In the USA, human infections are usually sporadic and small outbreaks occur each summer, mostly along the Atlantic and Gulf coasts. Peak incidence is in August and September. EEE mainly affects children and elderly persons.

The illness usually begins with constitutional symptoms lasting for several days, with fever, headache, nausea, and vomiting. About 8% of infected people develop encephalitis. Neurological symptoms usually occur abruptly with a fulminant course. Seizures and focal neurological deficits occur in approximately 90% of patients. Many will become comatose or stuporous. EEE is one of the most severe mosquito-transmitted diseases in the USA with approximately 33% mortality and significant brain damage in most survivors.

The diagnosis of EEE infections is generally accomplished by testing serum or CSF to detect virus-specific IgM and neutralizing antibodies.

Treatment

Treatment is supportive

Western Equine Encephalitis (WEE) Virus

WEE disease is found in North America (west of the Mississippi) and South America. Transmission occurs through mosquito vectors with birds acting as the reservoir. WEE mainly affects children and adults (age >50 years). The incidence of the disease is markedly reduced in the USA secondary to equine vaccination, vector control, and the decreased number of horses.

Clinical symptoms usually are headache, backache, altered consciousness, and seizures.

Diagnosis is by serologic testing with detection of IgM in serum and the CSF.

Treatment

Treatment is supportive.

Rocky Mountain Spotted Fever (RMSF) Encephalitis

RMSF is a tick-borne disease, and is the most common rickettsial infection in the USA. It is caused by *Rickettsia rickettsii*, an obligate intracellular bacterium. RMSF occurs throughout North America, Central, and South America. In the USA the disease is prevalent in the southeastern and south central states. Most cases occur in the spring and early summer. Transmission usually occurs after a tick bite. It may rarely occur after exposure to infective tick tissues or feces, conjunctival contamination, transcutaneous transmission, or inhalation. Clinical symptoms in the early phase of the disease consist of nonspecific symptoms like malaise, severe headache, arthralgia. A rash usually develops between the third and fifth day of illness. The rash begins as maculopapular and becomes petechial. It starts on the ankles and wrists and spreads centrally to the palms and soles. Neurological symptoms occur late in the disease and are often the cause of death. A wide variety of neurological complications has been described, including cranial nerve palsies, complete paralysis, seizures, and coma.

Diagnosis is made usually through clinical features in the appropriate epidemiologic setting. Most patients have normal white blood cell counts at presentation. As the disease progresses, thrombocytopenia becomes more prevalent and may be severe. CSF analysis usually shows a high white blood cell count with a neutrophilic or lymphocytic predominance, moderately elevated protein, and normal glucose levels. The diagnosis is best confirmed using serum for serological testing. The indirect fluorescent antibody test has a sensitivity of 95%.

Treatment

As diagnosis of RMSF can rarely be confirmed in the early stage, the corner stone of management is empiric antibiotic treatment. Oral or intravenous doxycycline is the drug of choice, though pregnant women should be treated with chloramphenicol. Treatment should be continued at least for 3 days after the patient has become a febrile.

Human Ehrlichiosis

Ehrlichiosis is another tick-borne disease, and the first case of human ehrlichosis was described in 1986. This etiologic agent, which was identified as *Ehrlichia chafeenesis*, causes human monocytic ehrlichiosis (HME). Another agent, *Anaplasma phagocytophilum*, which was identified in 1994, causes human granulocytic anaplasmosis (HGA).

Ehrlichiae are obligate intracellular bacteria that grow within membrane-bound vacuoles in human and animal leukocytes. Transmission is through a tick bite with the white-tailed deer acting as the mammalian reservoir. Other modes of transmission have been suggested, such as blood transfusion, maternal–child transmission, and through direct contact with slaughtered deer. Most cases occur in the summer and the spring.

Common presenting symptoms are fever, headache, nausea, malaise, anorexia, and, rarely, a skin rash. CNS involvement is common, patients may develop confusion, stupor, hallucination, cranial nerve palsies, and eventually seizures and coma.

Peripheral blood counts show leucopenia. Thrombocytopenia and an elevated level of transaminases are also seen. CSF examination often reveals elevated protein and a moderate pleocytosis with lymphocytic or neurtrophilic predominance.

A diagnosis can be made on finding intraleukocytic morulae in the peripheral blood or buffy coat. Serology can be tested using the indirect fluorescent antibody (IFA) test and reagents specific for HME and HGA or enzyme-linked immunosorbent assays (ELISA). The PCR for HME and HGA is also widely used currently.

Treatment

Treatment should be initiated in all patients suspected of having ehrlichiosis.The drug of choice is doxycycline and treatment should be continued for 10 days. Patients with a doxycycline allergy should be treated with Rifampin for 7–10 days. Pregnant women with severe infection should be treated with doxycycline, otherwise they can be treated with Rifampin.

Listeria Monocytogenes

Listeria monocytogenes is an uncommon cause of encephalitis in the general population but is an important pathogen in pregnant patients, neonates <1 month, elderly individuals greater than 50 years old, and immunocompromised individuals.

L. monocytogenes is a motile, nonspore-forming bacillus that has aerobic and anaerobic characteristics. It is typically a food-borne organism mostly from ingestion of unpasteurized milk and can also be found in water and soil.

Listeriosis symptoms include fever, headache, nausea, or diarrhea. Infected pregnant women may experience only a mild, flu-like illness; however, infections during pregnancy can lead to miscarriage or stillbirth, premature delivery, or infection of the newborn.

CNS infection generally develops as a diffuse meningoencephalitis, usually associated with bacteremia. In up to 24% of patients the encephalitis targets the brainstem (rhombencephalitis). Rhombencephalitis was first described in 1957 as an unusual form of listeriosis. It appears to occur predominantly in previously healthy patients without any predisposing conditions. The clinical course is usually biphasic, with a prodrome of nonspecific symptoms consisting of headache, malaise, nausea, vomiting, and fever, followed by progressive brainstem deficits with asymmetric cranial nerve palsy, cerebellar dysfunctions, hemi- or tetraparesis, sensory deficits, respiratory insufficiency, impairment of consciousness, and seizures. Blood and spinal fluid cultures are positive in 60 and 40% of patients, respectively. The condition is fatal unless treated early. Survivors commonly have significant neurological sequelae.

Diagnosis is always established by a culture of organism from the blood or CSF. The analysis of CSF shows pleocytosis ranging from polymorph nuclear cells to mononuclear cells with a substantial number of lymphocytes seen in the CSF. CSF protein is elevated and CSF glucose is reduced.

Treatment

Listeria is susceptible to common antimicrobial agents, such as ampicillin, penicillin, gentamicin, and trimethoprim-sulfamethoxazole. Ampicillin or penicillin G is the drug of choice. Gentamicin is also used to achieve synergy for Listeria CNS infection.

The duration of therapy varies, immunocompetent patients with CNS infection are usually treated for 2–4 weeks and immunocompromised patients for 3–6 weeks.

Noninfectious Causes
Acute Disseminated Encephalomyelitis (ADEM)

ADEM is an inflammatory demyelinating disease of the CNS which presents with a monophasic course associated with multifocal neurologic symptoms and encephalopathy. It usually occurs after bacterial or viral infection or immunization. The most common organisms associated with the ADEM prodrome are Corona virus, CMV, Epstein–Barr virus, and Herpes simplex. Neurological symptoms typically present 1–3 days after infection or immunization and the clinical course can progress rapidly over a few days. Neurological symptoms vary with the location of the white matter lesions, which can arise anywhere in the CNS. The disease usually presents in children and young adults, occasionally affecting older adults.

Presenting symptoms are frequently headache, vomiting, change in consciousness and motor deficits. Additionally, behavioral changes or psychosis can be seen on presentation. In older patients, there may be no obvious preceding infection or vaccination.

There is a characteristic pattern of extensive and diffuse hyperintense T2/FLAIR lesions affecting the brainstem and supratentorial regions with relatively small mass effect. Lesions not only affect the white matter but also gray matter and can cross the midline through the corpus callosum.

CSF findings are usually nonspecific and include lymphocytic pleocytosis with elevated protein levels and sterile cultures.

Treatment

Treatment is usually with high-dose corticosteroids, although no controlled trials have been performed. Additionally, there are reports of efficacy of plasmapheresis as well as intravenous immunoglobulins. Mortality is higher in adults than in children. In adults requiring ICU admission, mortality ranges between 8 and 25%.

Bibliography

Durand ML, et al. Acute bacterial meningitis in adults. A review of 493 episodes. *New Engl J Med* 1993; **328(1)**:21–28.

McLauchlin J. Human listeriosis in Britain, 1967–85, a summary of 722 cases. 2. Listeriosis in non-pregnant individuals, a changing pattern of infection and seasonal incidence. *Epidemiol Infect* 1990; **104(2)**:191–201.

Mylonakis E, Hohmann EL, Calderwood SB. Central nervous system infection with Listeria monocytogenes. 33 years' experience at a general hospital and review of 776 episodes from the literature. *Medicine (Baltimore)*, 1998; **77** **(5)**:313–336.

Polage CR, Petti CA. Assessment of the utility of viral culture of cerebrospinal fluid. *Clin Infect Dis* 2006; **43(12)**:1578–1579.

Siegman-Igra Y, et al. Listeria monocytogenes infection in Israel and review of cases worldwide. *Emerg Infect Dis* 2002; **8(3)**: 305–310.

Tunkel AR, et al. The management of encephalitis: clinical practice guidelines by the Infectious Diseases Society of America. *Clin Infect Dis* 2008; **47(3)**:303–327.

Part IV

Neuromuscular Complications Encountered in the Intensive Care Unit

Practical Management of Guillain–Barré Syndrome and Myasthenic Crisis

Alejandro A. Rabinstein

Department of Neurology, Mayo Clinic College of Medicine, Rochester, MN, USA

Introduction

Guillain–Barré syndrome (GBS) and myasthenia gravis (MG) constitute the two most common causes of primary neuromuscular respiratory failure in daily practice. They share some characteristics, including their typically self-limited course and response to immune therapies. However, they are also quite different in some important aspects. These differences have crucial practical implications and, therefore, should be known by clinicians caring for these patients. This chapter provides succinct and practical information to guide the management of patients with GBS and myasthenic crisis in the intensive care unit (ICU).

Basic Principles of Management of Neuromuscular Respiratory Failure

The diagnosis of primary neuromuscular respiratory failure should be suspected in any patient presenting with mixed (hypoxic-hypercapneic) or predominantly hypercapneic respiratory failure and signs of muscle weakness (bulbar or appendicular). At times, this may be difficult in patients presenting very acutely and in whom a recent history of progressive weakness is not available. GBS may be preceded by infections and MG can be exacerbated by any acute systemic illness. These possibilities are important to bear in mind when faced with cases in which the respiratory failure appears to be out of proportion to the severity of the systemic disease.

Once neuromuscular respiratory failure is suspected, the next step is to confirm the primary diagnosis. Characteristic features of GBS and MG will be discussed in the respective following sections of this chapter. Inability to determine the primary neuromuscular diagnosis is a very strong predictor of poor prognosis, probably because specific treatment cannot be provided in such cases. The next step is to search for precipitants (e.g. infections, medication changes in myasthenics), which should be addressed. These steps should be accomplished while assessing the adequacy of airway safety, ventilation and oxygenation. Systemic complications, such as aspiration pneumonia, atelectasis, and cardiac arrhythmias can occur early and demand prompt diagnosis and treatment.

SCIENCE REVISITED

Neuromuscular respiratory failure can be precipitated by bulbar muscle weakness or respiratory muscle weakness. In fact, both types of muscle weakness are most often combined.

Emergency Management in Neurocritical Care, First Edition. Edited by Edward M. Manno.
© 2012 John Wiley & Sons, Ltd. Published 2012 by John Wiley & Sons, Ltd.

Bulbar muscle weakness can lead to airway obstruction by oral and respiratory secretions due to the inefficiency of protective mechanisms, most notably cough. Aspiration can rapidly accelerate the clinical decline. Respiratory muscle weakness first produces microatelectases in the lung bases; the consequent shunting is responsible for the mild hypoxia observed early in the course of the disease. As weakness becomes more severe due to worsening muscular fatigue, tidal volumes get progressively smaller and hypercapnia supervenes. Rapid and profound hypoxia develops shortly thereafter as the compensatory action of accessory breathing muscles becomes overwhelmed.

The clinical signs of neuromuscular respiratory failure include dyspnea, tachypnea, restlessness, tachycardia, diaphoresis (drops of sweat often seen on the forehead), staccato speech, recruitment of accessory muscles (best objectified by palpating the sternocleidomastoid muscles), and, most importantly, paradoxical breathing pattern. The paradoxical breathing pattern is characterized by the inward (rather than the normal outward) movement of the abdominal wall with each inspiration and it is a reliable marker of diaphragmatic failure. Its presence signifies impending respiratory failure and should prompt consideration of ventilatory assistance.

Apart from the physical examination, the initial assessment of patients with acute neuromuscular respiratory failure should include bedside testing of respiratory volumes and pressures by spirometry, measurement of arterial blood gases, and performance of a chest X-ray to exclude pulmonary complications.

★ TIPS & TRICKS

Bedside respiratory tests provide very useful information to assess the initial severity and monitor the evolution of neuromuscular respiratory failure. Forced vital capacity (FVC), maximal inspiratory pressure (MIP, also known as negative inspiratory force), and maximal expiratory pressure (MEP) are the most valuable and commonly employed measures. However, they should never be interpreted in isolation; instead, they should

be regarded as a helpful complement to the clinical examination and arterial blood gases.

Some caveats should be kept in mind when performing and evaluating bedside respiratory tests in patients with acute neuromuscular weakness. The contributing role of pre-existent or intercurrent pulmonary disease should be considered when interpreting the results. Tests are strictly effort-dependent, thus it is crucial to ensure that the patient is providing maximal effort during testing. The best of three consecutive measurements should be used to optimize reliability. Careful coaching by an experienced respiratory therapist is essential before commencing the test, since repeated suboptimal efforts may be misleading due to increasing fatigue. Poor mouth sealing around the spirometer due to facial weakness may be another cause of deceivingly poor results and this problem should be noted when present. Suctioning of respiratory secretions should always precede these measurements. Finally, any overt discrepancy among FVC, MIP, and MEP (e.g. preserved FVC and MEP with very poor MIP) measured at the same time should alert the physician about the possibility of a spurious result.

Arterial blood gases revealing hypoxia or hypercapnia should be considered an indication for intubation in GBS. Myasthenic patients with progressive exacerbations might present with mild hypoxia and compensated hypercapnia. These patients must be admitted to the ICU and often require ventilatory support. The presence of acidosis before the initiation of mechanical ventilation portends a poor prognosis regardless of the cause of acute neuromuscular respiratory failure.

GBS and MG respond to immune therapy with plasma exchange (PE) and intravenous immunoglobulin (IVIg). In both conditions the early initiation of therapy maximizes the benefit. It is important to realize that the therapeutic effect of these interventions is not immediate when discussing expectations with patients and families. The mechanisms of action of PE and IVIg are incompletely understood. Clearing of pathogenic antibodies would be the most obvious

Table 16.1. Adverse events related to plasma exchange and intravenous immunoglobulin

Plasma Exchange	Intravenous Immunoglobulin
Venous catheter-related	Infusion-related
Infection	Headache
Pneumothorax	Shivering
Local hematoma	Myalgias
Hemodynamic instability (hypotension)	Chest pain
Hemoconcentration	Hyperviscosity (risk of thrombosis, including arterial events)
Coagulopathy (mild)	Aseptic meningitis
Hypocalcemia	Renal failure (tubular toxicity)
Removal of highly protein-bound drugs	Anaphylaxis (if IgA deficiency)

property of PE; however, there is only a limited correlation between the decrease in anti-acetylcholine receptor antibody titers and the clinical improvement after PE in MG patients, signaling that other mechanisms of action could also play a role. GBS patients who respond less favorably to IVIg, however, have lower serum IgG titers 2 weeks after the infusion, which suggests that the efficacy of IVIg may depend at least in part on its ability to achieve sustained elevations in serum IgG levels.

A treatment course of PE typically consists of exchanges of 1.5 to 2 liters per session on alternate days for a total of 5 exchanges. Lower volume exchanges can be safely performed on consecutive days. The usual recommended dose of IVIg is 400 mg/kg per day for 5 days (i.e. total dose of 2 g/kg). However, in patients in whom the anticipated risk from increased serum viscosity is not high, administering 1 g/kg IVIg per day for 2 days appears to be a safe option.

Given the lack of conclusive evidence that one type of immune therapy is better that another for either GBS or MG, the choice of PE or IVIg is often based on local preferences and experience and, especially, on the anticipated risk of adverse events in the individual case. Quantitatively, the frequency of adverse events with PE is greater than with IVIg. However, this difference is related to complications from the placement of central venous catheters. The main adverse events related to PE and IVIg are summarized in Table 16.1.

SCIENCE REVISITED

GBS is typically caused by an autoimmune demyelinating polyradiculoneuropathy (the nosological entity known as acute inflammatory demyelinating polyradiculoneuropathy). A more severe axonal form is often preceded by diarrhea most frequently provoked by Campylobacter jejuni (because this microorganism can trigger an antiganglioside response due to molecular mimicry).

The first symptoms of GBS are often back pain and distal leg paresthesias, but the hallmark of the syndrome is the rapid development of ascending weakness associated with the loss of deep tendon reflexes. Bulbar weakness usually occurs only after the weakness has progressed from the legs to the arms. Yet, severe cases exhibit bilateral facial weakness, ptosis, ophthalmoplegia, oropharyngeal muscle weakness, and respiratory failure. Diaphragmatic failure can develop very suddenly, demanding emergency intubation. The other major characteristic of GBS is autonomic dysfunction due to the involvement of autonomic nerves. Cardiac arrhythmias, hemodynamic instability, gastroparesis, paralytic ileus, and bladder retention are the principal manifestations. Clinical variants of GBS have been described; the best known is the Miller Fisher variant which features ataxia, arreflexia, and ophthalmoparesis as its defining triad.

The diagnosis of GBS relies on clinical criteria supported by electrophysiological and cerebrospinal fluid changes. The criteria that support the diagnosis of GBS most strongly are progression of symptoms and signs over days to 4 weeks (fluctuations or decline after 8 weeks indicates the diagnosis of acute-onset chronic inflammatory demyelinating polyradiculoneuropathy), symmetric weakness affecting the legs more than the arms (at least initially), mild or absent sensory symptoms and signs, cranial nerve involvement (especially of both facial nerves), increased protein content in the cerebrospinal fluid without associated cellular reaction (albumino-cytological dissociation), and electrophysiological signs of impaired nerve conduction, including conduction blocks, F wave abnormalities, and prolonged distal latencies.

☝ CAUTION

Any patient suspected of having GBS who presents with rapidly progressive weakness should be admitted to the ICU. As emergency intubation can induce life-threatening complications from dysautonomia, it is crucial to proceed with elective intubation in patients expected to require ventilatory assistance.

The main clinical factors associated with higher risk of requiring ventilatory assistance are a fast progression of weakness, the presence of facial and bulbar weakness, and a greater severity of generalized weakness. Serial bedside respiratory measurements also provide reliable information to predict which patients with GBS will require mechanical ventilation.

★ TIPS & TRICKS

Admission FVC or a decrease in FVC to less than 20 mL/kg, or a reduction in FVC, MIP, or MEP greater than 30% from the baseline should be considered indications for ICU monitoring and possible elective intubation. In addition, the combination of FVC lower than 20 mL/kg, MIP worse than −30 cm H_2O,

and MEP less than 40 H_2O predict requirement of mechanical ventilation ("20–30–40 rule").

Patients with electrophysiological signs of axonal dysfunction are more susceptible to developing respiratory failure. Figure 16.1 delineates a decision tree for the initial assessment of respiratory function in patients with GBS.

Overall, one-third of patients hospitalized for GBS will require mechanical ventilation. In patients with GBS, ventilatory assistance should always be invasive (i.e. delivered by means of an endotracheal tube). Noninvasive ventilation with a bilevel positive airway pressure (BiPAP) mask is not a safe option in GBS for several reasons: (1) patients who develop diaphragmatic failure usually remain extremely weak and require full ventilatory assistance for many days (more than a week); (2) diaphragmatic failure in GBS is due to denervation, a situation completely different from MG in which early respiratory insufficiency due to fluctuating neuromuscular transmission failure produces a respiratory muscle fatigue that can be substantially helped by timely institution of noninvasive ventilation; and (3) the manifestations of dysautonomia get worse as respiratory failure becomes more severe.

Once patients are intubated, initial ventilation should be delivered using assist-control (AC) to rest the patient. However, switching promptly to synchronized intermittent mandatory ventilation (SIMV) is advisable to avoid diaphragmatic atrophy from disuse. When ventilating with SIMV, adequate pressure support and positive end-expiratory pressure (PEEP) should be provided. Daily bedside respiratory measurements may be useful to monitor the evolution of respiratory muscle weakness. It is crucial to ensure that the patient receives adequate chest physiotherapy to prevent pulmonary complications.

The main manifestations of dysautonomia in GBS are listed in Table 16.2. It is very important to keep these in mind when prescribing medications. Beta blockers should be used very cautiously because they can provoke sudden hypotension and bradycardia. When blood pressure is very elevated, we prefer to use other options

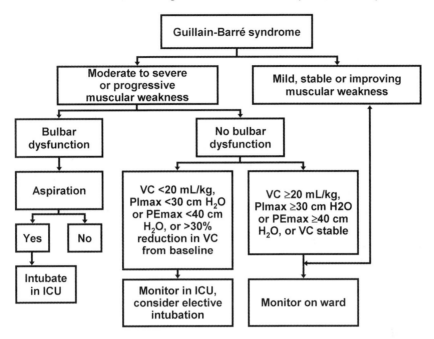

Figure 16.1. Proposed algorithm for the initial evaluation of respiratory function in patients with GBS.

(such as hydralazine or nicardipine), always starting at low doses. Hypotensive spells frequently respond to fluid boluses; when vasopressors are administered, low initial doses are again preferred. Treatment of gastroparesis and adynamic ileus is challenging because metoclopramide and neostigmine can induce dangerous arrhythmias in GBS patients. Unless it is unsafe because of very high gastric residuals and severe abdominal distension, enteral feeding should be continued. If enteral feeding needs to be decreased or stopped, parenteral feeding should be started without delay to prevent malnutrition. We initiate antineuropathic pain medications early and prefer those with antidepressant action since depression is a very common complication in these patients with severe weakness from GBS.

Table 16.2. Main features of dysautonomia in GBS

Labile blood pressure
• Hypertension
• Hypotension
Cardiac arrhythmias
• Tachycardia
• Bradycardia
• AV blocks
• Asystole
Gastroparesis
Adynamic ileus
Bladder dysfunction
• Retention
• Incontinence
Neuropathic pain

AV = atrioventricular

Immune therapy with PE or IVIg is considered the standard of care in patients with GBS and it should be ideally initiated within 2 weeks of symptom onset.

There is indirect evidence that higher doses of IVIg (i.e. more than the usual total dose of 2 g/kg) could be justified in patients with severe GBS. Studies have shown that corticosteroids are not useful in GBS and the administration of high doses of intravenous corticosteroids is associated with increased systemic complications.

The mortality rate of severe GBS causing neuromuscular respiratory failure may still reach 5–10%. In addition, 20% of survivors may suffer from long-term disability. Markers of poorer prognosis include older age, axonal changes on electrophysiological studies, diarrhea at onset (seen commonly in axonal forms), and degree of disability at 2 weeks. However, young patients may recover fully even if they develop extremely severe weakness with prolonged requirement for mechanical ventilation. The most common residual symptoms are fatigue, mild distal paresthesias, and weakness.

Myasthenic Crisis

> **⚘ SCIENCE REVISITED**
>
> MG is a neuromuscular transmission disorder most often caused (except for some rare genetic forms) by an autoimmune reaction that interferes with the activation of the post-synaptic muscle fiber.

In the majority of cases the mediators of this autoimmune disease are antibodies against the acetylcholine receptors; when these antibodies are present the cases are categorized as seropositive. Other autoantibodies can be observed in MG, most notably antimuscle specific tyrosine kinase (MuSK) antibodies. Patients with anti-MuSK antibodies tend to have a more severe bulbar weakness and they appear to be at increased risk of developing myasthenic crisis.

MG is clinically characterized by fluctuating weakness and fatigability with the early involvement of facial and bulbar muscles. Consequently, a worsening weakness in the late afternoon and evening, ptosis, diplopia, and nasal voice (from oropharyngeal muscle weakness) are conspicuous features. Patients presenting with MG exacerbation or crisis typically have a history of worsening weakness over the preceding days. Common triggers of these exacerbations include infections and medication changes.

The diagnosis of MG can be confirmed by serology, electrophysiology, or a therapeutic trial with a cholinesterase inhibitor (most often edro-

phonium). Decremental response with repetitive nerve stimulation is the electrophysiological hallmark of the disease. Increased jitter is seen in single-fiber electromyography.

Although frequently used to monitor the progression of weakness in patients with myasthenic crisis, the value of pulmonary function tests in MG is much less well established than in GBS. The fluctuating nature of weakness in patients with MG may render serial spirometric measurements more variable and unpredictable. In addition, the weakness of bulbar and facial muscles is often a predominant feature early in the course of a myasthenic crisis. In these cases, testing may become impracticable because of insufficient mouth sealing. Furthermore, patients with impaired swallowing and a weak cough may become unable to clear their secretions and require intubation for airway protection before they develop frank respiratory muscle weakness.

> **✫ TIPS & TRICKS**
>
> Prompt initiation of noninvasive ventilation with the BiPAP mask may avert the need for endotracheal intubation in patients with respiratory insufficiency from MG. This is the best strategy to treat failing MG patients and should be combined with administration of PE or IVIg very shortly after admission.

Even patients with severe bulbar weakness can tolerate noninvasive ventilation as long as they receive diligent respiratory care with frequent suctioning of oral and respiratory secretions. In fact, patients who are successfully treated with BiPAP have less pulmonary complications (atelectasis and pneumonia) than those who get directly intubated. However, it is crucial to start noninvasive ventilation with BiPAP early; once patients are already hypercapneic, the rate of BiPAP success diminishes markedly. Figure 16.2 illustrates a management strategy for patients with MG exacerbation/crisis evaluated in the Emergency Department.

When patients are intubated, the general principles of ventilation and chest physiotherapy

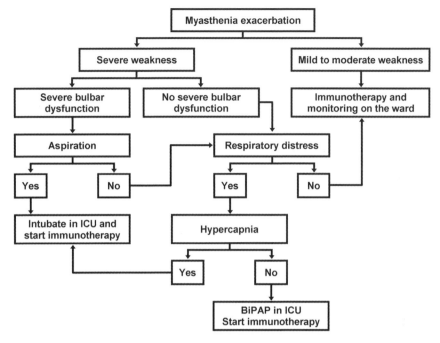

Figure 16.2. Proposed algorithm for the early management of patients with myasthenic exacerbation/crisis.

previously discussed for GBS also apply for MG. As gradual weaning proceeds, it is advisable to avoid reaching muscle fatigue.

☝ CAUTION

Extubation may fail in up to one-quarter of MG patients. Presence of atelectasis is strongly associated with extubation failure.

Noninvasive support with BiPAP may be extremely useful to prevent reintubation. BiPAP should be initiated immediately if patients have any signs of even mild respiratory insufficiency shortly after extubation. Otherwise patients may be closely watched, but it is prudent to have them wear the BiPAP mask the first night after extubation as this is the critical time when most patients fail – due to loss of muscle tone during REM sleep – and require reintubation.

The pharmacological treatment of myasthenic crisis should include immunomodulatory agents, anti-inflammatory/immunosuppressant drugs, and cholinesterase inhibitors.

Cholinesterase inhibitors (usually oral pyridostigmine, but parenteral neostigmine can be prescribed when the enteral route is not safe, such as in the rare cases of concurrent gastrointestinal bleeding or recent abdominal surgery) can be transiently discontinued after intubation to minimize the production of respiratory secretions, but should never be stopped when the patient is being treated with noninvasive ventilation and should always be restarted in adequate doses before weaning is initiated. If oral and respiratory secretions are excessive, low doses of atropine, glycopyrrolate, or scopolamine can be safely administered.

The ideal form of administration of corticosteroids (oral versus intravenous, optimal dose) in myasthenic exacerbation/crisis is not well established. As a principle, all these patients should receive corticosteroids. However, caution should be exercised when considering the prescription of high-dose intravenous methylprednisolone in nonintubated patients because one-third to one-half of patients will experience a clinically meaningful exacerbation of weakness within days of starting this treatment. Although daily dosing of prednisone (with a usual initial dose of 1 mg/kg of ideal body weight) is necessary at first, it is advisable to switch to alternate day dosing whenever feasible to reduce the risk of side effects. It is also reasonable to start a steroid-sparing immunosuppressant (such as azathioprine) during acute hospitalization to facilitate an earlier reduction in steroid dose and to reduce the risk of recurrent crises. All patients receiving high-dose corticosteroids should also receive gastric protection to avoid peptic ulcers.

EVIDENCE AT A GLANCE

Administration of PE or IVIg is considered standard of care for patients with myasthenic crisis. These immunomodulatory strategies have been shown to improve the muscle strength in patients with MG exacerbations and to reduce the risk of post-operative crisis when administered presurgically. However, they have never been specifically tested in myasthenic crisis (i.e. not specifically in patients with neuromuscular respiratory failure due to MG) and there is no proof that they shorten the duration of mechanical ventilation.

In the only randomized-controlled trial that compared PE versus IVIg in MG patients, the efficacy of both treatments was similar and both were safe, although IVIg was slightly better tolerated. The choice of immunomodulatory modality typically depends on local preference and experience. There is a lack of evidence that combining PE and IVIg confers any additional benefit.

The outcome of myasthenic crisis has improved over the decades due to refinements in critical care and, perhaps, the advent of better immune therapies. Mortality in recent series is lower than 5%. Still, ICU admissions spanning 10–14 days are the norm if patients require intubation. Only those treated successfully with BiPAP have a shorter and less complicated clinical course. The most common systemic complications are atelectasis, pneumonia, diarrhea, and venous thromboembolism. Recurrent crises are not uncommon; close outpatient monitoring and adequate pharmacological management, including immunosuppressive therapy, are necessary to prevent their occurrence.

Bibliography

Cabrera Serrano M, Rabinstein AA. Causes and outcomes of acute neuromuscular respiratory failure. *Arch Neurol* 2010; **67(9)**:1089–1094.

Fletcher DD, Lawn ND, Wolter TD, Wijdicks EF. Long-term outcome in patients with Guillain–Barré syndrome requiring mechanical ventilation. *Neurology* 2000; **54(12)**:2311–2315.

Gajdos P, Chevret S, Toyka K. Plasma exchange for myasthenia gravis. *Cochrane Database Syst Rev* 2002; **4:**CD002275.

Gajdos P, Chevret S, Toyka K. Intravenous immunoglobulin for myasthenia gravis. *Cochrane Database Syst Rev* 2008; **1:**CD002277.

Hiraga A, Mori M, Ogawara K, et al. Differences in patterns of progression in demyelinating and axonal Guillain–Barré syndromes. *Neurology* 2003; **61(4)**:471–474.

Hughes RA, Swan AV, van Doorn PA. Intravenous immunoglobulin for Guillain–Barré syndrome. *Cochrane Database Syst Rev* 2010; **6:**CD002063.

Kuitwaard K, de Gelder J, Tio-Gillen AP, et al. Pharmacokinetics of intravenous immunoglobulin and outcome in Guillain–Barré syndrome. *Ann Neurol* 2009; **66(5)**:597–603.

Lawn ND, Fletcher DD, Henderson RD, et al. Anticipating mechanical ventilation in Guillain–Barré syndrome. *Arch Neurol* 2001; **58(6)**:893–898.

Rabinstein AA, Wijdicks EF. Warning signs of imminent respiratory failure in neurological patients. *Semin Neurol* 2003; **23(1)**:97–104.

Raphaël JC, Chevret S, Hughes RA, Annane D. Plasma exchange for Guillain–Barré syndrome. *Cochrane Database Syst Rev* 2002; **2:** CD001798.

Seneviratne J, Mandrekar J, Wijdicks EF, Rabinstein AA. Noninvasive ventilation in myasthenic crisis. *Arch Neurol* 2008; **65(1)**:54–58.

Seneviratne J, Mandrekar J, Wijdicks EF, Rabinstein AA. Predictors of extubation failure in myasthenic crisis. *Arch Neurol* 2008; **65(7)**:929–933.

Thomas CE, Mayer SA, Gungor Y, et al. Myasthenic crisis: clinical features, mortality, complications, and risk factors for prolonged intubation. *Neurology* 1997; **48(5)**:1253–1260.

van Koningsveld R, Steyerberg EW, Hughes RA, et al. A clinical prognostic scoring system for Guillain–Barré syndrome. *Lancet Neurol* 2007; **6(7)**:589–594.

Walgaard C, Lingsma HF, Ruts L, et al. Prediction of respiratory insufficiency in Guillain–Barré syndrome. *Ann Neurol* 2010; **67(6)**:781–787.

Part V

Neurological Complications and Consultations in General Intensive Care Units

17

Metabolic Encephalopathies

Edward M. Manno

Neurological Intensive Care Unit, Cleveland Clinic, Cleveland, OH, USA

Introduction

Metabolic encephalopathies are disorders of brain function that do not have a structural source. They represent a group of entities that lead to neurological deterioration through a variety of mechanisms; however, their diagnosis is crucial in differentiating deterioration due to structural causes from more global disturbances seen with diffuse encephalopathies. Encephalopathies encountered in the intensive care unit are problematic and are associated with increased mortality and long-term cognitive deficits. The terminology "metabolic encephalopathy" is antiquated and probably too limited to encompass the scope of cognitive difficulties encountered in the modern-day intensive care unit. The syndromes of acute cerebral dysfunction have been housed under a number of terminologies and include acute confusional state, ICU psychosis, organic brain syndrome or failure, and cerebral insufficiency. Newer terminologies have been proposed such as "critical illness brain syndrome" or "critical illness associated cognitive dysfunction". All of these conditions have an acute onset, deterioration in consciousness, and cognitive function, and an underlying metabolic or structural etiology that can distinguish these disorders from psychiatric illness. Specific terminology such as "metabolic encephalopathy" presumes a known etiology. The spectrum of cognitive difficulties or encephalopathies encountered in the intensive care unit can be broad ranging from a mild delirium to coma. As this chapter is limited in context, the discussion will be limited to the description of delirium and the more commonly encountered encephalopathies attributed to sepsis and hepatic failure.

Delirium

Delirium is described as a fluctuating disturbance in consciousness characterized by impaired attention and disorganized thinking. The *Diagnostic and Statistical Manual of Mental Disorders* (DSM) 4th edition of the American Psychiatric Association defines delirium as an acute disturbance of consciousness with an impairment in cognition, attention, or perception. The disturbance cannot be accounted for by a general medical condition or a pre-existing dementia.

Hyperactive, hypoactive, and the mixed forms of delirium that have been described are based on the behavioral pattern of psychomotor activity. Hyperactive patients may be agitated and combative while hypoactive patients may appear calm and appropriate. The latter are subsequently underdiagnosed unless a thorough mental status examination is performed. The frequency and significance of these subtypes is incompletely characterized, however there is growing evidence to suggest that patients with the hypoactive form of delirium may have worse cognitive outcomes.

Emergency Management in Neurocritical Care, First Edition. Edited by Edward M. Manno.
© 2012 John Wiley & Sons, Ltd. Published 2012 by John Wiley & Sons, Ltd.

A number of clinical tools have been developed to detect and monitor delirium in critical care patients. The Confusion Assessment Method for the Intensive Care Unit (CAM-ICU) and the Intensive Care Delirium Screening Checklist (ICDSC) are the best validated against the DSM criteria. A recent comparison suggested increased sensitivity and a negative predictive value of the CAM-ICU.

Delirium is reported in as many as 90% of critically ill patients, depending upon the clinical assessment used. Most patients that are mechanically ventilated will have some period of delirium. The consequences of delirium in the ICU are significant. It is associated with increased mortality, length of stay, and unplanned catheter removal and extubation.

Management focuses on the treatment of the underlying diseases or physiological disturbances, and treatment of symptoms. Prevention strategies have been developed in an attempt to minimize factors that appear to exacerbate the risk of worsening delirium. These include reorientation of the patient, early mobilization, removal of catheters and physical restraints, sleep enhancement protocols, and the provision of eyeglasses and hearing aids. These nonpharmacologic measures have proved useful in the short term; however, the long-term impact on morbidity and mortality is unclear.

Benzodiazepines and opioids are thought to worsen delirium and are generally avoided or at best minimized during sedation of the critically ill patient. The exception is obviously benzodiazepine withdrawal. The preferred agents are antipsychotic agents: Haldol has been advocated for its efficacy and safety profile, and magnesium replacement should be adequate in patients receiving Haldol. Serial electrocardiograms monitoring the QT interval should be followed. Torsades de pointes has been reported with higher doses of Haldol and a small but growing body of literature is suggesting that continuous sedation with dexetomidate may be preferable to benzodiazepines or propofol in the prevention of delirium.

Septic Encephalopathy

Septic encephalopathy refers to the encephalopathy encountered in the acutely ill or septic patient. The terminology is imprecise since less than half of patients will have an identifiable infecting organism. A more appropriate term may be sepsis-associated encephalopathy or delirium. Since the encephalopathy is a consequence of systemic inflammation, some authors have advocated the term "systemic inflammatory response encephalopathy".

Whatever terminology is used, acutely ill patients with an encephalopathy have worse outcomes. Outcome appears to parallel the severity of the encephalopathy, which can be quantified on EEG monitoring. Mild encephalopathies are reversible but more recent findings of long-term neuropsychological changes after sepsis argue for more permanent structural neuronal damage.

Pathophysiology

The exact etiology of this sepsis or inflammatory-associated encephalopathy remains speculative. However, experimental evidence suggests that inflammatory mediators, either directly or indirectly, affect neurological function. Systemic and visceral inflammation is detected by vagal afferents through their axonal cytokine receptors. These afferents terminate in the nucleus tractus solitarius which modulate baroreflexes and connect to the paraventricular nuclei of the hypothalamus. The circumventricular organs lacking a blood–brain barrier are similarly exposed to inflammatory cytokines. The response of these exposed centers is an induction and escalation of other inflammatory mediators, including interleukins 2, 1b, 6, and tumor necrosis factors.

Inflammatory mediators can directly affect neurological function. Prostaglandins released during this process can directly interfere with neurotransmission and decrease the release of neurohormones. Specifically, prostaglandins, cytokines, and nitric oxide can directly modulate cholinergic transmission and the secretion of corticotrophic-releasing hormone, ACTH, and vasopressin.

Inflammatory mediators will greatly increase the oxidative stress encountered by neurons during sepsis and can lead to apotosis. This has been documented in the highly metabolic brain regions of the hippocampus and cortex in septic rats. Similarly, mitochondrial dysfunction through impairment of mitochondrial respiratory chain enzymes has been induced by nitric oxide in the medullary autonomic centers of a septic rat.

The escalation of inflammatory mediators can also lead to the disruption of the blood–brain barrier, subsequently exposing the internal millieu of the brain to neurotoxic substances. In a rat and pig model of sepsis, microvessel edema resulted in the displacement of astrocytic foot processes from the vasculature. This can possibly account for the development of the cerebral edema commonly found in the septic patient. Blood–brain barrier disruption and alterations in the astrocytic foot process may account for the pathological findings of microhemorrhages and the clinical presentation of posterior reversible encephalopathies.

The encephalopathy encountered during sepsis rarely occurs in isolation. Multi-organ dysfunction is common and an alteration in other organ functions can lead to electrolyte disturbances and hypoglycemia. Ischemia secondary to hypotension is common. Cerebral autoregulation can be maintained or can be severely affected. PET studies, however, suggest that decreased cerebral perfusion is matched to decreased cerebral metabolism.

Clinical Features

The encephalopathy attributed to inflammation appears to affect the cerebral hemispheres bilaterally. This nonfocal encephalopathy can range from mild agitation and/or delirium to coma. Cranial nerve examination reveals small minimally reactive pupils. Brainstem reflexes remain largely intact. Roving conjugate eye movements are common. Neurological findings are symmetrical and focal findings should prompt an investigation for a structural cause.

EEG findings parallel the depth of the encephalopathy. Mild slowing is followed by progression to theta and delta waves; and burst suppression patterns have an ominous prognosis. Somatosensory-evoked potentials are not affected by sedation but have limited utility in the septic patient.

The plasma levels of biomarkers (neuron-specific enolase, S-100B) have been studied in sepsis but the sensitivity and specificity for detecting brain dysfunction and morbidity are poorly characterized. Cerebral spinal fluid analysis is reserved for patients where meningitis is a consideration.

Magnetic resonance imaging of the brain is the most useful imaging modality in sepsis. Case reports have documented subtle infarctions in the basal ganglia and other highly metabolic brain regions. Diffusion imaging has been used to detect cerebritis and early changes for the posterior reversible encephalopathy syndrome.

Treatment

No specific treatment exists for the encephalopathy associated with critical illness. The treatment for this inflammatory mediated encephalopathy is treatment of the underlying illness. Inhibition of nitric oxide reduces lipopolysaccharide-induced neuronal apotosis in a rat model of sepsis. Calcium channel blockers and the removal of circulating cytokines through plasma filtration have been proposed. Various antioxidants have been used in experimental models to reduce the cerebral edema associated with sepsis. All treatments, however, remain experimental.

Hepatic Encephalopathy

Hepatic encephalopathy refers to the neuropsychiatric abnormalities that develop in chronic liver disease. It is also the principal feature of fulminant hepatic failure. The encephalopathy can be classified on the basis of the underlying etiology of the hepatic failure. The World Congress of Gastroenterology classified type A as being attributed to acute liver failure, type B to portosystemic bypass, and type C as chronic or persistent due to cirrhosis or portal hypertension. The encephalopathy can be further categorized by the severity of the encephalopathy and neurological findings. Morbidity and mortality are directly related to the severity of the encephalopathy. The West Haven criteria for classification of the encephalopathy attributed to hepatic failure is listed in Table 17.1.

Pathophysiology

The pathologic changes in hepatic encephalopathy have been well described. Pathologically, there is a direct increase in the number and size of protoplasmic astrocytes found predominantly in the deep layers of the cortex, thalamus, substantia nigra, and pontine nuclei. The degree of glial abnormalities appears to parallel the intensity and duration of the illness. These swollen

Table 17.1. West Haven criteria for altered mental status in hepatic encephalopathy

Grade 0	Minimal hepatic encephalopathy, lack of detectable changes in personality or behavior; no asterixis.
Grade 1	Trivial lack of awareness, shortened attention span, sleep disturbance, altered mood, and slowing the ability to perform mental tasks; asterixis may be present.
Grade 2	Lethargy or apathy, disorientation to time, amnesia of recent events, impaired simple computations, inappropriate behavior, and slurred speech; asterixis is present.
Grade 3	Somnolence, confusion, disorientation to place, bizarre behavior, clonus, nystagmus, and positive Babinski sign; asterixis usually absent.
Grade 4	Coma, lack of verbal, eye, and oral response to stimuli.

astrocytes display enlarged nuclei with displaced chromatin and are labeled Alzheimer type II astrocytes.

There have been many theories to explain the encephalopathy encountered with hepatic failure. The direct neurotoxic role of ammonia was forwarded in the 1950s when patients using ammonia-cation resins exchange resins as diuretics were found to develop an encephalopathy and EEG changes that were remarkably similar to those seen in patients with hepatic failure. Evidence supporting this contention has been substantial but this theory fell into disfavor as direct correlation of the encephalopathy with ammonia levels were lacking. The observation of increased production aromatic amino acids in liver disease raised speculation that the formation of false neurotransmitters may account for the encephalopathy. This theory has been supported by the finding of increased levels of octopamine – an end product of aromatic amino acid metabolism – in the CSF of patients with hepatic encephalopathy. However, octopamine directly injected into the CSF of animals does not produce an encephalopathy. Similarly, clinical trials evaluating the effects of diets rich in branched chain amino acids on hepatic encephalopathy have been inconsistent. The GABA benzodiazepine theory suggests that endogenously produced benzodiazepines (probably from gut microorganisms) during liver failure account for the encephalopathy. Pathologically, serum and CSF from animals with liver failure inhibit binding of benzodiazepines in cortical preparations. Similarly, human CSF chromatography and postmortem brain samples have revealed several benzodiazepine-like substances that act as ligands. These are markedly increased in autopsied samples of patients with hepatic encephalopathy. The ability of benzodiazepine antagonists to reverse the encephalopathy has also been inconsistent.

The most recent theory suggests that that intracytoplasmic glutamine is necessary for the development of cerebral edema and the subsequent encephalopathy. Glutamine synthetase has a high affinity for ammonia and is found almost exclusively in astrocytes. Glutamine is subsequently formed from glutamate and ammonia. Intracellular concentration directly correlates with intracranial hypertension and CSF glutamine levels highly correlate with the degree of the encephalopathy. Intracellular glutamine is believed to affect the brain glucose metabolism and lead to the development of intracellular osmoles. In vitro studies have also revealed that elevated intracellular ammonia can increase the mitochondrial membrane permeability. Glutamine can subsequently enter the mitochondria and disassociate into glutamate and ammonia. Intramitochondrial ammonia will then directly increase the production of free radicals and impair the oxidative energy production. This "Trojan horse" hypothesis speculates that intracytoplasmic glutamine allows the entry of ammonia into the mitochondria.

Other theories that may be involved with the development of the encephalopathy include alterations in brain proteins, increases in inflammatory mediators, and increases in the blood–brain barrier permeability attributed to ammonia.

Clinical Presentation

The majority of patients in fulminant hepatic failure will be unconscious and display evidence for cerebral edema. The progression from a grade I to a grade IV encephalopathy may be rapid in the fulminant form of hepatic failure, however more chronic conditions will present with a slower and fluctuating course.

The encephalopathy due to chronic hepatic failure is variable and relapsing. Initially, patients present with mild disturbances in consciousness manifested by subtle changes in cognitive functions, and personality. Worsening delirium and lethargy occur as the encephalopathy progresses. Interestingly, the irritability and restlessness seen in the early stages of fulminant hepatic encephalopathy is not seen in the more chronic condition. Repeated bouts of hepatic failure can lead to dementia. Seizures are rare. Fluctuating neurological signs are common in acute liver failure. Asterixis, an intermittent relaxation of increased extensor tone, is a common sign. Historically, this was believed to be pathopneumonic for hepatic failure but is now known to be a relatively nonspecific sign. Frontal release signs are common. Parkinsonian rigidity may be seen but paratonia is more common. The cranial nerves are generally spared. Cerebellar signs, such as ataxia cerebellar speech, dysarthria, ocular bobbing and dysconjugate gaze, are not uncommon.

★ TIPS & TRICKS

Metabolic encephalopathies generally present with evidence for global cerebral hemispheric dysfunction. Focal neurological signs are not found with most encephalopathies. Hepatic encephalopathies are the exception, where focal signs may be present perhaps due to the involvement of cerebellar or deep gray matter. These findings, however, should prompt an investigation for a structural source.

Fulminant liver failure presents with an agitated delirium that can progress rapidly to coma. Seizures can occur in this syndrome, but may be related to hypoglycemia. Early coma is generally accompanied by hyperreflexia, which may disappear as the coma deepens. Decerebrate posturing and loss of oculomotor reflexes is a late and ominous sign.

Evaluation and Testing

Systemic findings in hepatic failure include spider nevi, signs of portal hypertension, enlarged or shrunken livers, fetor hepaticus, and palmar erythema. An evaluation for the source of hepatic failure should be undertaken if the underlying etiology for this is unknown.

Laboratory studies in liver failure reveal an increase in serum bilirubin, and transaminases (although the latter may not be elevated in severe cirrhosis). A chronic respiratory alkalosis presumably from the direct effect of gut peptides on the medullary respiratory centers is also common. The most sensitive measure to assess the functional degree of hepatic disturbance is the coagulation profile. In liver failure the prothrombin time, thrombin time, and partial thromboplastin times are elevated due to inadequate synthesis of several coagulation factors. Platelet counts are typically under 100,000 and display impaired function. In fulminant hepatic failure the serum glucose can drop precipitously. In these circumstances renal failure can occur.

Clinical outcome in hepatic failure correlates highly with the depth of the encephalopathy. An EEG is capable of monitoring the progression of mental status changes although a quantitative EEG may be more sensitive. EEG findings mirror the encephalopathy with the EEG initially displaying mild diffuse slowing. As the encephalopathy progresses, triphasic waves appear which are followed by diffuse delta wave activity. Burst suppression is seen in coma.

The P300 response to an auditory stimulus is helpful in detecting early changes in mental status although other brainstem- and somatosensory-evoked responses are less helpful.

Computed tomography (CT) can evaluate for intracerebral or subdural hemorrhages. A grading system has been developed to evaluate the degree of cerebral edema detected on CT that occurs in fulminant hepatic failure but direct correlation to intracranial pressure has failed. The globus pallidus in cirrhosis can show a reversible signal change on the T1-weighted MRI. The significance of this remains questionable, as this does not appear to correlate with the encephalopathy.

Similarly, increased changes in cerebral white matter can be detected with FLAIR imaging. This may reflect the early development of cerebral edema. These changes are reversible with improvement in liver failure. MR spectroscopy and other MR techniques are active areas of research in the evaluation of acute liver failure.

Treatment

The initial treatment for neurological worsening in liver failure is to identify and correct any precipitating factors. This may include new infections, medical noncompliance with medications or dietary restrictions, gastrointestinal bleeding, the use of sedative of analgesic medications or electrolyte disturbances.

✶ TIPS & TRICKS

Even very small doses of benzodiazepines can have a profound and prolonged effect in patients with hepatic failure. This may be secondary to the prolonged clearance of these medications, but endogenous benzodiazepines may themselves partially account for the encephalopathy. If Flumazenil is used (a benzodiazepine antagonist) it should be used with EEG monitoring. Several cases of subclinical status have been reported with its use in hepatic encephalopathy. In addition, subclinical improvement in EEG patterns may be detected.

The pharmacologic treatment for hepatic encephalopathy centers on decreasing the ammonia production and uptake as well as facilitating its elimination. Lactulose or lacitol are nonabsorbable disaccharides which facilitate the movement of ammonia from the portal circulation to the colon; they also interfere with the uptake of glutamine from the intestinal mucosa and lead to gut acidification which will result in the suppression of the formation of ammonia from gut bacteria. The laxative effect will additionally lower gut ammonia levels. Dosing is 15–45 mL orally 2 to 4 times a day and is titrated to 3 or 4 bowel movements a day. Rectal administration (300 mL) can be given every few hours until

an improvement in the mental status is seen. Electrolyte changes will need to be followed and corrected. Use can be limited by abdominal symptoms.

Antibiotics reduce the intestinal production of ammonia by decreasing the urase-producing bacteria. Neomycin and metronidazole are the main treatments despite little evidence to support any long-term improvement with their use. Neomycin is given orally 1–4 g daily for chronic hepatic encephalopathy. Dosing for acute liver failure is 1–2 g every 4–6 hours. Its long-term use is limited by renal and ototoxicity. Metronidazole dosing is 250 mg orally every 12 hours.

The use of Rifaximin has increased in recent years. It may be as effective as other antibiotics with a better safety profile. It is a nonabsorbable derivative of rifamycin with antimicrobial activity against aerobic and anaerobic Gram-negative and positive bacteria. It appears to be as effective as lactulose and other antibiotics. Combined treatment has not been effectively studied.

L-ornithine and L-aspartate are amino acid supplements which may increase the conversion of ammonia to urea and glutamine. A meta-analysis of three studies suggested an improvement in the encephalopathy and ammonia levels in patients treated with L-ornithine and L-aspartate. This treatment may be helpful in patients that do not respond to lactulose.

Other treatments that have been studied have limited information as to their effectiveness. Zinc supplementation and probiotic diets may help in mild encephalopathies. Branched chain amino acids are best given enterally. Liver support devices incorporating extracorporeal albumin dialysis, or molecular adsorbent recirculation systems, are used as a bridge to transplantation.

Treatment of Cerebral Edema in Fulminant Hepatic Failure

Cerebral edema occurs in approximately 75% of patients with Grade 4 hepatic encephalopathy. Complications secondary to intracranial hypertension and decreased cerebral perfusion account for the significant morbidity and mortality encountered with this condition.

The treatment of elevated intracranial pressure can be particularly problematic in this population.

Invasive monitoring of intracranial pressure has become common practice despite little supporting evidence

⚠ CAUTION

The placement of intracranial pressure monitoring devices can be difficult in the patient with hepatic failure. The international normalized ratio must be corrected and platelets may need to be given prior to insertion. Even with these precautions, bleeding complications can develop. Obviously, close monitoring of the patient is essential.

Hyperventilation has not proved to be an effective method to treat intracranial hypertension in hepatic failure. The mainstay of treatment has been osmotic therapy. Mannitol of hypertonic saline solutions may be given to increase the serum osmolality of the patient. Mild hypothermia has many theoretical benefits to treating intracranial hypertension in acute liver failure, and preliminary data has been promising. Barbiturates have been used historically but can complicate the diagnosis of brain death should the patient deteriorate despite treatment.

⌗ SCIENCE REVISITED

The failure of hyperventilation to lower intracranial pressure in hepatic failure may be attributed to the state of the ammonia ion. Ammonia circulates in the plasma as an ion NH_4^+, however the unprotonated form of the ion (NH_3) is permeable to the blood–brain barrier. The alkalosis induced by hyperventilation will favor the formation of the unprotonated form of the ion and thus may facilitate ammonia entry into the brain.

The definitive treatment for cerebral edema is transplantation, where remarkable recoveries have been reported even in dire circumstances.

Bibliography

Iacobone EI, Bailly-Salin J, Polito A, et al. Sepsis-associated encephalopathy and its differential diagnosis. *Crit Care Med* 2009; **37**(Suppl): S331–S336.

Manno EM. Evaluation and treatment of the patient with toxic-metabolic encephalopathies. In: *Textbook of Neurosurgery* (Batjer H, Loftus C, eds). Lippincott-Raven Publishers, 2002: pp. 259–267.

Maramattom BV. Sepsis associated encephalopathy. *Neurol Res* 2007; **29**:643–646.

Siami S, Annane D, Sharshar T. The encephalopathy in sepsis. *Crit Care Clin* 2008; **24**:67–82.

Stevens RD, Pronovost PJ. The spectrum of encephalopathy in critical illness. *Semin Neurol* 2006; **26**:440–451.

Sudaram V, Shaikh OS. Hepatic encephalopathy: Pathophysiology and emerging therapies. *Med Clin N Am* 2009; **93**:819–836.

Vaquero J, Butterworth RF. Mechanisms of brain edema in acute liver failure and impact of novel therapeutic interventions. *Neurol Res* 2007; **29**:693–690.

Delirium and Sedation in the ICU

Jennifer A. Frontera

Neuroscience Intensive Care Unit, Departments of Neurosurgery and Neurology, Mount Sinai School of Medicine, New York, NY, USA

Epidemiology of Delirium

Delirium is a descriptive term defined in DSM IV as a fluctuating level of attentiveness with a reduced ability to focus, sustain, or shift attention. Fluctuations in levels of consciousness and/or behavioral disturbances develop rapidly (over hours to days) and are not accounted for by a pre-existing dementia. Additionally, there must be evidence that the disturbance is caused by a medical condition, substance intoxication, or medication side effect. Delirium is common among hospitalized patients, particularly in the ICU setting, where it has been reported to occur in up to 70% of patients, compared to 10% of emergency department patients, 16% of post-acute care patients, and 42% of hospice patients. (Older patients are particularly susceptible to developing delirium, with up to 50% developing delirium at some point during their hospital stay.

Etiology and Pathophysiology of Delirium

It is important to recognize that delirium is not a disease, but rather a symptom of underlying pathology. The term "delirium" is sometimes used interchangeably with "acute confusional state" or "encephalopathy" and represents a cluster of different etiologies. Despite differing, or sometimes multifactorial, causes patients with delirium all have a disruption in attention and arousal centers of the brain. The ascending reticular activating system (ARAS), stretching from the midpontine tegmentum to the anterior cingulate, is primarily responsible for arousal and attentiveness. The ARAS receives widespread input from the spinal cord, visual and auditory centers, thalamus, hypothalamus, and hippocampus, as well as cortical feedback. Disturbances in any of these areas may lead to delirium. Abnormalities in neurotransmitters (such as acetylcholine, serotonin, dopamine, GABA, tryptophan, melatonin, and glutamate) and cytokines (such as interleukins and interferons), have been implicated in the pathogenesis of delirium. Since the pathophysiology of delirium is so complex, it is not surprising that it is often multifactorial in nature. Some common etiologies of delirium are listed in Table 18.1. It is important to note that 50% of older patients with delirium have underlying diagnoses of stroke, Parkinson disease or dementia (that is often undiagnosed).

Emergency Management in Neurocritical Care, First Edition. Edited by Edward M. Manno.
© 2012 John Wiley & Sons, Ltd. Published 2012 by John Wiley & Sons, Ltd.

Table 18.1. Etiologies of delirium

Category	Example
Drugs	• Prescription: opiates, benzodiazepines, dexmedetomidine, barbiturates, antiepileptic medications, neuroleptics, anticholinergics, antihistamines, dopamine agonists, steroids, antibiotics, histamine-2 receptor blockers, Baclofen, cyclobenzepine, antidepressants, anti-arrhythmics, Beta-blockers, clonidine, digoxin • Illicit drugs • Seratonin syndrome • Neuroleptic malignant syndrome
Endocrine	• Hyper/hypothyroid • Hyper/hypoparathyroid • Hyper/hypoglycemia • Adrenal insufficiency
Infection	• Sepsis/SIRS • Hyperthermia • Hypothermia
Metabolic Disarray	• Hypoxia • Hypercapnia • Acidosis • Uremia • Acute liver failure (hyperammonemia) • Hyper/hypo Na, Ca, Mg, PO4
Neurological injury	• Seizures/status epilepticus (convulsive, nonconvulsive) • Ischemic stroke/TIA • Hypoperfusion syndrome • Intracranial hemorrhage (subdural, subarachnoid, intraparenchymal • CNS infection (meningitis, encephalitis, abscess) • Traumatic brain injury • Posterior reversible encephalopathy syndrome (due to hypertension, medications) • CNS vasculitis • CNS inflammatory lesion (multiple sclerosis, ADEM, neurosarcoidosis, Lyme disease, drug effect) • CNS tumor (primary CNS malignancy, metastasis) • Paraneoplastic syndrome
Nutritional	• Acute thiamine deficiency (Wernike's) • B12 deficiency • Niacin deficiency
Toxins	• Arsenic, lead, ethylene glycol, methanol, cyanide, carbon monoxide
Withdrawal states	• EtOH/benzodiazepine withdrawal • Opiate withdrawal
Other	• Poor pain control • Sleep deprivation • Sundowning • Sensory deprivation: low hearing, low vision, language barrier

✻ TIPS & TRICKS

Thirty percent of all delirium is due to medications. Stop all sedation to remove the drug effect from the equation. Simple laboratory tests can eliminate metabolic disarray and a focused neurological examination off sedation has a 97% negative predictive value for eliminating an underlying neurological etiology.

Evaluation of Delirium in the ICU

The CAM-ICU scale (used extensively in the trials mentioned above) was specifically developed to identify delirium as defined by DSM IV guidelines (Table 18.2). In a study of 96 mechanically-ventilated ICU patients, 471 CAM-ICU assessments were performed in patients with a RASS of −3 to +4 and compared with the gold standard DSM IV definition of delirium. The authors found that delirium, diagnosed by this tool, occurred in 83% of ICU patients for a mean of 2.4 days. The CAM-ICU had a 93–100% sensitivity and a 98–100% specificity when compared with the DSM IV guidelines.

A major limitation of the CAM-ICU scale is that it allows for the determination of delirium in the context of sedative use. In up to 30% of cases, the cause of fluctuating mental status is the sedation medication itself. In fact, though the CAM-ICU scale is meant to be repetitively used, patients may receive varying amounts of sedation during each evaluation. Though it is typical in a neuro-critical care setting for sedation to be held to examine a patient, this practice is not consistently applied in other specialty or mixed population ICUs. From a neurologist's and neurointensivist's perspective, without eliminating the obvious confounder of sedation upon a patient's mental status, it is impossible to: (1) identify if delirium is present (or levels of sedation are simply different), (2) determine the underlying cause of the delirium, and (3) address the underlying etiology. Additionally, in the setting of sedation, serious neurological events may be occurring and go undetected and untreated. For example, in a neuro-ICU setting, the rates of nonconvulsive status epilepticus are as high as 35%.

Table 18.2. Confusion Assessment Method (CAM-ICU)[21]

1	*Acute onset and fluctuating course* • Identify an acute change in mental status from the baseline exam OR • Identify fluctuating changes in mental status or behavior over the past 24 hours that may vary in severity
	AND
2	*Inattention* • Identify an inability to focus attention, easy distractibility or inability to process components of conversation (e.g. count backwards, say months backwards)
	AND
3	*Disorganized thinking* • If the patient is verbal (and not aphasic): identify illogical or incoherent thought processes, inability to understand proverbs or inability to perform simple calculations (e.g. How many things are in a dozen? Where does a cactus grow?) • If the patient is intubated or nonverbal (and not aphasic): use yes/no questions or letter board to identify illogical or incoherent thought processes (e.g. Can a cat sing? Does wool come from an alligator?)
	OR
4	Altered level of consciousness • Identify if the patient's level of consciousness is anything other than alert (i.e. drowsy, lethargic, stuporous, comatose or agitated/combative)

Even in patients with no underlying neurological diagnosis, it has been shown that 8–10% of medical ICU patients have seizures, the majority of which are nonconvulsive. Seizures in this population are particularly common in patients with sepsis. Similarly, stroke is not uncommon among ICU patients with a primary medical diagnoses. In a study of 123 medical ICU patients with "altered mental status," new CT findings were present in 26 (21%), including ischemic infarction in 13 (11%), intracerebral hemorrhage in 2 (2%), and tumor in 3 (2%).

Subtle or nonconvulsive seizures are impossible to diagnose without continuous EEG monitoring. Patients with an unexplained altered mental status or coma should undergo 24–48 hours of continuous EEG monitoring to evaluate for seizures or status epilepticus since this can be easily treated if diagnosed, but catastrophic if missed.

A solution to the problem of identifying delirium, but missing a serious underlying neurological condition, is to replace the CAM-ICU with serial neurological examinations performed off sedation. While it has been shown that nurses,

physicians, and other healthcare staff can quickly become proficient at the CAM-ICU, an argument can be made that this time would be better spent learning a basic neurological examination (Table 18.3). A neurological examination not only identifies fluctuations in attentiveness, but also identifies, or rules out, acute neurological injury. In a retrospective study of 127 ICU patients who received a neurological consult for an isolated change in mental status, 7% had an ischemic stroke and 1% had a subarachnoid hemorrhage. In this study, the neurological examination had a 97% negative predictive value for ruling out acute neurological injury. Most neurointensivists and neurocritical care nurses utilize an abbreviated neurological examination on a serial basis to track a patient's progress.

Table 18.3. Neurological assessment of delirium in the ICU Delirium is present when there is fluctuation in level of arousal, attentiveness and/or orientation. The cranial nerve and motor exam help to identify and localize an underlying neurological injury that may be contributing to delirium

Step 1	Assess for fluctuations in mental status	Mental status assessment*
	Arousal	• Spontaneously awake, eyes open and alert • Opens eyes to voice • Opens eyes to physical stimuli • No eye opening
	Attentiveness	• Able to say months backwards from December to January • Able to count backwards from 20 to 1, but cannot do months backwards • Able to count from 1 to 10, but cannot do either of the above • Able to follow complex 2–3 step verbal commands, but cannot do any of the above • Able only to follow simple verbal commands • Able only to follow mimicked commands • Cannot follow commands, but can track visual stimuli • Cannot track visual stimuli, but saccades to voice • Does not saccade to voice, but saccades to physical stimuli • No response to examiner
	Orientation	• Oriented to person, place and time • Oriented × 2 • Oriented to self only

Step 2	Identify localizing abnormalities in the neurological exam	
		Cranial nerve exam
	CN II/III	• Pupil symmetry and reactivity to light • Visual field assessment, blink to threat (II, VII, visual pathways)
	CN III/IV/VI/VIII	• Extraocular movements • If patient cannot track test Oculocephalic reflex (Doll's eyes maneuver) • Vesibulo-ocular reflex, hearing
	CN V/VII	• Corneal response, facial sensation, facial movement
	CN IX/X/XII	• Gag, tongue movement
		Motor exam*
	Strength	Test all 4 limbs: • No drift holding arm or leg out for 10 seconds • Drift; limb moves before 10 seconds, but does not hit bed or support • Able to move limb against gravity (MRC[60] 3/5) • Unable to move limb against gravity, but some movement if force of gravity eliminated (MRC[60] 2/5) • No movement to command
	Response to physical stimuli	If patient cannot comply with above motor exam, test response to physical stimuli[a]: • Localizes to physical stimuli • Withdraws from physical stimuli • Flexor posturing (decorticate) • Extensor posturing (decerebrate) • Plegia (no movement to physical stimuli) or triple flexion (stereotyped flexion at hip, knee and ankle)

Exam should be performed in patient's native language after sedation has been discontinued for a reasonable amount of time
*Within each category responses are listed from best to worst.
**Patient can have mixed responses.

In patients who are other than neurologically intact, a leading indicator can be identified, which demonstrates the patient's best examination (i.e. the patient can reliably count from 20 to 1). If the patient becomes unable to perform this task, then efforts should be mounted to determine why the patient has changed neurologically. It is possible to label this fluctuation in attentiveness as "delirium," but irrespective of the label applied, the cause of the alteration must be identified and treated.

The following is a rational approach to evaluating delirium in the ICU. First, sedating and toxic medications should be discontinued, if possible. After an appropriate washout period, a neurological examination should be performed to identify any focal features that might lead to localization or etiology. Basic laboratory tests to evaluate for metabolic disarray (e.g. uremia, hyperammonemia, hypoxia, hypercarbia, hypoglycemia, endocrine dysfunction) should be sent. Based on the examination and laboratory results, imaging such as head CT or MRI and vascular imaging, such as CT or MR angiography, should be considered. Continuous EEG to evaluate for seizures or nonconvulsive seizures should be entertained in all patients with unexplained delirium. For patients undergoing continuous EEG monitoring who are able to follow commands, 24 hours of monitoring will capture 95% of seizures, but only 80% of seizures were detected in comatose patients monitored for 24 hours. For this reason, 48 hours of continuous EEG may be required in comatose patients. New onset meningitis is exceedingly uncommon in hospitalized patients; however, lumbar puncture should be considered in patients with fever and meningismus or patients who have had neurosurgical procedures that might predispose them to CNS infection.

Impact of Delirium in the ICU

The implications of delirium in the ICU were explored in a prospective study of 275 mechanically-ventilated patients in a medical and cardiac ICU setting. Delirium was diagnosed in patients with a Richmond Agitation and Sedation Scale (RASS) of −3 to +4 (Table 18.4) who were CAM-ICU + (Table 18.2) for delirium. Coma was defined as response to physical stimuli, but no eye opening, or no response to physical stimuli (RASS −4 or −5). There was no stipulation as to the amount or type of sedation a patient could receive when evaluated. Delirium occurred in 82% of patients and was significantly associated with 6-month mortality (Hazard Ratio 3.2, 95% CI 1.4–7.7, p = 0.008), hospital length of stay (Hazard Ratio 2.0, 95% CI 1.4–3.0, P < 0.001) and post-ICU length of stay (Hazard Ratio 1.6, 95% CI 1.1–2.3, p = 0.009). Each additional ICU day spent in delirium was associated with a 10% increased risk of death (Hazard Ratio 1.1, 95% CI 1.0–1.3, p = 0.03). Being in a "coma" in addition to delirium further increased the mortality rates and prolonged the length of stay. Indeed, 18.5% of the patients in this study remained in a persistent "coma" and died, though neither the cause of "coma" nor the cause of death was reported. This study also found that the use of lorazepam and the cumulative lorazepam dose was directly associated with the presence of delirium. This was not the case for propofol, fentanyl, or morphine. It remained unclear from this study whether delirium was a marker for lorazepam use or if, indeed, lorazepam was responsible for increased mortality and prolonged length of stay, or even if lorazepam was a causal factor in the development of delirium.

This question was addressed, in part, by the MENDS trial. This randomized-controlled trial of

Table 18.4. Richmond Agitation and Sedation Scale (RASS)[20]

Score	Rating	Description
+4	Combative	Violent, immediate danger to self and staff
+3	Very agitated	Aggressive, removes devices, tubes, catheters
+2	Agitated	Ventilator dyssynchrony, frequent nonpurposeful movement
+1	Restless	Anxious but no aggressive movements
0	Alert and calm	
−1	Drowsy	Sustained eye opening and eye contact to voice (>10 seconds) but not fully alert
−2	Light sedation	Brief eye opening and eye contact to voice (<10 seconds)
−3	Moderate sedation	Movement or eye opening to voice but no eye contact
−4	Deep sedation	No response to voice, but movement or eye opening in response to physical stimulation
−5	Unarousable	No response to voice or physical stimulation

106 mechanically-ventilated medical/surgical ICU patients examined the impact of dexmedetomidine (up to 1.5 µg/kg/h) compared to lorazepam (up to 10 mg/h) during the first 120 hours of ICU stay on the development of delirium, diagnosed by the CAM-ICU. Both medications could be titrated to a RASS level dictated by the treating physician and a sedation cessation period was not mandated. The addition of fentanyl to treat pain was allowed. This study excluded those with a history of neurological disease, learning disability, dementia, seizure, liver failure, alcohol abuse, MI, second- or third-degree heart block, as well as moribund and pregnant patients. Compared to patients who received lorazepam, those randomized to dexmedetomidine had significantly more days without delirium and coma and a trend toward shorter mechanical ventilation time, shorter length of stay (7.5 vs. 9 days, p = 0.92) and lower 28-day mortality (17% vs. 27%, p = 0.18). There was a lower prevalence of "coma" in the dexmedetomidine group (63% vs. 92%, P < 0.001). Though patients on dexmedetomidine spent less time delirious, there was no difference in the incidence of delirium between the two groups (79% vs. 82%, p = 0.65). Other factors that may have contributed to delirium in either group were not adjusted for in the analysis.

The SEDCOM trial, published 2 years later, randomized 375 medical/surgical ICU patients to dexmedetomidine (0.2–1.4 µg/kg/h) vs. midazolam (0.02–0.1 mg/kg/h) titrated to RASS −2 to +1 from enrollment until extubation or 30 days. Patients with acute stroke, uncontrolled seizures, liver failure, dementia, renal insufficiency requiring dialysis, acute MI, second- or third-degree heart block, EF < 30%, bradycardia, or hypotension were excluded. Though the primary outcome measure was the percentage of time within the target sedation range (RASS −2 to +1), delirium was examined as a secondary endpoint using the CAM-ICU. A "daily arousal assessment" was performed during which RASS −2 to +1 patients were asked to open their eyes to voice, track the examiner, squeeze the examiner's hand or stick out their tongue and were graded as "awake" if they could perform 3 of the 4 tasks. There was no mandated sedation vacation time and CAM-ICU assessments could be performed while the patient was receiving sedation.

This study found a lower prevalence of delirium in those receiving dexmedetomidine (54%) compared to those receiving midazolam (76.6%, P < 0.001) and, similarly, increased delirium-free days (2.5 vs. 1.7, p = 0.002) and shorter time to extubation (3.7 days vs. 5.6 days, p = 0.01). Though this trial found an association of increased delirium rates in midazolam compared to dexmedetomidine, it did not control for other possible causes of delirium that may have differed between the two groups. Since patients were never examined off sedation, it is not clear that acute neurological injury (stroke, seizure, etc.) was excluded as an etiology of delirium.

In a substudy of SEDCOM, mortality was found to be significantly lower in patients without delirium (11.9% vs. 30.3% in those with delirium, P < 0.001) and the median time to extubation and length of stay were shorter in those without delirium (P < 0.001). There was a dose response effect for the duration of time spent in delirium and the risk of mortality, prolonged ventilation time, and prolonged length of stay. Interestingly, 30-day mortality did not differ between the dexmedetomidine and midazolam groups in the larger SEDCOM study (22.6% vs. 25.4%, p = 0.60), suggesting that the association of delirium and mortality cannot be explained by a sedation effect alone. This poses the tantalizing question: What was the etiology of delirium in these patients? Unfortunately, none of the trials mentioned thus far addressed this crucial issue. Is delirium a marker for undiagnosed acute neurological injury (stroke, seizure, etc.), sepsis, or something else?

In ICU survivors, delirium in the ICU has been associated with long-term cognitive dysfunction. In a prospective cohort study of 99 mechanically-ventilated ICU patients surviving ≥3 months enrolled in the Awakening and Breathing Controlled trial, cognitive outcomes were assessed at 3 and 12 months by a blinded neuropsychologist administering a battery of nine neuropsychological tests measuring: attention and concentration, information processing speed, verbal memory, visual-spatial construction and delayed visual memory, executive function, language and global mental status. Cognitive impairment occurred in 79% of patients at 3 months and 71% at 12 months. After adjusting for age, education, baseline cognitive status, APACHE II scores, severe sepsis and exposure to sedative medications in the ICU, increasing days of delirium was associated with worse age-adjusted cognitive scores at 3 months (p = 0.02) and 12 months (p = 0.03). Duration of mechanical ventilation, however, was not significantly associated with cognitive scores. This study is unique because after adjusting for causes of delirium such as sepsis, exposure to sedative medication, and severity of illness, the duration of time with delirium was significantly associated with worse cognitive outcomes. Though this study excluded patients with cardiac arrest and neurological deficits that prevented them from living independently (e.g. large stroke, severe dementia), it did not account for any new neurological injury that may have occurred during the ICU stay. Since only 4% of patients in this cohort had the admission diagnoses of hepatic or renal failure or alcohol withdrawal, it is possible that undiagnosed neurological injury was a contributor to the development of delirium. In fact, the patients enrolled in this study were all at high risk for adverse neurological complications of their primary illness. Fifty percent of patients in this study had severe sepsis, which is a risk factor for seizures and status epilepticus. Additionally, 20% of patients had an admitting diagnosis of myocardial infarction or CHF. The risk of ischemic stroke is increased 5-fold during the first month after diagnosis of CHF. The risk of stroke after MI is 4.6% over 42 months and the risk of seizure after MI is nearly doubled compared to age- and gender-matched controls.

The above literature has identified the fact that delirium is associated with an increased risk of death and poor cognitive outcome. While sedation use is associated with the development of delirium, other unspecified factors are clearly contributing. The diagnosis of delirium may, in fact, be a marker for unrecognized neurological events (i.e. stroke or seizure). Though it is possible that an entirely different or novel mechanism for acute brain injury is occurring in delirious ICU patients, common and treatable adverse neurological events should be evaluated. Determining the underlying mechanism for delirium is critical if adequate treatment strategies are to be addressed.

★ TIPS & TRICKS

Delirium is a descriptive diagnosis and gives no information about the underlying etiology. General ICU patients (even those that do not have a primary neurological diagnosis) are at risk of neurological complications that may manifest as delirium. Stroke and seizure are particularly common comorbidities of critical illness.

The Argument for Limiting Sedation in the ICU

Though evidence suggests that delirium is associated with worse outcomes independent of sedative effect, the MENDS and SEDCOM trials suggest that sedation can contribute to the prevalence of delirium and the duration of time spent delirious. Furthermore, in order to drill down on the etiology of delirium, it is critical that the contribution of sedation be eliminated from the equation. Frequent arguments for sedating patients include the concept that sedation prevents patients from accidentally harming themselves or self-extubating, or that it is more "humane" to keep an intubated patient sedated. In fact, that literature does not support either of these concepts. Daily interruption of sedation has been shown not only to be safe, but to improve outcomes and is now a routine component of most ventilator weaning protocols. In a landmark trial of 128 mechanically-ventilated medical ICU patients randomized to daily sedation interruption until the patient awakens versus sedation interruption at the discrepancy of the treating physician, those receiving a sedation vacation spent 2.4 fewer days on the ventilator (p = 0.004) and had a significantly shorter length of stay (6.4 days vs. 9.9, p = 0.02) Though this study included agitated and uncomfortable patients, there was no difference in the rates of accidental extubation. Stopping sedation also allowed physicians to identify neurological injury. Significantly more patients in the control group never awakened from a coma (20%) and died in a coma (17%) compared to the sedation interruption group (9 and 8%, respectively). This may be because serious neurological illness went undiagnosed and untreated in the control group.

Conversely, more head CTs and MRIs were performed on the control group than on the sedation interruption group, presumably because these studies were unnecessary in the context of a reassuring, unsedated, neurological examination.

This study was followed by the multicenter Awakening and Breathing Controlled trial, which randomized 336 mechanically-ventilated patients to either sedation interruption followed by a spontaneous breathing trial or continued sedation with a spontaneous breathing trial. As in the Kress trial, those in the intervention group had significantly more ventilator-free days and a shorter ICU and hospital length of stay. In addition, 1 year mortality rates were lower in the intervention group (44% vs. 58%, p = 0.01). The number of patients needed to treat to prevent one mortality was only 7. Though there were more self-extubations in the treatment group (10% vs. 4%, p = 0.03), there was no difference in re-intubation rates, and the rate of tracheostomy was lower in the intervention group (13% vs. 20%, p = 0.06).

Aside from improved performance during spontaneous breathing trials, sedation interruption can allow patients to participate in other tasks, such as physical therapy. In a randomized trial of 104 mechanically-ventilated ICU patients, 49 received sedation interruption followed by a standardized physical therapy protocol (which included an escalating pathway of passive ROM followed by active supine activities, followed by transfers, and finally performance of routing activities of daily living), while 55 patients underwent sedation interruption and physical therapy at the discretion of the treating physician. Significantly more patients in the intervention group had a return to independent functional status at hospital discharge (59% vs. 35%, p = 0.02). The time from intubation to achieving ADL milestones such as getting out of bed, standing, marching in place, transferring to a chair, and walking, were also significantly shorter in the intervention group. Similarly, patients who received the physical therapy protocol had higher Barthel index scores (measure of activities of daily living), shorter duration of mechanical ventilation and a trend toward a shorter ICU length of stay. This study was also able to demonstrate significantly less delirium in the ICU and hospital in the intervention group. Along with the Kress and Awakening and Breathing Controlled trial, this study demonstrates that sedation interruption is not only safe, but also improves outcomes and may ameliorate delirium.

Though continuous sedation has long been the paradigm in most ICU settings, this concept was recently challenged in a single center randomized trial of 140 mechanically-ventilated patients who received either no continuous sedation, but as-needed morphine or Haldol (which could be converted to a continuous infusion if necessary) or continuous sedation with daily sedation interruption until awakening. Those not receiving continuous sedation had significantly more days off the ventilator, and a shorter ICU and hospital length of stay. Additionally, there was a trend toward lower ICU mortality (22% vs. 38%, p = 0.06), though there was no difference in hospital mortality rates. Although data was analyzed on an intention to treat basis, 18% of patients in the noncontinuous sedation group required a continuous infusion at some point during the study. Agitated delirium occurred in 20% of the nonsedation group and 7% in the continuous sedation group (p = 0.04), but there may be a diagnosis bias reflecting the difficulty of diagnosing delirium in sedated patients. It is important to note that this study was conducted with 1:1 nurse to patient staffing. Since using as-needed medication dosing is labor intensive, the results of this study may not be generalizable to ICUs with less generous staffing models. Nevertheless, the cost savings in shorter length of stay and fewer mechanical ventilation days may offset the expense of higher staffing ratios.

Overall, limiting sedation allows for faster liberation from mechanical ventilation, shorter length of stay, better functional outcome at discharge, lower mortality rates, and possibly less delirium. Use of intermittent, as-needed sedation appears to be efficacious and may further limit the total duration of exposure to sedation compared to continuous infusions.

Treatment of Delirium in the ICU Setting

Delirium has traditionally been treated with sedative medications; however, as mentioned above, these same medications may induce or worsen delirium. Old paradigms for treating delirium have promulgated the use of lorazepam infusions, though more recent data from the MENDS and SEDCOM trials would suggest that this is an outdated approach. In fact, a prospective study of ICU patients found that lorazepam increased the risk of incident delirium by 20%. It should be mentioned, however, that benzodiazepines are the most appropriate treatment for alcohol or benzodiazepine withdrawal.

First-generation antipsychotics, such as Haldol, have also been commonly used to treat delirium in doses that are alarmingly high. Some studies have advocated Haldol 5 mg IV followed by doubling of the dose every 20 minutes. Others have suggested infusion rates of 10 mg/h with increases of 5 mg/h every 30 minutes as needed. In fact, Haldol doses of 1200 mg/day and >200 mg/day for 15 days have been reported. Safety data for these doses of typical neuroleptics is based on only a handful of case reports. In one case series, 8 patients with agitation refractory to benzodiazepines and narcotics were treated with 3–25 mg/h of Haldol. Of this group, 5 patients survived, 2 developed a tremor, 1 developed third-degree heart block, and 1 developed ventricular tachycardia. Adverse reactions to antipsychotics include extrapyramidal movement disorders, neuroleptic malignant syndrome, and sudden death. Extrapyramidal side effects are higher with high-dose typical neuroleptics and include akathesia, acute dystonic reaction (more common in young men), Parkinsonism (more common in older women), and tardive dyskinesia (more common in older patients receiving first-generation antipsychotics for a prolonged period of time). Additionally, antipsychotic medications carry a black box warning of sudden death. In a study of 90,000 Medicaid patients, both typical and atypical antipsychotics were found to double the rate of sudden death compared to non-use. This study also found a dose-related effect on the risk of death, presumably due to the cardiac repolarization effects, prolonged QTc, and risk of arrhythmia. Other studies have found an increased risk of mortality in elderly and demented patients when antipsychotics are used to treat delirium. In these studies, risk seems to be greater soon after initiation of antipsychotics and more pronounced with conventional neuroleptics.

Typical and atypical neuroleptic use for the treatment of delirium has been compared in an ICU setting in two small well-designed studies; however, the utility of these agents remains unclear. When Haldol and ziprasidone were compared to placebo in a randomized-controlled trial of 100 mechanically-ventilated ICU patients, there was no difference in the number of days spent in delirium or coma, nor was there a difference in mechanical ventilation days, ICU length of stay, or mortality. In this study, the average daily doses of Haldol and ziprasidone were 15 and 113 mg/day, respectively. At these doses, there was no difference in the incidence of akathesia or extrapyramidal syndrome compared to placebo. In another randomized, placebo-controlled study, 36 patients with delirium in the ICU received either quetiapine at escalating doses up to 200 mg every 12 hours, or placebo. Patients receiving quetiapine (median daily dose of 110 mg) spent significantly less time delirious or agitated and had a trend toward better functional status at discharge. More somnolence was observed in the quetiapine group. Interestingly, it is not uncommon for physicians to use quetiapine in low doses (below antipsychotic thresholds, such as 25–50 mg) to promote restoration of normal sleep–wake cycles. It is possible that simply restoring normal sleep may attenuate delirium.

While benzodiazepines may induce or worsen delirium (except in the case of alcohol or benzodiazepine withdrawal), and the role of antipsychotics in treating ICU delirium is unclear, pharmacologic pain control is an important component of managing delirium. It has been long recognized that inadequate analgesia is a strong risk factor for delirium. In one study, severe pain increased the risk of delirium ninefold. Pain control is also important for limiting post-ICU conditions such as post-traumatic stress disorder (PTSD). In a study of 696 ICU military patients without serious traumatic brain injury, 35% developed PTSD. In a multivariate analysis, adequate pain control with morphine significantly reduced the risk of developing PTSD.

Nonpharmacologic strategies can also be effective in limiting the incidence of delirium. Sleep deprivation may contribute significantly to delirium. Not only do ICU patients spend fewer hours sleeping, but sleep quality, architecture, and circadian rhythms are also altered. Since up to 40% of ICU patients are sleep deprived, simple strategies to increase sleep include keeping shades open and the lights on during the day and off at night, and limiting night-time examinations and interruptions in sleep. These strategies are also helpful to reduce sundowning. Limiting sensory deprivation by providing patients with glasses, hearing aids, calendars, and clocks can also mitigate against delirium. In non-English speaking patients, having ready access to staff or family members for translation can be important for reorientation. In a study of 852 elderly hospitalized patients, a protocol of orientation, cognitive stimuli, nonpharmacologic sleep aids, early mobilization, minimization of restraints, visual and hearing aids, and prevention of dehydration resulted in a significant reduction in the number of delirium episodes and the number of days spent in delirium compared to a control group.

☆ TIPS & TRICKS

Agitated delirium can be initially addressed using nonpharmacologic methods such as restoring sleep–wake cycles, or by providing vision and hearing augmentation to the impaired. Restraints and chemical sedation can often worsen agitation. If continuous intravenous sedation is necessary, dexmedetomidine is a superior choice to benzodiazepines (except in the circumstance of alcohol withdrawal). Antipsychotics should be used with caution, due to side effects.

Conclusions

Fluctuating attentiveness, or delirium, is common in ICU patients. Delirium has been associated with increased mortality and poor cognitive outcome but, unfortunately, the etiology of delirium in the ICU has not been well characterized in major studies. Serious neurological insults, such as stroke or seizure, may be underdiagnosed or labeled as delirium in the general ICU setting. It is

incumbent upon the scientific community to adequately investigate the causes of delirium in the ICU and characterize the neurological and cognitive risks of ICU care. Limiting sedation and/or using dexmedetomidine, rather than midazolam or lorazepam, may help to attenuate the risk of developing delirium and allow for the identification of an acute neurological injury, as well as shorten mechanical ventilation time, improve length of stay, reduce mortality rates and improve functional outcome.

Bibliography

Ely EW, Shintani A, Truman B, et al. Delirium as a predictor of mortality in mechanically-ventilated patients in the intensive care unit. *J Am Med Aassoc* 2004; **291**:1753–1762.

Ely EW, Inouye SK, Bernard GR, et al. Delirium in mechanically-ventilated patients: validity and reliability of the confusion assessment method for the intensive care unit (CAM-ICU). *J Am Med Assoc* 2001; **286**:2703–2710.

Pandharipande PP, Pun BT, Herr DL, et al. Effect of sedation with dexmedetomidine vs lorazepam on acute brain dysfunction in mechanically-ventilated patients: the MENDS randomized controlled trial. *J Am Med Assoc* 2007; **298**:2644–2653.

Riker RR, Shehabi Y, Bokesch PM, et al. Dexmedetomidine vs midazolam for sedation of critically ill patients: a randomized trial. *J Am Med Assoc* 2009; **301**:489–499.

Shehabi Y, Riker RR, Bokesch PM, et al. Delirium duration and mortality in lightly sedated, mechanically-ventilated intensive care patients. *Crit Care Med* 2010; **38**:2311–2318.

Girard TD, Kress JP, Fuchs BD, et al. Efficacy and safety of a paired sedation and ventilator weaning protocol for mechanically-ventilated patients in intensive care (Awakening and Breathing Controlled trial): a randomised controlled trial. *Lancet* 2008; **371**:126–134.

Girard TD, Jackson JC, Pandharipande PP, et al. Delirium as a predictor of long-term cognitive impairment in survivors of critical illness. *Crit Care Med* 2010; **38**:1513–1520.

Kress JP, Pohlman AS, O'Connor MF, Hall JB. Daily interruption of sedative infusions in critically ill patients undergoing mechanical ventilation. *New Engl J Med* 2000; **342**:1471–2477.

Schweickert WD, Pohlman MC, Pohlman AS, et al. Early physical and occupational therapy in mechanically-ventilated, critically ill pa-tients: a randomised controlled trial. *Lancet* 2009; **373**:1874–1882.

Strom T, Martinussen T, Toft P. A protocol of no sedation for critically ill patients receiving me-chanical ventilation: a randomised trial. *Lancet* 2010; **375**:475–480.

Neurologic Complications of Cardiac Surgery

Cathy Sila

Department of Neurology, Case Western Reserve University School of Medicine, and Stroke & Cerebrovascular Center, Neurological Institute, University Hospitals–Case Medical Center, Cleveland, OH, USA

Neurological Complications of Cardiac Surgery

Coronary artery bypass graft (CABG) surgery for myocardial revascularization is the most frequently performed cardiac surgery with more than 500,000 procedures performed in the USA and 800,000 procedures world wide. Although percutaneous coronary revascularization procedures outnumber CABG surgery by at least three-fold, CABG remains the preferred therapy approach for left main or severe triple vessel disease, concomitant valvular, or aortic arch disease, and may be the only option for patients who have failed endovascular procedures. Neurologic complications of cardiac surgery and interventional procedures for cardiac disease are important determinants of patient outcome. Ischemic stroke following cardiac surgery increases mortality by three- to five-fold, increases critical care days and hospital length of stay, and increases the likelihood of discharge to a care facility. Since 1989, the Society of Thoracic Surgeons has sponsored a registry to collect key outcomes data on patients undergoing cardiac surgery and now more than 90% of US programs participate. Stroke, defined as a new post-operative neurologic deficit persisting for more than 24 hours, is one of the registry outcomes measures and is also one of the

11 performance measures endorsed by the National Quality Forum. Public reporting of these risk-adjusted outcomes for approximately 20% of the US cardiac surgery programs is currently available at: http://www.comsumerreportshealth.org.

The spectrum of neurologic complications includes encephalopathy, ischemic stroke, cognitive decline, coma, peripheral nerve injuries, optic neuropathy, and pituitary apoplexy. Postoperative neurologic complications may be classified by the clinical manifestation of the injury (e.g. stroke, encephalopathy, coma, etc.) or by the proposed mechanism of the injury (e.g. macroembolism, microembolism, hypoperfusion, hypoxic-ischemic injury, hemorrhage, etc.) but for many cases the relationship between the clinical picture and the presumed mechanism is either multifactorial or uncertain.

☝ CAUTION

Don't be too quick to attribute a patient's delay from awakening from anesthesia to a medication or metabolic effect. This is often the first clue to a perioperative neurologic complication.

Emergency Management in Neurocritical Care, First Edition. Edited by Edward M. Manno.
© 2012 John Wiley & Sons, Ltd. Published 2012 by John Wiley & Sons, Ltd.

Encephalopathy and Neurocognitive Deficits

The most common neurologic complication of cardiac surgery is a neurocognitive deficit ranging from post-operative encephalopathy to a more subtle cognitive decline noted by family members and confirmed by neuropsychometric testing. In prospective studies of patients undergoing CABG, post-operative encephalopathy was recognized in 3% of patients by ICU staff but diagnosed in up to 12% by neurologists. The majority of patients will improve during hospitalization, and 80% will recover to be able to perform normally on a bedside neurocognitive tests by the time of discharge. However, when more extensive neuropsychological test batteries are employed, 35–75% of patients have documented impairments in cognitive function within the first 7–10 days after surgery and 20% of these are rather severe. Deficits in attention, concentration, memory, and processing speed persist in 10–30% at 3–6 months. Risk factors for post-operative encephalopathy include post-operative intra-aortic balloon pump support or use of pressor agents, which are markers of systemic hypotension, as well as advanced age,

hypertension, diabetes, excessive alcohol consumption, post–operative atrial fibrillation, a history of peripheral vascular disease or prior CABG (Table 19.1). Patients with post–operative encephalopathy or cognitive decline are also more likely to have pre-operative cerebral atrophy or white matter changes on baseline neuroimaging. In one longitudinal neurocognitive study, 42% of patients developed progressive cognitive decline at 5 years, which was attributed to an underlying vascular or degenerative dementia. As post-operative cognitive decline is also a risk factor for late cognitive deterioration – particularly in patients who are older and with lower levels of education – it may be an unmasking of a pre-existing vascular or degenerative dementia.

Stroke

Stroke following cardiac surgery is almost invariably ischemic in nature. The risk of ischemic stroke following CABG is 2–5% but can be as high as 5–15% following more complex cardiac surgeries, such as valvular replacement or repair, ventricular aneurysm resection, or aortic arch reconstruction. Neuroimaging patterns include

Table 19.1. Risk factors for neurologic deficit after coronary artery bypass surgery

	Encephalopathy	Stroke
Medical History	Hypertension Diabetes History of Alcohol abuse Peripheral artery disease Prior CABG	Hypertension Diabetes Prior stroke Recent MI Left ventricular dysfunction Chronic renal insufficiency
Patient Features	Older age Cognitive impairment Cerebral atrophy	Older age Carotid stenosis Cerebrovascular disease
Intraoperative/Post-operative factors	IABP support Pressor support Atrial fibrillation Circulatory arrest	Aortic arch atheroma Atrial fibrillation Prolonged cross-clamp time Prolonged CBP time Low cardiac output Complex cardiac surgery

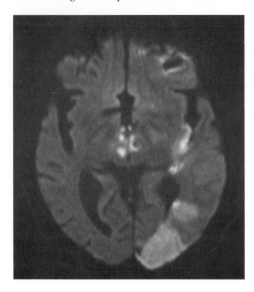

Figure 19.1. Neuroimaging patterns of stroke-MRI diffusion-weighted image of a major territory embolism in a patient with post-operative coma.

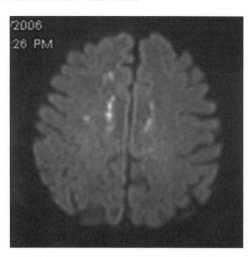

Figure 19.3. Neuroimaging patterns of stroke-MRI diffusion-weighted image of a bilateral border zone pattern of infarction. Whether this indicates poor clearance of emboli or hypoperfusion, this pattern is associated with a poor prognosis for survival.

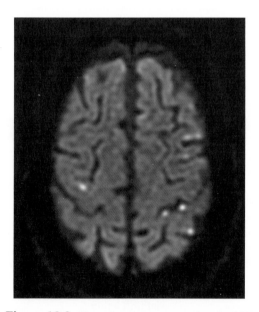

Figure 19.2. Neuroimaging patterns of stroke-MRI diffusion-weighted image of multifocal embolism in a patient with post-operative confusion. This pattern, characteristic of a proximal source of embolism, is best detected with MRI diffusion imaging and was not evident on CT.

major territory embolism, multifocal embolism characteristic of a proximal source of embolism, and a multifocal border zone pattern best detected with MRI diffusion imaging (see Figures 19.1–19.3). Risk factors for stroke after CABG include advanced age, aortic arch atheromatous disease, prior stroke or documented cerebrovascular disease, recent myocardial infarction, left ventricular dysfunction, hypertension, diabetes, chronic renal insufficiency, and post-operative atrial fibrillation (Table 19.1). Patients with post-operative stroke were also more likely to have longer cross-clamp times, total cardiopulmonary bypass (CPB) time and post-operative low cardiac output. An important cue to a postoperative neurologic deficit is a delay in awakening from anesthesia.

Intracranial hemorrhage within one week of cardiac surgery is rare and results from hemorrhagic transformation of bland infarcts or coagulopathies in the critically ill or after cardiac transplantation. Subdural hematomas have also been described, presenting as post-operative seizures or focal neurologic deficit. Neuroimaging features include both acute bleeding as well as acute chronic features and are likely related to the anticoagulation required by the cardiopulmonary bypass circuit.

Coma

Although many patients with a neurologic complication are slow to awaken from anesthesia, true post-operative coma or "failure to awaken" is uncommon, occurring in less than 1% of patients. For these patients, neuroimaging is essential as many are due to major territory cerebral infarction with a risk of life-threatening brain swelling that may warrant surgical intervention. Other causes include smaller territory but multifocal cerebral infarction affecting brainstem or thalamic nuclei, bilateral border zone patterns, or a diffuse global hypoxic–ischemic insult. The sensitivity of MRI diffusion-weighted imaging in identifying cerebral infarction is at least twice that of CT. The prognosis of post-operative non-metabolic coma is extremely poor with an 85% mortality and a < 5% chance of useful neurologic recovery.

Seizures

Seizures occur in about 3% of patients following cardiac surgery and are often indicative of an underlying ischemic injury.

Peripheral nerve injuries

Peripheral nerve injuries following CABG occur in 2–13%. Injury to the brachial plexus is probably the best known and the most problematic. Lower trunk injuries are the most common and present with weakness and sensory loss in the ulnar-C8-T1 distribution. Causalgic pain is often a major presenting feature and although many improve during hospitalization, 0.8% are chronic. Involvement of the overlying sympathetic chain produces a Horner syndrome with miosis, ptosis, and anhidrosis. Injury to the lower trunk plexus and the sympathetic chain are attributed to stretch injuries related to chest wall retraction or fracture or dislocation of the first or second ribs. Upper trunk brachial plexus injures are uncommon and there is controversy whether these result from jugular vein cannulation.

Myocardial cooling techniques employing ice slush or cold saline solutions in the pericardium can result in thermal injuries to the phrenic and recurrent laryngeal nerves. In a prospective study, injury to the phrenic nerve, most commonly the left, could be demonstrated in up to 70% of patients. As an elevated left hemidiaphragm is a common and nonspecific radiographic finding in the post-operative period, addition testing with fluoroscopy or ultrasound is often required to establish the diagnosis of a phrenic neuropathy. Minor injuries resolve during hospitalization although more significant injuries require 3–6 months. The orthopnea and reduced ventilation of a unilateral phrenic neuropathy may be well tolerated in patients with otherwise normal pulmonary function, but in the setting of underlying chronic obstructive pulmonary disease, it is associated with significant prolongation of ICU and hospital stay, rehospitalizations, and reduced survival. Injury to the recurrent laryngeal nerve may also occur during intubation and central venous line placement. Presenting as hoarseness and a weak cough, it may also cause dysphagia, increasing the risk of aspiration pneumonia.

Local injury to the saphenous and radial nerves during the harvesting of veins and arteries for the bypass grafts range from the common, localized neuralgia and peri-incisional sensory deficit to rare severe injuries from traction and laceration. Lastly, positional compression neuropathies affecting the peroneal and ulnar nerves can affect any patient with prolonged immobility and bedrest, weight loss, and nutritional deficits.

Other Rare Complications

Ischemic optic neuropathy following cardiopulmonary bypass is rare, reported to occur in 0.01–0.1%. The proposed mechanism is reduced posterior ciliary artery blood flow in the setting of hypotension, and some case-control studies have also suggested post-operative anemia as a risk factor. Pituitary apoplexy is a rare complication of pituitary adenomas but its occurrence, precipitated by recent cardiopulmonary bypass surgery, is recognized by multiple case series in the literature.

Presentations include ptosis, mydriasis, multiple oculomotor nerve palsies and visual loss, but the presentation can be less obvious with headache, malaise, unexplained hyponatremia. Less severe cases missed in the post-operative period may present later with malaise and pituitary insufficiency. Off-pump surgery has been proposed as a superior alternative for patients with a known untreated pituitary adenoma warranting CABG surgery.

Mechanisms of Neurologic Injury

In most institutions, cardiac surgery is performed with CPB or the "heart-lung machine." The cardiopulmonary bypass circuit can contribute to cerebral injury by a variety of potential mechanisms: cerebral embolization of atheromatous material and other debris, cerebral hypoperfusion, or from cerebral edema resulting from a systemic inflammatory response. The CPB circuit constructs an extracorporeal course encompassing cannulation of the proximal ascending aorta and the right atrium through a median sternotomy exposure. Cardiac arrest is achieved after systemic heparinization and occlusion of the ascending aorta either by external cross-clamping or internal balloon occlusion, and systemic blood flow is then supported by the CPB pump. Oxygenated blood is supplied to the body though approximately 6 feet of tubing and adjusted for target pump flows, perfusion pressure, temperature, and in-line venous saturation. Surgeries which require opening of the cardiac chambers, such as valvular repair or replacement or resection of a ventricular aneurysm, are associated with a significant increase in the risk of stroke. This increased risk is related to prolongation of the cross-clamp time and total bypass time, reflecting the complexity of the case, potential for embolism of valve debris, and embolism of air and particulates during mechanical de-airing of the heart.

Combining clinical information with neuroimaging data, the proposed mechanism of ischemic stroke after cardiac surgery performed with cardiopulmonary bypass is largely embolic; nearly half are attributed to emboli from atheromatous debris from the aortic arch, from the heart, or from the bypass pump. Less than one-third are attributed to hypoperfusion with or without concomitant cerebrovascular disease with the remainder cryptogenic. Much of the data supporting the major role of aortic arch atheromatous disease as a source of cerebral embolism comes from transcranial Doppler (TCD) monitoring of high-intensity signals (HITS) and transesopha-

geal echocardiography (TEE) monitoring of microemboli during cardiac surgery. Several prospective studies have correlated the burden of HITS on TCD during CPB with cognitive deficits on neuropsychological testing. The majority of HITS occur during aortic arch cross-clamping and other manipulation, and at the initiation of bypass. These studies have also been instrumental in guiding technologic improvements to limit embolization from the CPB circuit. In-line filtration with 40 micron filters and membrane oxygenators were introduced to filter such macroemboli as air, fat, glove powder, PVC tubing debris, and silicone antifoaming agents. Heparin-bonded and closed circuits have been developed to reduce activation of the inflammatory and coagulation system while on bypass.

Around 1995, "off-pump" coronary artery bypass surgery was introduced in an effort to reduce the risk of embolization from the CPB circuit or from the aortic arch. Performed on the "beating heart" using specialized stabilizers that limit coronary vessel motion, off-pump surgery does not require aortic cross-clamping and does not use CPB. However, off-pump techniques are often performed under induced bradycardia and relative hypotension, and although flow is pulsatile, relative hypotension may increase the risk of cerebral hypoperfusion in patients with a poor vascular reserve or an underlying small vessel disease. To test the relative efficacy of these new techniques, investigators have employed neurocognitive testing results as a primary endpoint since the incidence of stroke is too infrequent to reasonably power a trial. Although off-pump surgery has demonstrated a substantial reduction in the number of cerebral microemboli as well as a reduced severity of the inflammatory response compared to surgery performed with CPB, there has been no significant impact on neurocognitive testing results or composite endpoints that include stroke events. The topic remains controversial among experts and institutions, and studies continue to investigate the subsets and evolution of hybrid PCI-CABG surgery, endovascular and robotic procedures.

Cardiopulmonary bypass is performed under mild hypothermia at 32 °C, which provides a neuroprotective state by lowering the cerebral neuronal metabolism. At this temperature, autoregulation is preserved and cerebral blood flow is more than adequate to meet demands; this state is proposed as the major contributor to the good neurologic outcome of the majority of patients undergoing these complex surgeries. Cerebral autoregulation remains preserved until the temperature drops to less than 22 °C or when mean arterial pressures are less than 20 mmHg or greater than 100 mmHg, particularly in patients with diabetes. When the aortic arch is too diseased to permit cross-clamping, or when the aorta itself requires repair or reconstruction, circulatory arrest with deeper hypothermia at 18 °C is employed, which carries a higher risk, ~20% risk, of neurocognitive impairment. Various studies have demonstrated that cognitive deficits increase with older age and circulatory arrest time over 25 minutes with up to one-third demonstrating significant deficits with circulatory arrest times of 50 minutes or longer. When prolonged circulatory arrest is anticipated, cerebral circulation can be supported by selective antegrade or retrograde cerebral perfusion. The benefits of these techniques are offset by the risks associated with cannulation of the great vessels, including dissection, vessel occlusion, distal atheroembolism, and delayed stenosis.

Many neuroprotective agents, efficacious in animal models when administered prior to an ischemic insult, were not demonstrated to have any clinical benefit in the treatment of acute ischemic stroke. Several of these have been studied as a prophylactic therapy prior to cardiac surgery and have not shown promise although the small trials and low risk of stroke overall make the results difficult to interpret.

Concomitant Carotid Stenosis and Cerebrovascular Disease

Carotid stenosis is an important risk factor for stroke during CABG. Patients at highest risk include those with symptomatic and severe stenosis of the extracranial or intracranial cerebral arteries, carotid occlusion bilateral greater than 50% carotid stenosis, and significant intracranial stenosis. Despite this, there is no evidence that a routine protocol of prophylactic carotid revascularization reduces the perioperative stroke risk

of 3–19%. A meta-analysis of 16 nonrandomized studies comparing combined versus staged CABG and carotid endarterectomy (CE) reported a significantly higher risk of stroke, death, and stroke or death when the surgeries were combined (6.0, 4.7, and 9.5%) compared to staged surgery (3.2, 2.9, and 5.7%), respectively. Several nonrandomized studies analyzing the neuroimaging features of post-CABG ischemic stroke indicate that approximately 5% are consistent with a large-artery mechanism, but 60% are not confined to a single carotid territory and at least 75% occur in the absence of significant carotid stenosis. In one retrospective single-center cohort study, the perioperative stroke risk with CE + CABG was 15% and determined to be in excess of the risk of stroke experienced by patients with a similar degree of carotid stenosis who underwent CABG alone. After this study was reviewed, their institution abolished routine pre-operative carotid ultrasound screening of patients anticipating CABG surgery.

EVIDENCE AT A GLANCE

Meta-analysis of nonrandomized studies indicate a significantly higher risk of poor outcomes with combined CABG + CE when compared to staged surgeries.

Clinical trials of carotid angioplasty and stenting (CAS) have demonstrated a lower risk of periprocedural myocardial ischemia than CE. CAS is approved for patients with symptomatic carotid stenosis with high-risk criteria, such as coronary heart disease. A single-center experience, comparing combined coronary and carotid revascularization with either CAS or CE, reported a significantly lower risk of stroke or myocardial infarction at 30 days in those managed with CAS + CABG compared to CE + CABG (5% vs. 19%, $p = 0.01$). However, the majority in both groups had asymptomatic carotid stenoses, 54% vs. 77% and as there was no control group without carotid revascularization, it is uncertain whether this strategy would reduce stroke risk compared to CABG alone. Until the requisite data is available, a reasonable approach to patients with carotid and coronary disease using existing clinical trials results is to attempt to view the carotid disease independently. Patients with asymptomatic carotid stenosis should undergo CABG alone but be followed carefully in the post-operative period as symptoms related to a perioperative carotid plaque rupture can occur. For patients with recently symptomatic ≥ 70% carotid stenosis, CAS would be the preferred revascularization strategy prior to CABG based on the single-center study. Aggressive medical risk factor management is also warranted, as the long-term prognosis of patients with symptomatic carotid and coronary disease is poor, with 36% mortality at 3.4 years.

Evaluating an Acute Neurologic Deficit in a Cardiac Surgical Patient

The evaluation and management of a suspected acute ischemic stroke in the setting of a recent cardiac surgery is not fundamentally different from other situations, but this situation poses several challenges that warrant a tailored approach. The first challenge is establishing the time of onset or when the patient was last known to be neurologically at the baseline. If the consult is requested when the patient is slow to awaken from anesthesia, the time last known well was prior to the induction of anesthesia. Determining whether a stroke has occurred or whether a revascularization strategy is an option will require more sophisticated imaging than the usual CT scan without contrast. In the setting of non-transplant cardiac surgery, stroke is almost exclusively ischemic in nature. The most useful imaging modality is MRI with diffusion-weighted imaging to establish the presence and distribution of infarction, MR angiography to evaluate for arterial occlusion, and MR perfusion to evaluate the tissue at risk. If MR imaging is contraindicated due to the presence of a permanent pacemaker or temporary pacing wires, the alternative is to combine CT with CT angiography and CT perfusion to evaluate for a substantial mismatch in the cerebral blood flow deficit from the cerebral blood volume imaging.

The majority (as much as 60%) of strokes noted in the first post-operative days are complete at the time of evaluation and are not eligible for revascularization strategies. The focus of neurologic

Table 19.2. Bleeding complications of intra-arterial thrombolytic therapy for acute ischemic stroke complicating cardiac surgery (aggregate data, less than 100 cases in the literature)

17%	Bleeding requiring transfusion
12%	Perivascular or catheter intervention site
6–10%	Symptomatic hemorrhagic transformation of the cerebral infarct
5%	Tamponade from hemopericardium
5%	Operative site hemorrhage-thoracic or mediastinal
5%	Nasal, pharyngeal, or esophageal hemorrhage

care is then on the appropriate diagnosis, evaluation for potential life-threatening brain swelling, supportive care, prevention of medical complications, assessment for rehabilitation therapies, and neuroprognostication. The remainder of post-operative strokes have their onset rather equally distributed throughout the post-operative period and should be evaluated aggressively for potential revascularization options. The ideal patient is one recovering from successful cardiac surgery with an acute deficit witnessed by their healthcare team who is otherwise hemodynamically stable and off anticoagulants.

Thrombolytic therapy options are still limited by the post-operative state or presence of concomitant antithrombotic therapies which increase the risk of bleeding. Limited case series of patients with acute focal ischemic stroke treated with mechanical revascularization, intra-arterial thrombolysis and combined therapies have suggested similar revascularization outcomes with somewhat increased risks of systemic bleeding (Table 19.2).

★ TIPS & TRICKS

The majority of strokes noted in the first post-operative days are complete at the time of evaluation but the remaining 40% that occur in the post-operative period should be evaluated aggressively for potential revascularization options.

Bibliography

Barbut D, Yao FS, Hager DN, et al. Comparison of transcranial Doppler ultrasonography and transesophageal echocardiography to monitor emboli during cardiopulmonary bypass. *Stroke* 1996; **27**:87–90.

Borger MA, Fremes SE, Weisel RD, et al. Coronary bypass and carotid endarterectomy: does a combined approach increase risk? A meta-analysis. *Ann Thorac Surg* 1999; **68**:14–20.

Breuer AC, Furlan AJ, Hanson MR, et al. Central nervous system complications of coronary artery bypass graft surgery: prospective analysis of 421 patients. *Stroke* 1983; **14**:682–687.

Diegler A, Hirsch R, Schneider F, et al. Neuromonitoring and neurocognitive outcome in off-pump versus conventional coronary bypass operation. *Ann Thorac Surg* 2000; **69**:1162–1166.

Katzan I, Masaryk TJ, Furlan AJ, et al. Intra-arterial thrombolysis for perioperative stroke after open heart surgery. *Neurology* 1999; **52**: 1081–1084.

Lederman RJ, Breuer AC, Hanson MR, et al. Peripheral nervous system complications of coronary artery bypass graft surgery. *Ann Neurol* 1982; **12**:297–301.

Li Y, Walicki D, Mathiesen C, et al. Strokes after cardiac surgery and relationship to carotid stenosis. *Arch Neurol* 2009; **66**:1091–1096.

Moody DM, Brown WR, Challa VR, et al. Brain microemboli associated with cardiopulmonary bypass: a histologic and magnetic resonance imaging study. *Ann Thorac Surg* 1995; **59**: 1304–1307.

Murkin JM, Newman SP, Stump DA, Blumenthal JA. Statement of consensus on assessment of neurobehavioral outcomes after cardiac surgery. *Ann Thorac Surg* 1995; **59**:1289–1295.

Newman MF, Grocott HP, Stanley TO, et al. Longitudinal assessment of neurocognitive function after coronary artery bypass surgery. *New Engl J Med* 2001; **344**:451–452.

Roach GW, Kanchuger M, Mangano CM, et al. Adverse cerebral outcomes after coronary bypass surgery. *New Engl J Med* 1996; **335**:1857–1863.

Stamou SC, Hill PC, Dangas G, et al. Stroke after coronary artery bypass: incidence, predictors, and clinical outcome. *Stroke* 2001; **32**:1508–1513.

Svensson LG, Crawford ES, Hess KR, et al. Deep hypothermia with circulatory arrest. Determinants of stroke and early mortality in 656 patients. i 1993; **106**:19–28.

Wolman RL, Nussmeier NA, Aggarwal A, et al. Cerebral injury after cardiac surgery: identification of a group at extraordinary risk. Multicenter Study of Perioperative Ischemia Research Group (McSPI) and the Ischemia Research Education Foundation (IREF) Investigators. Stroke 1999; **30(3)**:514–522.

Ziada KM, Yadav JS, Mukherjee D, et al. Comparison of results of carotid stenting followed by open heart surgery versus combined carotid endarterectomy and open heart surgery (coronary bypass with or without another procedure). *Am J Cardiol* 2005; **96**:519–523.

Neurological Complications of Medical Illness: Critical illness Neuropathy and Myopathy

Edward M. Manno

Neurological Intensive Care Unit, Cleveland Clinic, Cleveland, OH, USA

Introduction

Technological advancements and improvements in the management of critically ill patients have increased patient survival after prolonged bouts of critical illness. This has led to the recognition of limb and respiratory weakness that can commonly occur after a bout of sepsis. These neuromuscular complications of severe illness have been recognized for a long time but were poorly characterized. Osler (1892) described a catabolic myopathy and diaphragmatic weakness that occurred in patients after a bout of sepsis. Mertens (1961) described a group of polyneuropathies that occurred in patients that had been in a prolonged coma. Bolton and colleagues, however, provided the best characterization of this illness. From 1977 to 1983 Bolton and colleagues described 19 cases of a polyneuropathy that they attributed to the mediators of sepsis. This neuropathy accounted for the difficulties in weaning from mechanical ventilation.

It became immediately apparent that this neuropathy was not an isolated phenomenon. Around the same time Zochodne et al. (1994) described the first cases of a necrotizing myopathy that occurred in patients that had been treated with large doses of corticosteroids and were

pharmacologically paralyzed. Thus, the terminology of critical illness neuropathy and myopathy were used to describe the clinical, electrophysiological and pathological findings of critically ill patients. However, the neuropathy rarely occurs without simultaneous involvement of the muscle. Most authors now prefer the term "critical illness neuromyopathy" to describe the clinical features encountered after severe critical illness.

Clinical Presentation

Patients with critical illness neuropathy and myopathy typically present with flaccid areflexic limbs, with intact sensation, and a normal cranial nerve examination. Neurological consultation usually occurs for failure to wean from the ventilator long after cardiopulmonary conditions have resolved. The patient may grimace to noxious stimuli but will be unable to withdraw the involved extremity. The exam may be difficult to interpret since most patients will have a concurrent septic encephalopathy (see Chapter 17) and may be sedated.

The neuropathy is primarily axonal. It involves the motor axons to a greater degree than the sensory axons, but with advancement of the disease the sensory nerves will become progressively involved. The neuropathy also progresses distally to more proximally over time. Subsequently, muscle weakness and areflexia will progress from distally to more proximal.

Muscle atrophy will develop as the neuropathy progresses and leads to denervation of involved muscles. The atrophy is often more severe than can be accounted for by immobilization alone and most likely represents the simultaneous involvement of a critical illness myopathy. Cranial nerve and facial muscle involvement can occur late in the process but early involvement should prompt an investigation into other possible neuromuscular etiologies such as Guillian–Barre or myasthenia.

Critical illness myopathy may occur simultaneously or independently of the neuropathy. The exact onset may be difficult to determine because of a concurrent neuropathy or encephalopathy, or the use of neuromuscular blockade. A diffuse flaccid weakness involves the limbs, neck flexors, and diaphragm. Unlike the neuropathy, facial muscles are not spared. Reflexes become depressed as the myopathy worsens. Myalgias are uncommon.

The acute quadriplegic myopathy was originally described in young patients that were treated for a severe bout of status asthmaticus. Patients were treated with high-dose corticosteroids and were pharmacologically paralyzed to facilitate mechanical ventilation. As the patients improved and the paralysis was reversed, an acute quadriplegia was discovered. Initial concerns for cervical injury during intubation prompted radiological evaluation but the diagnosis was made electrophysiologically, which revealed a diffuse myopathic process.

Incidence

Both the neuropathy and myopathy due to critical illness are common to patients in the intensive care unit. The incidence is related to the severity of illness and time spent in the intensive care unit. About a third of all patients on mechanical ventilation will exhibit electrophysiological evidence for a neuropathy. Approximately 60% of patients in an intensive care unit will develop evidence for a neuropathy after one week. 75% of septic patients will develop a neuropathy and this will increase to almost all patients that develop multiorgan failure.

Predominant muscle involvement occurs in about a third of patients treated for status asthmaticus and 40% of critically ill patients. Over two-thirds are patients that are in an intensive care unit for greater than 1 week have some evidence of muscle involvement.

Electrophysiologic Studies

Conventional electrophysiological studies are the mainstay for identifying the presence of a neuropathy or myopathy. The predominant electrophysiological abnormality encountered in the critically ill patient is a reduction in amplitude of the compound muscle and sensory nerve action potentials. These findings are consistent with a progressive axonal sensorimotor degeneration of the peripheral nerves and represent a decrease in the total number of nerve fibers that can be stimulated. Conduction velocities are largely unaffected since the peripheral nerve myelin is spared until late in the course of the process. Needle electromyography typically will reveal fibrillation potentials or sharp waves indicative of muscle involvement.

Phrenic nerve conduction studies and electromyography of the diaphragm and the respiratory muscles can reveal respiratory muscle and nerve involvement which may account for the difficulty in weaning from mechanical ventilation. Phrenic nerve conduction velocities usually reveal normal latencies but diaphragmatic muscle action potentials may be reduced. Amplitudes increase as recovery ensues. Motor units in the diaphragm may reveal a myopathic appearance.

Differentiating involvement of the peripheral nerves found in critical illness neuropathy from the muscle involvement in critical illness myopathy can be challenging. Critical illness neuropathy and myopathy can both lead to a decrease in compound action muscle potentials. As mentioned, fibrillation potential and sharp waves are commonly found during needle examination. This, however, may represent denervation of the involved muscle. In the cooperative patient, low amplitude motor unit potentials with early recruitment is suggestive of direct muscle involvement. Bolton (2005) has suggested a set of criteria for diagnosis which is listed in Table 20.1.

However, in many cases the patient may not be able to cooperate with the examination, and in

Table 20.1. Diagnostic criteria of critical illness myopathy. For a definitive diagnosis, patients should have the first five features

- Sensory nerve action potential amplitudes >80% of the lower limit of normal.
- Needle EMG with short-duration, low amplitude muscle unit potentials with early or normal full recruitment, with or without fibrillation potentials.
- Absence of a decremental response on repetitive nerve stimulation; and
- Muscle histopathologic findings of a myopathy with myosin loss.
- Compound muscle action potential amplitudes <80% of the lower limit of normal in two or more nerves without conduction block;
- elevated serum creatine kinase and
- Demonstration of muscle inexcitability.

Source: Bolton 2005.

these circumstances direct muscle stimulation may be required. In direct muscle stimulation, compound muscle action potentials are measured after nerve stimulation and compared to compound muscle action potentials of direct stimulation of the muscle (Figure 20.1). If the muscle is relatively unaffected, nerve-stimulated compound muscle action potentials will be less than the muscle action potential that is directly stimulated. If a myopathy exists, the nerve-stimulated compound muscle potential will be the same or greater than the direct muscle-stimulated action potential. In situations where both a neuropathy and a myopathy exist, the ratio of nerve to muscle stimulation is usually greater than 0.5.

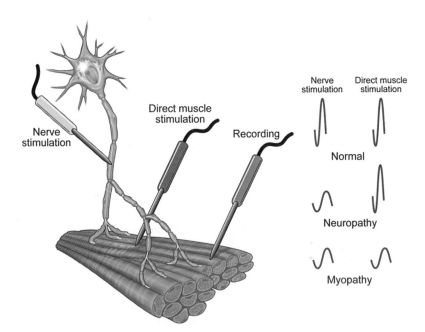

Figure 20.1. Determining muscle involvement with critical illness may require direct muscle stimulation. In this testing compound action muscle potentials are recorded at a site distal to stimulation. Stimulation occurs at the nerve and subsequently directly on the muscle proximal to the recording site. Compound muscle action potentials are recorded and compared. (Adapted from Zink et al. 2009; with permission from Nature.)

Histopathology

Nerve biopsy samples were performed by Bolton (2005), and colleagues, of patients with electrophysiological documented critical illness polyneuropathy. Samples revealed fiber loss and axonal degeneration. The distal nerve segments were more severely involved. No inflammation was noted. Muscle changes showed acute and chronic denervation. In a small number of cases nerve biopsies were normal despite electrophysiological evidence for a neuropathy. This was believed to reflect either the limitations of the biopsy itself or that functional change may precede pathological alterations.

There are a wide range of myopathic changes that can be found with muscle biopsy. Findings can range from normal to diffuse and severe muscle necrosis. This may represent a spectrum of pathology that exists from muscle inexcitability to necrosis.

Several subtypes of critical illness myopathies have been described, but are now generally grouped into three categories. The most common type of myopathy described is attributed to thick filament myelin loss. This is most commonly encountered after pharmacological paralysis and high-dose corticosteroids. A muscle biopsy reveals the loss of all fiber types; electron microscopy reveals the complete loss of myosin (Figure 20.2). Cachetic myopathies histologically reveal internalized nuclei, rimmed vacuoles, fatty degeneration, and fibrosis. A severe necro-

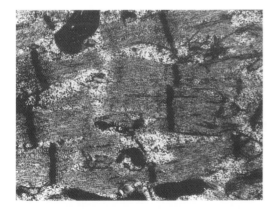

Figure 20.2. Electronmicrography of a biopsy in a patient with acute quadriplegic myopathy. Note the complete loss of myosin filaments.

tizing myopathy has also been characterized by the phagocytosis of myocytes. Selective muscle changes secondary to denervation (either functionally from pharmacological paralysis or physically due to critical illness neuropathy) are commonly encountered and can complicate the interpretation of the muscle biopsy.

Pathophysiology

The pathophysiologic mechanism involved in the development of critical illness polyneuropathy is complex and incompletely understood. The severity of the neuropathy, quantified by electrophysiological studies, correlates directly with intensive care length of stay, glucose levels, and hypoalbuminemia.

Sepsis itself is believed to directly affect the peripheral nerve function. Since blood vessels to peripheral nerves lack autoregulation, mediators of sepsis may gain direct access to the peripheral nerves. Cytokines exhibit histamine-type qualities and can increase the microvascular permeability to the nerves. Endovascular edema is increased in hyperglycemia and hypoalbuminemia, which may account for the decreased peripheral neuropathies reported in critically ill patients with tight glucose control. Endoneural edema also is believed to increase the intercapillary distance. Capillary leakage is facilitated through the passage of neurotoxic substances into the endoneurium. Increased E selectin and leukocyte adhesion molecules found in sepsis have been documented in the endothelium of peripheral nerves. Both are known to increase permeability. Similarly, metabolites of pharmacologic paralytics known to be neurotoxic may gain access to the peripheral nerves with increased permeability.

Bioenergetic studies of muscle have revealed an impaired mitochondrial function in muscle in sepsis. It is speculated that bioenergetic failure would lead to a decrease in energy-dependent ATP-ase necessary for axonal transport of nutritional substances and structural proteins. This may account for the distal to proximal involvement of the peripheral nerves.

The processes involved with the development of the myopathy are multifactorial. Proteolytic pathways are activated by proinflammatory cytokines (interleukin 1 and 6, tumor necrosis factor, interferon γ) and are released during systemic inflammation or sepsis. Degradation targets the myosin heavy chains. Proteins are also degraded by a proteosome, apoptosis is increased, and intrinsic anabolic processes are impaired through the interleukin suppression of myosin repair genes. Similarly anabolic hormones are decreased during critical illness.

A channelopathy has been speculated to develop during sepsis which could inhibit muscle membrane excitability. An overall drop in cortisol levels may lead to an inactivation of sodium channels. Nitric oxide is crucial to maintaining muscle membrane excitability; and an impaired gene expression of nitric oxide synthetase is reported in sepsis. Calcium entry into the sarcoplasmic reticulum necessary for muscle contraction is also decreased in critical illness. An unidentified myotoxic substance is also believed to be released in critical illness.

Changes in metabolic pathways may account for bioenergetic failure determined by nuclear magnetic resonance studies. During sepsis, gluconeogenesis is increased and muscle develops a relative resistance to insulin. Subsequently, muscle can become relatively starved of metabolic substances and will initiate processes that will lead to intrinsic muscle breakdown.

Infiltration of the muscle with activated leukocytes has been well documented and strongly suggests a role for inflammation in the development of the myopathy.

The reason for the preferential degradation of myosin is unknown; however, the role of pharmacologic or functional denervation has been implied. Denervated rat muscle myosin rapidly develops increased corticosteroid receptors. High doses of corticosteroid could subsequently lead to severe preferential catabolism of myosin. Similarly, a neuromuscular blockade increases the corticosteroid receptors in muscle cytoplasm.

A direct myotoxic effect of neuromuscular blockers themselves has been speculated. An increased capillary permeability during sepsis may allow direct access to muscle membranes.

Treatment

The best treatment is the aggressive treatment of sepsis. Limiting the systemic inflammatory response to sepsis is the highest priority. Similarly, a judicious use of pharmacologic paralysis may decrease the incidence of the myopathy.

There are no specific treatments for either the myopathy or neuropathy secondary to critical illness, and there have been several attempts to specifically treat or prevent the development of the neuropathy. Trials of corticosteroids, plasma exchange, and intravenous immunoglobulin have all been unsuccessful in arresting or slowing the development of the neuromyopathy. Nutritional supplements and antioxidants have similarly not been helpful. Patients treated with testosterone or growth hormone supplementation actually did worse than their respective placebo arms, presumably due to increased hyperglycemia.

Tight glucose control, however, may have a role in preventing the development of the neuropathy. A planned subanalysis of an intensive insulin trial in critically ill patients (Van den Berghe et al., 2005) was suggestive of a decrease in both critical illness neuropathy and myopathy in patients with tight glucose control. For patients in the intensive care unit longer than 1 week, the incidence of the neuromyopathy was 39% for tight glucose control group compared to 50% of the nonintensive insulin group (p >0.02). There was also an improved 3-month mortality (but not 1 month) in the intensive insulin group. This has been attributed to the better rehabilitation potential of patients that survived a bout of sepsis. Concerns have been raised about the safety of intensive insulin treatment due to an increase in the number of hypoglycemic episodes. Thus the decision to initiate tight glucose control remains a clinical one. Future studies focusing on patients projected to have a prolonged bout with sepsis may be warranted.

There is a growing body of evidence to suggest that exercise and early mobilization can decrease both the incidence and severity of the neuromyopathy. Prospective clinical trials are currently under debate.

Prognosis

The prognosis for critical illness neuropathy is dependent upon the length and degree of axonal loss. The severity of the illness can range from mild, with recovery within weeks, to significant permanent functional loss. Recovery has been reported in about 50% of patients although rehabilitation may be extended for patients that have been in the intensive care unit longer than 1 month. In more severe (about a third) cases patients may be para- or tetraplegic and experience severe impairment in their quality of life.

> ★ **TIPS & TRICKS**
>
> Serial electrophysiological studies can be performed and used to assess prognosis. The length of the neuropathy and the muscles involved can be determined. Also which muscles are denervated can be determined.

Patients with an isolated myopathy may have a better prognosis; however, little data exists to support this supposition.

> ★ **TIPS & TRICKS**
>
> An important differentiation, that will affect both recovery and weaning from mechanical ventilation, is determining if muscle is primarily affected or secondarily from disuse. For patients with a functional denervation due to complete axonal loss there will be little reason to attempt weaning from mechanical ventilation until the nerves are reconnected to muscle. Disuse atrophy can benefit from weaning trials.

Conclusions

Critical illness neuropathy and myopathy represent a spectrum of neuromuscular disorders affecting both peripheral nerve and muscle found in critically ill patients. The process appears to be mediated through inflammatory cytokines released during the systemic inflammatory syndrome or sepsis. The incidence and severity of the process is directly related to the severity of illness and length of stay in the intensive care unit. Treatment focuses on early recognition and treatment of sepsis. A limited use of neuromuscular blockade may also prove useful. Prognosis is related to the degree of axonal loss and muscle involvement. Tight glucose control may limit the severity of the neuropathy. Early mobilization is hoped to improve rehabilitation.

Bibliography

Bolton CF. Neuromuscular manifestations of critical illness. *Muscle Nerve* 2005; **32:** 140–163.

Hermans G, De Jonghe B, Bruuyninckx F, Van den Berghe G. Interventions for preventing critical illness polyneuropathy and critical illness neuropathy. *Cochrane Database Syst Rev* 2009; **Issue 1:** Art.No. CD006832.doi:10.1002/14651858.CD006832.pub2(2009).

Hermans G, Wilmer A, Meersseman W, et al. Impact of intensive insulin therapy on neuromuscular complications and ventilator-dependency in MICU. *Am J Resp Crit Care Med* 2007; **175:** 480–489.

Lacomis D, Giuliani MJ, Van Cott A, Kramer DJ. Acute myopathy of intensive care: clinical, electromyographic, and pathological aspects. *Ann Neurol* 1996; **40:** 645–654.

Latronico N, Shehu I, Guarneri B. Use of electrophysiologic testing. *Crit Care Med* 2009; **37(Suppl):** S316–S320.

Maramattom BV, Wijdicks EFM. Acute neuromuscular weakness in the intensive care unit. *Crit Care Med* 2006; **34:** 2835–2841.

Mertens HG. Disseminated neuropathy following coma. On the differentiation of so-called toxic polyneuropathy. *Nerve-nartz* 1961; **32:** 71–79.

Needham DM. Mobilizing patients in the intensive care unit: improving neuromuscular weakness and physical function. *J Am Med Assoc* 2008; **300:** 1685–1690.

Osler W. *The Principles and Practices of Medicine.* D. Appleton: New York, 1892.

Van den Berghe G, Schoonheydt K, Becx P, et al. Insulin therapy protects the central and peripheral nervous system of intensive care patients. *Neurology* 2005; **64:** 1348–1353.

Zink W, Kollmar R, Schwab S. Critical illness polyneuropathy and myopathy in the intensive care unit. *Nat Rev Neurol* 2009; **5:** 372–379.

Zochodne DW, Ramsey DW, Saly V, et al. Acute necrotizing myopathy of intensive care: electrophysiological studies. *Muscle Nerve* 1994; **17:** 285–292.

Hypothermia: Application and Use in Neurocritical Care

Edward M. Manno

Neurological Intensive Care Unit, Cleveland Clinic, Cleveland, OH, USA

Introduction

Reducing core body temperature to treat neurological injury is not a new concept. The observation that hypothermia could be beneficial after neurological injury was initially described in the 1940s. Intraoperative hypothermia was applied during cardiac and neurological surgery in the 1950s and Peter Safar's initial description of cardiac resuscitation included hypothermia as one of its treatment modalities. Development and widespead use did not occur primarily because of the intensity of care needed to manage patients on the hospital floors and the multiple complications encountered with moderate to deep hypothermia (26–32 °C).

In the 1990s several factors converged to support the application of hypothermia. One was the development and refinement of intensive care which could allow for resources to manage these complex patients. Similarly, preclinical research suggested that the use of mild hypothermia could accomplish the beneficial effects of hypothermia while avoiding many of the deleterious side effects of more aggressive hypothermia. Basic science work from Myron Ginsberg's laboratory and others began to outline the deleterious effects of fever and the therapeutic benefits of mild hypothermia on ischemic neurons. Animal models utilizing mild hypothermia during cardiac arrest and low flow states began to show significant neurological benefit. These results, coupled with several reports of excellent neurological outcomes after prolonged submersion in ice water in children playing ice hockey, invigorated the search for the clinical application of therapeutic hypothermia.

Hypothermia: Mechanisms of Action and Therapeutic Targets

A complex series of events occur after neurological injury and have been the source of a number of reviews. In brief, cerebral ischemia leads to the development of cellular energy failure at the level of the mitochondria. The loss of ATP production inhibits the activity of Na-K membrane pumps. Loss of cellular integrity occurs as increases in extracellular glutamate leads to NMDA receptor-mediated calcium entry into the cell. Intracellular mediated excitotoxicity leads directly to cell death through the production of free radicals with subsequent membrane peroxidation and DNA fragmentation.

Reperfusion prior to cell death can also lead to the production of free radicals which can worsen neurological injury. Many cells that are initially viable will also suffer subsequent death due to apoptotic mechanisms. Secondary injury is common in many types of neurological injury beyond

Emergency Management in Neurocritical Care, First Edition. Edited by Edward M. Manno.
© 2012 John Wiley & Sons, Ltd. Published 2012 by John Wiley & Sons, Ltd.

cerebral ischemia and may include direct trauma, cerebral edema, diffuse axonal injury, and continued seizure activity.

Hypothermia affects several areas not only in the ischemic cascade of events but in multiple other secondary events (Table 21.1). Cellular oxygen and glucose requirements are uniformly lowered with decreased temperature. Blood–brain barrier permeability is reduced with hypothermia, as is reperfusion injury. Epileptic activity, microthrombus formation, and post-injury inflammation is similarly reduced with decreasing temperature.

Induced Hypothermia After Cardiac Arrest

In 2002, two randomized-controlled trials confirmed the benefit of therapeutic hypothermia after cardiac arrest. All of the patients enrolled had witnessed events, with initiation of resuscitation within 15 minutes and the return of spontaneous circulation within 1 hour. Patients needed to have a GCS score < 8 after the return of spontaneous circulation and the initial rhythm had to be either ventricular fibrillation or ventricular tachycardia. On average, approximately 10% of patients screened were eligible for study.

The largest study included 275 patients from nine European hospitals; the patients were randomized to therapeutic hypothermia (defined as 32–34 °C) or normothermia after resuscitation from cardiac arrest. The trial excluded patients older than 75, presenting cardiac arrhythmia of asytole and pulseless electrical activity (PEA), and patients with prolonged periods of post-resuscitation hypoxia or hypotension.

The protocol initiated hypothermia upon arrival to the hospital and used refrigerated cooling blankets to induce (goal within 4 hours) and maintain hypothermia for 24 hours. This was followed by a slow rewarming period over 12 hours. Midazolam and vecuronium were used for sedation and paralysis to prevent shivering.

The results were impressive with an improvement in 6 month mortality from 55 to 41% (RR, 0.74; CI: 0.58–0.95) and favorable neurological outcome from 39 to 55% (RR 1.4; CI: 1.08–1.81).

The second study randomized 77 patients from four Australian hospitals to either hypothermia (33 °C) for 12 hours or normothermia. Cooling was initiated immediately by paramedics applying cold packs to the head and torso. Midazolam and vecuronium were used to prevent shivering and aid temperature modulation. This study did not exclude older patients or those with prolonged hypoxia. The primary outcome variable of favorable outcome (defined as hospital discharge to home or a rehabilitation facility) was improved from 26 to 49% (p < 0.05) After adjustments for age, baseline characteristics, and time for return of spontaneous circulation, the odds ratio for good outcome improved to 5.25 (CI: 1.47–18.76, p = 0.011).

On the basis of these studies the American Heart Association and the Task force of the International Liaison Committee on Resuscitation (ILCOR) recommended therapeutic hypothermia (33 °C) for 12–24 hours post-cardiac resuscitation in patients with a presenting cardiac arrhythmia of ventricular fibrillation or ventricular tachycardia. A meta-analysis concluded that 6 patients would need to be treated to allow for 1 patient to leave the hospital in good condition.

Therapeutic Hypothermia in Hospital Arrest and for Nonventricular Fibrillation Arrest

Given the success of these studies, there is considerable interest in expanding the use of hypothermia after cardiac arrest beyond the inclusion criteria of the initial studies. The majority of patients after cardiac arrest present in either asystole or PEA. There is increased risk of neurological injury in patients presenting with asystole or PEA since these rhythms most likely degenerated from preceding ventricular tachycardia or fibrillation. Thus, asystole or PEA in these circumstances will represent an agonal end stage arrhythmia with a longer period of cerebral ischemia or anoxia. In addition, asystole and PEA will most likely represent a no-flow condition while ventricular tachycardia and fibrillation may represent a persistent low-flow state.

Small pilot trials appear to confirm these suspicions with only 7% of patients surviving after the return of spontaneous circulation in patients presenting with either asystole or PEA. Given the low survival rate and poor outcome in this population, the number of patients needed to achieve

Table 21.1. Potential mechanisms for the beneficial effect of hypothermia

Prevention of apoptosis*	Ischaemia can induce apoptosis and calpain-mediated proteolysis Hypothermia can prevent or reduce this process	Hours to many days or even weeks
Reduced mitochondrial dysfunction, improved energy homoeostasis[†]	Mitochondrial dysfunction is a frequent occurrence in the hours to days after an episode of ischaemia, and might be linked to apoptosis Hypothermia reduces metabolic demands and might improve mitochondrial function	Hours to days
Reduction of excessive free radical production[†]	Production of free radicals such as superoxide, peroxynitrite, hydrogen peroxide, and hydroxyl radicals is typical in ischaemia Mild-to-moderate hypothermia (30–35°) is able to reduce this event	Hours to days
Mitigation of reperfusion injury[†]	Cascade of reactions following reperfusion, partly mediated by free radicals but with distinctive and a range of features Suppressed by hypothermia	Hours to days
Reduced permeability of the blood-brain barrier and the vascular wall; reduced oedema formation*	Blood-brain barrier disruptions induced by trauma or ischaemia are moderated by hypothermia. The same effect occurs with vascular permeability and capillary leakage	Hours to days
Reduced permeability of cellular membranes (including membranes of the cell nucleus)[†]	Decreased leakage of cellular membranes, with associated improvements in cell function and cellular homoeostasis, including decrease of intracellular acidosis and mitigation of DNA injury	Hours to days
Improved ion homoeostasis[†]	Ischaemia induces accumulation of excitatory neurotransmitters such as glutamate and prolonged excessive influx of Ca^{2+} into the cell. This activates numerous enzyme systems (kinases) and induces a state of permanent hyperexcitability (exitotoxic cascade), which can be moderated by hypothermia	First minutes to 72 h
Reduction of metabolism*	Cellular oxygen and glucose requirements decrease by an average of 5–8% per degree Celsius decrease in temperature	Hours to days
Depression of the immune response and various potentially harmful proinflammatory reactions*	Sustained destructive inflammatory reactions and secretion of proinflammatory cytokines after ischaemia can be blocked or mitigated by hypothermia	First hour to 5 days

Table 21.1. (*Continued*)

Reduction in cerebral thermopooling*	Some areas in the brain have significantly higher temperatures than the surrounding areas and measured core temperature. These differences can increase dramatically during injury, with up to 2–3°C higher temperatures in injured areas of the brain. Hyperthermia can increase the damage to injured brain cells; this is mitigated by hypothermia	Minutes to many days
Anticoagulant effects*	Microthrombus formation might add to brain injury after CPR. Anticoagulant effects of hypothermia might protect against thrombus formation. Thrombolytic therapy has been shown to improve outcome after CPR[7]	Minutes to days
Suppression of epileptic activity and seizures*	Many patients experience seizures after ischaemic episodes or trauma, or both, which might add to injury. Hypothermia has been shown to mitigate epileptic activity	Hours to days

On the basis of observations in animal studies, with some support from clinical observations (e.g., reduction in inflammatory response and pro-inflammatory cytokine levels associated with hypothermia after traumatic brain injury and CPR: decrease in excitatory transmitters measured using microdialysis probes in human beings; decrease in local brain hyperthermia). CPR-cardiopulmonary resuscitation. *Some supporting clinical evidence. †Animal studies only.
Reproduced from Polderman KH, 2008 with permission from Elsevier.

statistical significance in a randomized trial would be unfeasible. Nevertheless, given the safety of therapeutic hypothermia there appears little reason not to consider initiating a protocol.

An in-hospital cardiac arrest differs from an out-of-hospital arrest in several features. The response time and return of spontaneous circulation may be faster during in-house resuscitation. Patients in cardiac care units can often have their circulation restored immediately with little neurological effect. Out-of-hospital cardiac arrest is primarily attributed to underlying cardiac disease, while in-hospital cardiac arrest can be secondary to a number of factors, including respiratory insufficiency, sepsis, pulmonary embolism, electrolyte abnormalities, etc.

The rate of survival to hospital discharge after in-hospital cardiac arrest is only 18% according to data obtained from the National Registry of Cardiopulmonary Resuscitation. Given this poor survival rate, the feasibility of performing a con-

trolled trial is unlikely. However, in selected patients where neurological injury is probable, the use of therapeutic hypothermia seems warranted. The Post Cardiac Arrest Care Section of the 2010 *American Heart Association Guideline for Cardiopulmonary Resuscitation and Emergency Cardiovascular Care* suggests that induced hypothermia may be considered for comatose patients with a return of spontaneous circulation after in-house cardiac arrest or out-of-house cardiac arrest with an initial rhythm of asytole or PEA.

Application of Therapeutic Hypothermia: Technical Aspects

The optimal timing, technique, and duration of therapeutic hypothermia are currently unknown. Animal studies suggest that hypothermia should be initiated as soon as possible post-cardiac arrest. Better neurological outcomes are achieved in laboratory animals if cooling is initiated during resuscitation; however, clinical studies have yet to verify this observation. In fact, even delayed hypothermia may provide some benefit. In the European study, the target temperature was not attained for 16 hours in many patients. Various methods to achieve hypothermia have, however, been developed since the initial studies. The European study applied forced-air-cooling blankets upon arrival at the hospital. The Australian study applied ice packs to the head and torso. Cooling was initiated by emergency personnel during transport to the hospital. Each technique has selected advantages and disadvantages: cooling blankets took longer to achieve therapeutic target temperatures, however ice packs may be more cumbersome and make the titration of exact temperatures difficult.

Newer cooling devices applied directly to the limbs and torso have been developed. The temperature can be closely regulated through a feedback mechanism from bladder thermometers. These devices are noninvasive and can be applied by nursing or auxiliary personnel. Skin care is also important since devices left in place for extended periods can lead to burns.

Invasive cooling devices that have also been developed are placed in a central vein using the same technique for central line placement. Temperature control is modulated through iced saline infused into a bladder which is in contact with venous blood. The procedure is invasive, requires physician placement, and carries all the risks of an invasive line. The technique, however, may achieve faster times to target temperatures and can be placed during other procedures such as cardiac catheterization.

Other methods currently being studied are nasopharyngeal cooling through the use of perfluorochemical evaporation administered via nasal prongs. This is effective in decreasing forebrain temperature in animal studies and is currently being investigated in clinical trials. The infusion of large volumes of intravenous iced crystalloids is also effective in lowering the body temperature quickly. Clinical trials to date suggest that pulmonary edema has not been problematic with the use of iced crystalloids.

The optimal duration of hypothermia is also unknown. Preclinical studies suggest that longer hypothermic time may improve outcome but will need further study for clinical verification.

Another question not addressed by the current state of the literature is whether noncomatose survivors of cardiac arrest may benefit from therapeutic hypothermia. These studies will require a long-term follow up and more sensitive measures of cognitive outcome.

Shivering will greatly increase the cerebral metabolic rate and can actually impair the neuroprotective effects of therapeutic hypothermia. Care to prevent and manage shivering is crucial for the induction and maintenance of hypothermia. In the European and Australian studies, patient shivering was prevented through heavy sedation and paralysis, using both midazolam and vecuronium. Sedation and paralysis were continued during the rewarming phase.

In practice, a series of medications and maneuvers can be used to prevent shivering. The highest number and density of skin temperature receptors are found on the face, hands, and feet. Surface counter rewarming with attention to the hand, feet, and face can provide sufficient hypothalamic feedback in many instances to prevent shivering. This approach may seem counterintuitive since surface or intravascular cooling may occur with surface warming of the hands and face. Rewarming of these thermoregulators can suppress shivering while allowing the maintenance of hypothermia.

A number of medications are also used to suppress shivering. Traditional measures using acetaminophen and/or ibuprofen are largely ineffective in temperature control and the prevention of shivering in the brain-injured patient. The most effective medication to prevent shivering is meperedine; however, it must be used judiciously, given its multiple metabolites and poor side effect profile (most notably, lowering the seizure threshold). Intravenous magnesium lowers the shivering threshold and may provide some neuroprotective effects. Some authors suggest maintaining magnesium levels between 3 and 4 mg/dL. Buspirone is a serotonin 1A partial agonist often used to prevent shivering. It is less sedating than many of the other medications listed and can be used in combination with other agents. Dexetomidate used as a drip or in combination with meperidine or buspirone can be particularly effective in controlling shivering. A stepwise protocol with increasing measures to decrease shivering can also be employed. Shivering management is reviewed in Mahmood (2007).

There are many potential complications that can develop with the use of therapeutic hypothermia. The most worrisome are bleeding and sepsis. Multiple metabolic derangements are also common with induced hypothermia and can include the development of a metabolic acidosis, hyperglycemia, and hypokalemia. Lactate levels are commonly elevated during hypothermia, however levels above 5–6 mmol/L should raise concern for sepsis or worsening cardiac function.

Rewarming is performed slowly to avoid rapid electrolyte shifts (hyperkalemia can occur in the rewarming stage as potassium shifts into the extracellular space), vasodilation, shivering, and potential worsening neurological injury. The European study allowed for passive rewarming over 8 hours while the Australian study initiated controlled rewarming over 6 hours.

Neurological Prognostication after Therapeutic Hypothermia

Determining neurological prognosis after cardiac arrest may be more difficult with the use of therapeutic hypothermia. In 2006 the American Academy of Neurology developed practice parameters for the prediction of neurological outcome in comatose patients after cardiac arrest. Almost 400 publications were reviewed and recommendations were based and categorized on a progressive classification scheme. Clinical features that were predictive of poor outcome included: myoclonic status epilepticus within the first 24 hours, absent pupillary or corneal responses within the first 3 days, or absent or extensor posturing after 3 days. The bilateral absence of the N20 component of the somatosensory-evoked potential recorded 1–3 days post event was similarly predictive of poor outcome. The biochemical marker, neuron-specific enolase, was predictive of poor outcome if a level of 33 µg/L or greater is recorded 1–3 days post event.

Therapeutic hypothermia confounded normal neurological prognosis after cardiac arrest from many potential mechanisms. One possible mechanism is through the effect on drug metabolism. A systematic review of 21 studies evaluated the effects of hypothermia and rewarming on metabolism and drug disposition. These studies suggested that the clearance of medications metabolized by the enzyme cytochrome P450 were decreased 7–22% for each change in degree Celsius. This would have considerable influence on many sedative medications commonly used in patients' post-cardiac arrest.

The prognostic significance of biochemical markers and physiological studies in cardiac arrest patients treated with therapeutic hypothermia has also been studied in small series. In one study a decrease in neuron-specific enolase obtained 24–48 hours post event was associated with good neurological outcome. This was more commonly found in patients treated with therapeutic hypothermia. In another study a neuron-specific enolase level of >33 µg/L had a false positive rate of 29%.

The utility of somatosensory-evoked potentials has also been questioned in the setting of therapeutic hypothermia. Two out of 36 patients tested with bilateral absence N20 responses had good outcomes. While the majority of patients had poor outcomes, the authors concluded that absent N20 responses alone should not be used to limit therapies. Similarly, 4 of 6 patients with post-anoxic status treated with therapeutic hypothermia had moderate recoveries. One patient was described as having a complete neurological recovery.

The neurological examination continues to be the most useful for prognostic guidance in patients treated with therapeutic hypothermia after cardiac arrest. Rosetti et al. (2010) studied 111 patients treated with hypothermia post-cardiac arrest. The clinical findings of incomplete brainstem reflexes, myoclonus, and absent motor responses obtained 3 days post-arrest individually had a false positive rate that varied between 4 and 24%. Interestingly, two of these findings in combination continued to have prognostic significance for poor outcome. A nonreactive EEG was also incompatible with a good functional outcome. A retrospective series from the Mayo Clinic compared neurological findings in 103 patients treated with hypothermia post-cardiac arrest and compared them with 89 patients that were not treated with therapeutic hypothermia. In this series the findings of absent pupillary, corneal, or motor responses 3 days post-cardiac arrest remained predictive of poor neurological outcome. More work will need to be done in this area.

The Use of Therapeutic Hypothermia in other Neurological Diseases

Traumatic Brain Injury

The application of therapeutic hypothermia has not been limited to cerebral anoxic damage. Over the past 20 years several clinical studies have assessed the efficacy of therapeutic hypothermia after traumatic brain injury. There were significant variations in trial design and treatment protocols. Although results varied, there were enough positive trends in outcomes to fund larger clinical trials.

What appeared to be clear from these clinical studies was that hypothermia was effective in lowering intracranial pressure. What was unknown was whether the induction of hypothermia could improve long-term patient outcome. In 2001 a controlled trial of 392 patients randomized patients to therapeutic hypothermia or normothermia. The target goal was to reach, and maintain, a temperature of 33 °C for 48 hours. There was no improvement in mortality or functional outcome. However, on subset analysis there was a trend for patients that were younger than 40, and patients that were hypothermic on presentation (that were randomized to the hypothermia group), to show significant improvement.

⚛ SCIENCE REVISITED

The decrease in intracranial pressure found with hypothermia is most likely accounted for by a decrease in cerebral metabolic rate. A decrease in cerebral metabolic rate will be accompanied by a decrease in cerebral blood flow and subsequent cerebral blood volume. Since the brain is enclosed within a fixed space (the skull), a decrease in blood volume will result in a decrease in pressure. Long-term benefits of hypothermia may be secondary to decreases in the formation of cerebral edema.

A subsequent trial of hypothermia initiated soon after injury also failed to show any benefit of therapeutic hypothermia. A subset analysis of this study, however, revealed that patients who were randomized to hypothermia and had had surgical evacuation of a subdural hematoma had a trend toward better outcomes that those who were maintained at normal temperatures. Currently the 2007 Guidelines for Severe Traumatic Brain Injury state that there is insufficient data to support the use of therapeutic hypothermia for traumatic brain injury. A review by the Cochrane data group in 2009 made similar recommendations.

Despite the failure of large clinical trials to reveal any benefit for hypothermia in traumatic brain injury, some enthusiasm for this treatment remains. One possible explanation for the failure of efficacy may be that the duration of treatment was insufficient. There is some preliminary data to suggest that maintaining hypothermia for greater than 48 hours may improve the outcome. A meta-analysis of several small series reported an improved outcome when hypothermia is continued for 2–5 days post-traumatic injury. The Eurotherm 3235 Trial is a multicenter randomized-controlled trial scheduled to enroll 1800 patients over 41 months. In this trial hypothermia will be maintained for an indefinite period to maintain an intracranial pressure below 20 mm/Hg.

Ischemic Stroke

Therapeutic hypothermia has been investigated for the treatment of ischemic stroke. The application of therapeutic hypothermia to noncomatose patients may be difficult since conscious patients may require significant amounts of sedation to induce hypothermia and prevent shivering.

The feasibility of inducing hypothermia in conscious patients with an ischemic stroke was initially tested in a phase I trial and was subsequently followed by a phase II study. In the Cooling for Acute Ischemic Brain Damage II study, 18 patients were randomized to a target temperature of 33 °C within 12 hours of onset and were compared to 22 patients with standard medical therapy. The target temperature was maintained for 24 hours. In the hypothermic group, mean diffusion-weighted imaging lesion growth was lower than in the nontreated group but the results were statistically insignificant. There was also no difference in the long-term outcome between treatment and control groups. Approximately 40% of the patients treated with hypothermia required endotracheal intubation. While these trials demonstrated the feasibility of applying hypothermia to this population, they were not powered sufficiently to address questions of efficacy.

A similar study analyzing CSF volumes on computed tomography scans as a surrogate for cerebral edema, demonstrated a tendency for decreased amounts of post-stroke cerebral edema in 18 patients treated with therapeutic hypothermia as compared to a control group. In this study, however, CSF volumes normalized within 30 days and infarct volumes and functional outcomes were no different.

Therapeutic hypothermia has been evaluated for the management of malignant cerebral edema in large hemispheric infarcts. Reported mortality rates were better than historical controls but worse than those reported with hemicraniectomy. These trials were hindered by medical complications and difficulties with managing rebound intracranial hypertension during the rewarming phase. Therapeutic hypothermia combined with hemicraniectomy was studied and 25 patients randomized to either hemicraniectomy alone or in combination with hypothermia. Mortality was 12% in both groups and there was a trend for improved NIH stroke scores for the hypothermia group.

The above studies appear to suggest that hypothermia alone may be ineffective in ischemic stroke; however, it may serve as an effective adjuvant treatment. To that end trials are currently underway, including hypothermia coupled with IV thrombolytic therapy (in an attempt to extend the window for administration of tPA) and other pharmacologic agent such as caffeine and ethanol. To date, however, the American Heart Association guidelines for the treatment of acute ischemic stroke cannot recommend the use of therapeutic hypothermia.

Subarachnoid Hemorrhage

A single study assessed the feasibility of applying and maintaining therapeutic hypothermia after subarachnoid hemorrhage for the treatment of recalcitrant cerebral edema. Twenty-one high-grade patients after subarachnoid hemorrhage (SAH) were treated with therapeutic hypothermia. One group was treated for less than 72 hours and another for greater than 72 hours. No difference was noted on functional independence after 3 months.

The success of intraoperative hypothermia in patients undergoing cardiopulmonary bypass or temporary circulatory arrest has led to an interest in expanding this modality to other neurosurgical procedures. The Intraoperative Hypothermia for Aneurysm Surgery Trial randomized 1001 good grade SAH patients to an intraoperative temperature of 33 °C or to a normothermia group with a temperature of 36.5 °C. No statistical difference was noted in ICU or hospital length of stay or 6-month functional outcome. The lack of difference in functional outcome may be attributed to the overall good clinical condition of these patients.

Intracerebral Hemorrhage

No study to date has assessed therapeutic hypothermia in the treatment of intracerebral hemorrhage.

Status Epilepticus

One small case series reported control of refractory status epilepticus when therapeutic hypothermia was added as an adjuvant therapy. No systematic trials have been studied.

Spinal Cord Injury

Animal models evaluating cooling strategies in thoracic and cervical contusions have reported improved locomotive function and forelimb grip strength after treatment with therapeutic hypothermia. To date no clinical studies have been undertaken. The American Association of Neurological Surgeons/Neurological and Spinal Surgery Joint Sections of the Disorders of the Spine and the Joint Section of Trauma state that there is no evidence to recommend either for or against the practice of therapeutic hypothermia as a treatment for acute spinal cord injury.

Conclusions

Significant preclinical and basic science work supporting the use of therapeutic hypothermia to treat neurological injury was verified in two studies reporting improved neurological outcomes after cardiac arrest with the use of induced mild hypothermia.

While the exact mechanism of action is unknown, therapeutic cooling is known to affect several steps in the ischemic cascade of neurological injury.

The implementation of therapeutic hypothermia requires initiation soon after resuscitation, and preclinical models suggest that cooling should start during resuscitation. The questions still remain as to the timing and duration of treatment and to whether this treatment can be extended to cardiac arrest if the initial discovered rhythm is a systole or pulseless electrical activity. Clinical work evaluating the effects of hypothermia on neurological prognostication after cardiac arrest is currently underway. The expansion of therapeutic hypothermia to other areas of neurological injury has been less successful. Enthusiasm continues for its use in traumatic brain injury, although clinical trials to date have not been able to provide evidence for a benefit. Further work is needed in neurological ischemia from subarachnoid hemorrhage and intracerebral hemorrhage. Therapeutic hypothermia may prove beneficial as an adjuvant treatment for acute ischemic stroke.

Bibliography

Badjatia N. Hyperthermia and fever control in brain injury. *Crit Care Med* 2009; **37(Suppl)**: S250–S257.

Bernard S. Hypothermia after cardiac arrest: Expanding the therapeutic scope. *Crit Care Med* 2009; **37:** S227–S233.

Bernard SA, Gray T, Buist MD, et al. Treatment of comatose survivors of out of hospital cardiac arrest with induced hypothermia. *New Engl J Med* 2002; **346:** 557–563.

Clifton GL, Valadka A, Zygun D, et al. Very early hypothermia induction in patients with sever brain injury (the National Acute Brain Injury Study: Hypothermia II): a randomized trial. *Lancet Neurol* 2011; **10:** 131–139.

Fugate JE, Wijdicks EFM, Mandreker J, et al. Predictors of outcome and patient surviving cardiac arrest. *Ann Neurol* 2010; **68:** 907–914.

Ginsberg MD, Sternau LL, Globus MY, et al. Therapeutic modulation of brain temperature: relevance to ischemic brain injury. *Cerebrovasc Brain Metab Rev* 1992; **4:** 189–225.

Holzer M, Bernard SA, Hachimi-Idrissi S, et al. (on behalf of the Collaborative Group in Induce Hypothermia for Neuroprotection after Cardiac Arrest). Hypothermia for neuroprotection after Cardiac arrest: Systematic review and individual patient data meta-analysis. *Crit Care Med* 2005; **33:** 414–418.

Linares G, Mayer SA. Hypothermia for treatment of ischemic and hemorrhagic stroke. *Crit Care Med* 2009; **37(Suppl):** S243–S249.

Mahmood MA, Zweifler RM. Progresss in shivering control. *J Neurol Sci* 2007; **261:** 47–54.

Polderman KH, Herold I. Therapeutic hypothermia and controlled normothermia in the intensive care unit: Practical considerations, side effects, and cooling methods. *Crit Care Med* 2009; **37:** 1101–1120.

Polderman KH. Induced hypothermia and fever control for prevention and treatment of neurological injuries. *Lancet* 2008; **371:** 1955–1969.

Rosetti AO, Oddo M, Logroscino G, Kaplan PW. Prognostication after cardiac arrest and hypothermia. A postoperative study. *Ann Neurol* 2010; **67:** 301–307.

The Hypothermia After Cardiac Arrest Study Group. Mild therapeutic hypothermia to improve the neurological outcome after cardiac arrest. *New Engl J Med* 2002; **346:** 549–556.

Etiologies of Posterior Reversible Encephalopathy Syndrome and Forms of Osmotic Demyelination Syndrome

J. Javier Provencio

Cerebrovascular Center, Cleveland Clinic, Cleveland, OH, USA

Introduction

Among the myriad of diseases that can cause acute neurological dysfunction, two which are commonly linked together, are the syndrome of posterior reversible encephalopathy (PRES) and osmotic demyelination syndrome (ODS). These two diseases have a number of things in common, which make them natural partners for this chapter.

First, they are both poorly named. PRES and its common subtypes have gone through a number of name changes, including hypertensive encephalopathy, eclampsia-associated encephalopathy, and transplant-associated encephalopathy. It has been recognized that all of these syndromes are probably the same process manifesting in a number of different disease states. The term "PRES" has largely been settled on in the literature despite the fact that the injury in PRES is not always (and not even commonly) posterior and is not always reversible. This leaves only the words "encephalopathy" and "syndrome" that are accurate, but they are so vague that they are not useful. There has been at least one call to change the name again to "neurotoxic vasogenic edema syndrome" based on a theory of the true cause of the edema

(Bartynski, 2008). As this theory is still not well tested, I suggest that we stick with PRES at the moment.

In the case of ODS, there have also been a number of names given to the syndrome, including central pontine myelinolysis and extrapontine myelinolysis. Again, when it was recognized that these were the same syndrome with different manifestations, the term "osmotic demyelination" was adopted. Unlike PRES, however, this name actually does represent what occurs in this disease.

Second, both of these syndromes reflect aberrations of control of water in the brain and both lead to edema. In the case of PRES the problem seems to be in the control of the blood–brain barrier leading to the development of vasogenic edema; in ODS, the central aberration is the loss of the ability to regulate the osmotic milieu of the brain parenchyma leading eventually to the development of cytotoxic edema.

In this chapter, we will take each syndrome in turn. We will discuss the prevailing theories about their causes because they inform our decisions for treatment. We will discuss the common presentations in the patients, including subgroups, that are most affected. We will discuss

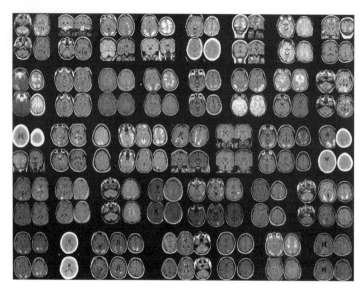

Figure 22.1. Neuroimages of 38 patients with reversible posterior leukocephalopathies. The top row represents the initial images while the bottom row represents repeat imaging at a later point. Note that not all leukoencephalopathies are posterior. (Reproduced from Lee et al., 2008. Copyright © (2008) American Medical Association. All rights reserved.)

imaging including the pitfalls to making the correct diagnosis. Finally, we will discuss treatment algorithms based on the prevailing theories.

It is important to note that as both of these entities are less common and, therefore, do not avail themselves to large clinical treatment trials, the algorithms will be based on small trials, common practices, and the theory of the cause of the insult. In addition, particularly in regard to PRES, there is still controversy surrounding the actual cause and, therefore, the treatment that should be implemented. The chapter will include the common treatment algorithm with the understanding that in the near future it may fall out of favor. An attempt will be made to highlight areas that are likely to change in the future.

Posterior Reversible Encephalopathy

PRES has been recognized in one form or another for decades but the initial published reports dealt exclusively with patients with a single instigating disease (reviewed in Hefzy et al., 2009). The earliest reports were from the obstetric literature where it was noticed that women with eclampsia occasionally developed an encephalopathic syndrome that, on computer tomography (CT) scans of the head, showed hypodensities suggesting edema in the occipital and parietal lobes. Not long after, reports in patients with accelerated hypertension surfaced. Because both of these original entities shared hypertension as a cardinal feature, it was assumed that the edema was due directly to the hypertension. The initial common theory was that the pressure induced locally by the hypertension caused damage to the blood–brain barrier and water was forced into the brain. This theory could be called into question for two reasons: (1) the amount of hypertension does not predict who will develop PRES, or its severity (in fact, most patients with PRES do not have sufficiently high blood pressure to overcome cerebral autoregulation); and (2) clinical scenarios would become apparent (including medication toxicities) in which hypertension was not a prominent feature. Despite the change in name and understanding of the links to hypertension, antihypertensive therapy remains an important pillar of therapy.

★ TIPS & TRICKS

PRES is not just a disease of hypertension. Thinking of the disorder as a toxic phenomenon will help determine and ameliorate the cause. At risk populations include chronic hypertension, pregnancy, solid organ transplantation particularly those on cyclosporine and tacralimus.

PRES has now been described in a multitude of disease processes. The most common include pre-eclampsia/eclampsia, accelerated hypertension with no other cause, allogenic bone marrow transplantation (allo-BMT), in patients taking cyclosporine (and occasionally tacrolimus), in patients with autoimmune diseases (with or without cyclosporine treatment), and in patients receiving chemotherapy. Interestingly, of the patients taking cyclosporine who develop PRES, those with hypertension seem to have less severe vasogenic edema than patients who do not have hypertension, calling into question whether hypertension is truly the cause of PRES.

If not hypertension, then it is clear that the process leading to PRES must have the ability to affect both the brain and be associated with hypertension in some patients. The obvious body systems that have the potential to affect the blood–brain barrier (BBB) integrity and lead to hypertension are the kidneys and the endothelial cells of the vasculature. It is still not certain if either of these systems is the ultimate cause of PRES but both deserve further discussion.

Interestingly, eclampsia, accelerated hypertension, cyclosporine, and autoimmune disorders all share renal failure as a common manifestation. The rennin angiotensin system is important in the regulation of blood pressure, and stenosis of the renal artery clearly leads to accelerated hypertension. How the renal system would affect the permeability of the cerebral vasculature to water is still not clear. The release of vascular endothelial growth factor from the kidney is one possible mechanism.

In regard to the vascular endothelium, there are more mechanisms to consider. It is clear that eclampsia leads to endothelial dysfunction and endothelial damage in some cases. Hypertension also has detrimental effects on the endothelium, as does cyclosporine and other chemotherapeutic agents. The effects of autoimmune diseases on the endothelium are less well studied, and have conflicting findings. There is also the possibility that this syndrome develops either independently or from the interplay between the above mechanisms.

The implication of this non-hypertension mediated alternative theory (that cyclosporine is directly toxic to blood vessels and is therefore the cause of PRES) is that our current therapy of lowering blood pressure may be detrimental. Hypertension and its associated vasoconstriction may decrease the amount of blood that crosses that damaged vasculature, subsequently decreasing the amount of edema (this may account for the finding in cyclosporine patients that hypertension is associated with more limited disease). In addition, hypertension may have the additional effect of helping to perfuse distal arterial beds, limiting damage to the blood vessels and preventing further edema (similar to findings in stroke).

Although water has previously been thought to transit across the BBB easily, this is now known to be mediated by a specific channel, aquaporin-4. Work in animals suggests that water transport across the BBB is regulated in large part by aquaporin-4, and recent work has identified aquaporin-4 as a possible agent in the development of PRES.

⚗ SCIENCE REVISITED

PRES has been thought of as hypertensive encephalopathy. There is considerable evidence that PRES presents itself in patients without hypertension or in patients in whom hypertension does not seem to be the culprit. Newer theories of PRES suggest that there are multiple mechanisms that may injure brain vascular endothelial cells. It is important to take nonhypertensive causes of PRES, even in patients with a history of hypertension.

Imaging

The imaging of PRES can be difficult for the nonradiologist. The common, textbook images show patients with occipital and parietal bilateral vasogenic edema affecting both the cortex and subcortical white matter on either CT or MRI of the brain. In fact, the other common sites for PRES include the frontal lobes, the inferior temporal-occipital junction, and the cerebellum. Although bilateral lesions are the most common finding, there are reports of mostly unilateral or asymmetrical patterns. In some patients, the occipital and parietal lobes are not involved. Some authors have attempted to categorize the localization into three subtypes: holocerebral, superior frontal, and occipital-parietal. This classification, although tempting, has many exceptions and may be an oversimplification.

★ TIPS & TRICKS

PRES was originally thought to only present in the occipital lobes. Although a significant number of patients have some occipital lobe involvement, lesions can appear anywhere in the white matter with edema extending to the cortex.

The vasogenic edema in PRES usually resolves completely within a week. In some patients, however, intracerebral hemorrhage and stroke have been noted in the areas of PRES. There are reports of permanent damage, particularly in patients with eclampsia. The one finding that is consistent in PRES is the presence of diffusion-weighted lesions without changes in the actual diffusion coefficient (ADC) suggesting vasogenic edema and not infarction. In less than classic cases, consultation with a radiologist with experience in neurologic imaging can be very helpful.

Treatment

Because of the lack of conclusive evidence for the causative agent for PRES, the treatment has centered on stopping the offending agent and controlling the blood pressure. In the case of eclampsia, there is evidence that the placenta may be the offending agent. If PRES occurs during the pregnancy, delivery of the baby is almost always curative. If it occurs after the birth of the child, retained placental products are often found and removal seems to be curative.

☠ CAUTION

Lowering blood pressure precipitously in patients with chronic hypertension may lead to ischemia due to the shift of the autoregulation curve toward hypertension.

In the case of cyclosporine toxicity, stopping the cyclosporine often helps to resolve the issue. This may not be a simple decision since patients often take cyclosporine to prevent organ rejection after solid organ transplant. The decision to stop cyclosporine may risk failure of the transplanted organ. Failure to stop the medicine, in our experience, has lead to a continuation of the edema. With the approval of tacrolimus, the decision whether to continue or stop cyclosporine was made easier. In many cases, changing to tacrolimus has helped to resolve the PRES. Although there are case reports of tacrolimus-induced PRES, they are less frequent.

☠ CAUTION

In patients with solid organ transplantation where cyclosporine or tacralimus are thought to be the culprit, stopping these drugs acutely may lead to acute organ rejection and death. Close consultation with the transplant physicians is important.

Autoimmune disorders pose a particular problem. Many patients with autoimmune disorders take immunosuppressive medications including cyclosporine. It can be a difficult to determine if the autoimmune disease or the treatment is the culprit. If the autoimmune disease is to blame, the rational treatment is to intensify therapy. The converse would be true if the treatment is to blame.

The second mainstay of therapy is hypertension control. As mentioned earlier, this may be of benefit or may be detrimental. In patients with accelerated hypertension as the cause of PRES, it seems reasonable to lower the blood pressure cautiously. It is important to remember that patients with prolonged untreated hypertension have a shifted cerebral autoregulation curve that may predispose them to ischemia at pressures that we would normally consider normotensive. For this reason, in our institution, we lower mean arterial blood pressure by about 15% from the highest recorded value. The exception to this rule is in patients who have significant enough edema to increase the intracranial pressure. In this situation, lowering the mean arterial pressure to a pressure that will keep the cerebral perfusion pressure (CPP) greater than 60 mm/Hg seems reasonable (although untested in this patient population).

Because the science behind PRES is still unclear, it is possible that the treatment strategy may change with new studies. Ultimately, supportive care with careful attention to complicating issues in the intensive care unit may offer the most benefit. Renal failure seems to be associated with many of the processes that lead to PRES. The monitoring of renal function and consultation with a nephrologist may be of particular benefit.

Osmotic Demyelination Syndrome

ODS was first described in 1959 in 4 patients with myelin loss in the central pons. At the time, the syndrome was associated with poor nutrition (particularly in alcoholic patients). The association with sodium correction was made definitively in 1981.

The pathophysiology of ODS is not well understood. Almost all physicians have had the experience of a patient who becomes hyponatremic in the hospital and is inadvertently corrected faster than expected by algorithms of sodium replacement. In these cases, ODS is uncommon. The response of the clinician is invariably surprise and a feeling of luck. A better understanding of the physiology that leads to ODS would reveal that this patient is unlikely to become ill.

To understand ODS, it is important to understand water and sodium balance in the brain. Because of the unique relationship between the vascular endothelial cells, astrocytes and neurons that make up the BBB complex, solute management in the brain is dissimilar from that of many other parts of the body. Sodium moves across the BBB through an energy-dependent channel (Na-K ATPase pump). When the blood becomes hypo-osmolar, the oncotic pressure difference favors entry of water into the brain (which moves freely across the BBB). This results in cerebral edema. The immediate response from the astrocytes and endothelial cells is to move the sodium out of the brain, thereby decreasing the osmolarity of the brain interstitium and force water out of the brain. If the blood osmolarity increases acutely at this stage, the brain is usually capable of shifting sodium ions across the BBB quickly enough to prevent damage to the myelin.

The risk of ODS increases the longer the hypo-osmolarity is present. The ability of the brain to manage osmolarity with sodium efflux in the setting is limited and can be expended over time. Once the ability of the brain to manage osmolarity changes (by moving sodium out of the brain) is expended, the brain resorts to moving proteins and other complex chemicals, collectively called organic osmoles (often referred to as idiopathic osmoles) across the BBB to prevent the brain swelling. Although this process is effective at normalizing the osmolar gradient between the brain and the blood, the complex nature of the organic osmoles makes transport back to the brain slow. This increases the risk that if the blood osmolarity is rapidly corrected, the brain (needing to reaccumulate organic osmoles) takes a long time to normalize the gradient. During the time between the normalization of osmolarity of the blood and the slower process of re-establishing the organic osmoles, the concentration of blood is higher than that of the brain, leading to water movement from the brain to the blood. The ensuing change in water content causes demylination of susceptible brain tissues.

For many years, it was thought that ODS was a disease of alcoholics. This is likely due to the chronic hyponatremia and hypo-osmolarity associated with chronic alcoholism. This led to hypotheses that there may be deficiencies in specific nutritional cofactors that contribute to the predisposition to ODS. No cofactors have been found to date, and the current theory of organic osmole loss accounts for the syndrome well enough that other factors need not be considered. It is now recognized that patients with cancer, severely malnourished patients, solid organ transplantation patients, and patients who take medicines that cause the chronic syndrome of inappropriate antidiuretic hormone (SIADH), as well as other causes of chronic hyponatremia, are at increased risk of ODS.

There is still debate whether rapid correction of sodium in nonchronically hyponatremic individuals can overwhelm the Na-K ATPase pump. There is no conclusive evidence that this is the case but most practitioners practice prudence in the acute situation because there are rarely times when rapid correction of sodium is necessary. The exceptions are cases of severe hyponatremia with seizures or cardiac arrhythmias.

✋ CAUTION

Remember hidden sodium sources in intravenous fluids, medications and food in patients in whom sodium is being repleted. It is imperative that serum sodium levels be monitored frequently with appropriate changes in therapy based on these results. Reliable bedside sodium analysis is most advantageous.

⚙ SCIENCE REVISITED

ODS is due to the inability of the brain to rapidly adjust to osmolarity changes in blood after compensatory changes in the brain to control brain edema in the setting of chronic hyponatremia. Once organic osmoles are transported out of the brain, rapid correction can cause cell contraction and demyelination.

Imaging

The initial description of ODS focused on demyelination of the central pons region leading to the name central pontine myelinolisis (CPM). Later reports coined the term extrapontine myelinolysis (EPM). The term ODS is an attempt to unify the diagnosis based on the

pathophysiology. It is clear that certain parts of the brain, particularly deep gray structures, are more susceptible to demyelination. The reasons for this are unclear.

Imaging with MRI is more sensitive than CT. The lesions are hypointense on T1-weighted images and hyperintense on T2 and FLAIR lesion. There may be the T2 shine-through phenomenon on diffusion-weighted images (DWIs). The diagnosis is made by the acute development of lesions in classic areas in a patient with hyponatremia and acute neurological deterioration. The areas most often seen in this syndrome are the central pons, thalamus, basal ganglia, and deep cerebellar nuclei. Occasionally, the subcortical white matter is also affected. In some cases, this syndrome can be confused with PRES.

Treatment

There are no effective treatments for ODS, so prevention is the most important strategy. With reported mortality ranging from 6% to greater than 90% and permanent morbidity common, the careful and slow correction of sodium has become the norm. Most guides suggest correcting hyponatremia no faster than 10–12 mEq/L per day. There are clearly patients who survive rapid correction without demyelination and some patients who develop the syndrome at slower correction rates. There are reports that hypokalemia may potentiate the effects of rapid correction.

★ TIPS & TRICKS

ODS is better prevented than treated. Replete sodium no faster than 10–12 mEq/L/day particularly in patients susceptible to ODS: chronic alcoholics, severely malnourished patients, transplant and cancer patients.

There are a number of theoretical treatments that have been proposed. Acutely lowering serum sodium in a patient with symptoms of ODS could theoretically reverse some of the cellular contraction and may decrease morbidity. Administration of myoinositol, a naturally occurring intracellular osmole, could be taken up by the brain and mitigate the oncotic stress. Steroids and plasma pheresis have also been tested with good results in very small studies.

★ TIPS & TRICKS

It is prudent to cautiously replace sodium in all patients regardless of risk factors. Aggressive potassium replacement may also help prevent ODS.

Prognosis

There is a prevailing sentiment among neurologists that this syndrome has a very poor prognosis. This is partly due to the fact that the majority of patients encountered are alcoholic, and a neurological disability with limited home support structure entails a poor prognosis. The mortality in more recent studies may be as low as 6%, and there are cases that many neurologists see that do quite well. Good early rehabilitation may be important for good recovery.

Bibliography

Adams RD, Victor M, Mancall EL. Central pontine myelinolysis: a hitherto undescribed disease occurring in alcoholic and malnourished patients. *AMA Arch Neurol Psychiat* 1959; **81(2):** 154–172.

Adler S, Verbalis JG, Williams D. Effect of rapid correction of hyponatremia on the blood–brain barrier of rats. *Brain Res* 1995; **679(1):** 135–143.

Bartynski WS. Posterior reversible encephalopathy syndrome, part 1: fundamental imaging and clinical features. *Am J Neuroradiol* 2008; **29(6):** 1036–1042.

Bartynski WS. Posterior reversible encephalopathy syndrome, part 2: controversies surrounding pathophysiology of vasogenic edema. *Am J Neuroradiol* 2008; **29(6):** 1043–1049.

Bartynski WS, Boardman JF. Distinct imaging patterns and lesion distribution in posterior reversible encephalopathy syndrome. *Am J Neuroradiol* 2007; **28(7):** 1320–1327.

Hefzy HM, et al. Hemorrhage in posterior reversible encephalopathy syndrome: imaging and clinical features. *Am J Neuroradiol* 2009; **30(7):** 1371–1379.

King JD, Rosner MH. Osmotic demyelination syndrome. *Am J Med Sci* 2010; **339(6):** 561–567.

Kleinschmidt-DeMasters BK, Norenberg MD. Rapid correction of hyponatremia causes demyelination: relation to central pontine myelinolysis. *Science* 1981; **211(4486):** 1068–1070.

Lee VH, Wijdicks EFM, Manno EM, Rabinstein AA. Clinical spectrum of reversible posterior leukoencephalopathy syndrome. *Arch Neurol* 2008; **65:** 205–210.

Lien YH. Role of organic osmolytes in myelinolysis. A topographic study in rats after rapid correction of hyponatremia. *J Clin Invest* 1995; **95(4):** 1579–1586.

Mount DB. The brain in hyponatremia: both culprit and victim. *Semin Nephrol* 2009; **29(3):** 196–215.

Silver SM, et al. Myoinositol administration improves survival and reduces myelinolysis after rapid correction of chronic hyponatremia in rats. *J Neuropathol Exp Neurol* 2006; **65(1):** 37–44.

Sterns RH, Silver SM. Brain volume regulation in response to hypo-osmolality and its correction. *Am J Med* 2006; **119(7 Suppl 1):** S12–S16.

Verbalis JG, et al. Hyponatremia treatment guidelines 2007: expert panel recommendations. *Am J Med* 2007; **120(11 Suppl 1):** S1–S21.

Yang B, Zador Z, Verkman AS. Glial cell aquaporin-4 overexpression in transgenic mice accelerates cytotoxic rain swelling. *J Biol Chem* 2008; **283(22):** 15280–15286.

Part VI

Acute Neuroimaging and Neuromonitoring in Neurocritical Care

Application of MR Diffusion, CT Angiography and Perfusion Imaging in Stroke Neurocritical Care

Carlos Leiva-Salinas[1], Wade Smith[2] and Max Wintermark[3]

[1]Department of Radiology, Neuroradiology Division, University of Virginia, Charlottesville, VA, USA
[2]Department of Neurology, University of California, San Francisco, CA, USA
[3]Department of Radiology, Neuroradiology Division, University of Virginia, Charlottesville, VA, USA

Introduction

Stroke is one of the leading causes of mortality world wide. In the United States more than 750,000 new strokes occur each year and, approximately every 3 minutes, someone dies from a stroke. Furthermore, stroke is the leading cause of adult disability in North America; indeed, a significant portion of stroke victims are left with a devastating disability for the rest of their lives. The direct and indirect costs of a stroke represent a major economic burden to society and healthcare systems, and this is likely to increase in the years to come.

An ischemic stroke results from a reduction of the blood supply to the brain parenchyma, usually caused by the occlusion of an intracranial artery. Ischemic strokes account for more than 80% of strokes. Rapid determination of the cause and degree of existing brain injury, and of the vascular status, can be critical in making the correct therapeutic decision and limiting the extent of irreversible brain damage. In particular, thrombolytic agents and mechanical thrombo-

lytic devices have provided a means to improve the clinical outcome of acute ischemic stroke patients and to reduce the proportion of patients with disability and death.

The imaging evaluation of patients with suspected acute ischemic stroke has markedly changed over the past few years. With the advent of functional imaging modalities such as perfusion-CT (PCT), perfusion-weighted magnetic resonance (MR) imaging, and the development of fast and robust noninvasive angiographic techniques, neuroimaging is no limited to just anatomy. Routine imaging now includes vascular and perfusion imaging, which are used to guide therapy.

Therefore, it is important for all physicians caring for stroke patients to be familiar with current multimodal CT and MR stroke imaging. They should be familiar with the different components, strengths and limitations, and their role in stroke diagnosis, ischemic tissue characterization, and selection of patients for reperfusion therapies.

Emergency Management in Neurocritical Care, First Edition. Edited by Edward M. Manno.
© 2012 John Wiley & Sons, Ltd. Published 2012 by John Wiley & Sons, Ltd.

Why Image an Acute Stroke Patient?

Modern neuroimaging targets six main aspects of the initial assessment of patients suspected of an acute ischemic stroke: (1) exclusion of intracerebral hemorrhage, (2) exclusion of other stroke mimics, (3) confirmation and localization of ischemia, (4) localization of the clot, (5) differentiation of infarct core and penumbra, and (6) assessment of bleeding risk.

Perfusion imaging allows differentiation between infarcted brain tissue and potentially salvageable penumbra in acute cerebral ischemia. The presence and extent of an ischemic penumbra is time and patient dependent. A growing number of clinical trials have used the concept of penumbra to select patients for reperfusion therapy beyond 3–4.5 hours from symptom onset.

Vascular imaging provides an additional dimension to the understanding of individual stroke pathophysiology. Current noninvasive angiographic techniques allow for an acute assessment of the patient's vascular status, detecting both intracranial arterial occlusions and cervical artery pathology. Finally, imaging may also help to identify patients at an increased risk of hemorrhagic transformation after thrombolysis.

CT and MR Imaging of Acute Stroke

Exclusion of Intracranial Hemorrhage and Other Stroke Mimics

Up to 30% of patients initially diagnosed with ischemic stroke are later diagnosed with a stroke mimic. Three-quarters of these mimicking conditions are neurologic disorders, and many of them

can be diagnosed with imaging techniques. The most common include intracranial and subarachnoid hemorrhage, subdural hematoma, seizures, toxic/metabolic disturbances, and space-occupying lesions Interestingly, most patients with stroke mimics have a disorder that is likely to benefit from an urgent neurologic intervention.

Gradient-recalled echo (GRE) and other T2* sequences are equally sensitive for the detection of acute intracranial hemorrhage. For the evaluation of frequent nonhemorrhagic stroke mimics, MR imaging is clearly superior to NCT. In particular, conventional T2 and fluid attenuation inversion recovery (FLAIR) images can depict post-ictal changes, mass lesions, and some metabolic disorders, thus avoiding potentially harmful reperfusion stroke therapies.

Location of Ischemia

Diffusion-weighted MR imaging is the most sensitive imaging method for the depiction of hyperacute ischemia (see Plate 23.1). Although DWI lesions can be partially reversible in the very early phase of ischemia, baseline diffusion-weighted imaging (DWI) is useful in predicting the outcome and lesion volume in the majority of stroke patients. Direct visualization of the infarct core and assessment of the brain tissue viability is probably the main advantage of MR over CT in stroke patients.

Signs of cerebral ischemia on T2-weighted and FLAIR images are not visible until 3 hours post-stroke (see Plate 23.2). A "mismatch" between positive DWI and negative FLAIR allows for the identification of patients within the 3-hour time window with high specificity and positive predictive value.

The presence of early ischemic signs on NCT should not be considered a contraindication to thrombolytic treatment.

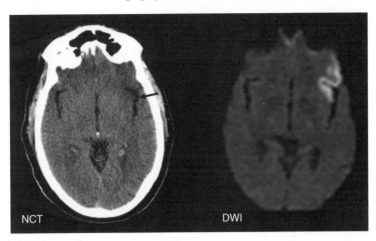

Figure 23.1. Insular ribbon sign in a 62 year-old man with suspected left MCA stroke. Noncontrast CT of the head (NCT) obtained 3 hours after the onset of symptoms shows loss of the definition of the left insular white-grey matter differentiation (black arrow). DW MR image (DWI) obtained 6 hours later shows the acute ischemic injury as a region of relative hyperintensity.

CT is comparable to T2-weighted or FLAIR magnetic resonance images in its ability to detect early signs of ischemic stroke. However infarct detection with NCT in the first 3 hours after onset has low sensitivity (25%), when compared with DWI-MR. CT sensitivity increases in the 6-hour time window to 40% or 60%. Early CT signs of ischemia include:

1. *Insular ribbon sign.* The insular cortex is supplied by the insular segment of the MCA and its branches. When the proximal middle cerebral artery is occluded, the insular ribbon is particularly vulnerable as it is the most distal region from the anterior and posterior cerebral collateral circulations. When ischemic, this region shows loss of definition of its gray–white interface (Figure 23.1).
2. *Obscuration of the lentiform nucleus.* Due to its blood supply through end-arteries, the basal ganglia are particularly vulnerable to early infarction, with obscuration of its contour (see Plate 23.2).
3. *Hyperdense artery sign.* Contrary to other CT signs of early brain ischemia, the dense artery sign hallmarks an acute thrombo-embolic event. This will be discussed later (Figure 23.2).

⚠ CAUTION

Unlike these subtle findings, areas of frank hypoattenuation are highly specific for infarct, and their extent is predictive of the clinical outcome and the risk of hemorrhagic transformation. As such, a frank hypoattenuation represents a contraindication to thrombolysis.

Location of Clot

CTA images demonstrate arterial abnormalities in up to 95% of patients with acute ischemic infarcts. MRA demonstrates abnormalities in 75% of cases.

3D time-of-flight (TOF) noncontrast MR angiography (MRA) is the preferred technique for the MR evaluation of intracranial vessels. This noncontrast MR sequence provides image contrast that is dependent on the flow of blood protons through a selected slab of brain (see Plate 23.2). For the evaluation of the extracranial arteries, additional contrast-enhanced sequences may be required. CT angiography (CTA) allows for the evaluation of both intra- and extracranial

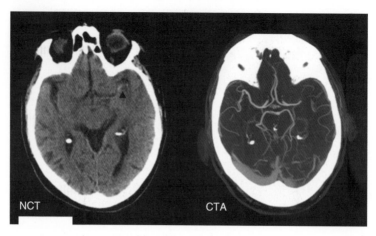

Figure 23.2. Hyperdense middle cerebral artery sign in a 76-year-old woman admitted to the emergency department after sudden onset of right face-arm-leg hemisyndrome. Non-contrast CT of the brain (NCT) shows a hyperdense left MCA (black arrowhead). Concurrent CTA maximum intensity projection (MIP) image shows a filling defect of the left MCA, consistent with an intraluminal thrombus.

vasculature, using one single contrast injection (see Plates 23.1, 23.3, and Figure 23.2).

Analysis of the source images is the most accurate approach to characterize the site of occlusion. An area on CTA that reveals a paucity of vessels has been shown to represent the infarct core with a sensitivity of 72% and a specificity of 98%. Analysis of the maximal intensity projection (MIP) images is the most accurate approach to characterize the degree of collateral circulation. The collateral flow estimate on MIP CTA images has been shown to be inversely related with the final infarct volume.

Patients that may benefit from recanalization should be differentiated on the basis of the amount of ischemic penumbra and the location of clots that can be treated with reperfusion therapies. The location of the clot has been shown to predict recanalization success. Patients with proximal MCA branch occlusion, tandem lesions, or significant thrombus burden, might be poor candidates for intravenous thrombolytics, and may be better candidates for intra-arterial or mechanical thrombolysis. Moreover, the pattern of vascular obstruction has a prognostic value in terms of the clinical outcome after recanalization. For example, early recanalization in a patient with an isolated middle cerebral artery occlusion has a higher rate of clinical response than a patient with a tandem ICA-MCA occlusion.

Conventional imaging can sometimes detect arterial clots. Due to the high concentration of deoxyhemoglobin in the acute thrombus, $T2^*$-weighted images are able to detect intraluminal clots as linear or dot-shaped low signal areas of magnetic susceptibility (Figure 23.3). Similarly, the presence of a hyperdense thrombus or embolus in the MCA creates a linear hyperattenuation on NCT. This has been labeled the "hyperdense middle cerebral artery sign." This sign is seen in approximately one-third of acute stroke patients and it is associated with poor clinical and radiologic outcome.

Differentiation of Infarct Core and Penumbra

In cerebral ischemia blood flow to a certain brain territory is compromised. The central core of tissue that dies initially is labeled the infarct core.

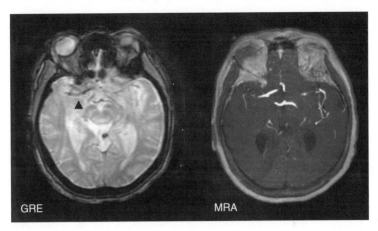

Figure 23.3. Thrombus detection of with gradient-recall echo (GRE) images in a patient with right MCA ischemic stroke. The linear black signal in the right MCA illustrates the susceptibility artifact crated by an acute thrombus (black arrowhead). The time-of-flight MR angiography (MRA) identify the site of occlusion in the M1 segment of the right MCA.

Surrounding this core is an area of brain that is hypoperfused but still viable. This area of brain, which is ischemic but potentially salvageable, is called the ischemic penumbra.

Brain imaging allows for the distinction of infarct core and penumbra by measuring capillary perfusion. In MR imaging, the method most commonly used in clinical practice is the dynamic susceptibility contrast-enhanced perfusion-weighted imaging (PWI) technique. In this technique a bolus of gadolinium-based paramagnetic contrast agent is injected and the signal change is tracked by susceptibility-weighted, T2*-weighted MR sequences. Relative semiquantitative measures reflecting cerebral blood volume (CBV), mean transit time (MTT), Tmax, and cerebral blood flow (CBF) can be derived from the signal intensity-over-time curve.

MR delineation of the infarct core and ischemic penumbra rely on the assumption that DWI reflects irreversibly damaged tissue, whereas PWI represents an overall area of hypoperfusion. The volumetric difference between these abnormal areas, called the PWI/DWI "mismatch," represents the MR correlate of the ischemic penumbra (see Plate 23.2). If there is no difference in the volumes of PWI and DWI, this is termed a PWI/DWI "match." This occurs in patients who do not have penumbral tissue. It is not yet clearly demonstrated which parameter gives the best approximation to critical hypoperfusion and allows for differentiation of infarct from penumbra. However, Tmax and MTT seem to give the best results.

PCT imaging relies on the analysis of the signal density curve produced by the entry and washout of a bolus of standard iodinated contrast injected into a peripheral vein. The linear relationship between contrast concentration and CT tissue density allows for quantitative brain capillary information. Characterization of ischemic tissue with PCT requires intact cerebral autoregulation. In the penumbra, where autoregulation is intact or mildly jeopardized, MTT is prolonged due to arterial occlusion but CBV is maintained or increased due to this compensatory vasodilatation. On the other hand, in the infarct core where autoregulation is damaged, MTT is prolonged and CBV is reduced. Therefore, by combining MTT and CBV results, PCT has the ability to reliably identify reversible ischemic penumbra and irreversible infarct core in acute stroke patients (see Plates 23.1 and 23.3). Quantitatively, the parameter that most accurately describes tissue at risk of infarction is the relative MTT. The optimal threshold for describing tissue at risk is 145%. The parameter that most accurately describes the infarct core on admission is the absolute CBV. The optimal threshold for this parameter is 2.0 mL/100 g.

SCIENCE REVISITED

Both CT and MR estimates of infarct core and ischemic penumbra have been validated by prospective studies and a comparison with positron emission tomography (PET) or Xenon CT.

Prediction of the Risk of Bleeding

SCIENCE REVISITED

Thrombolysis in acute stroke increases the risk of cerebral hemorrhage. Severe hemorrhage with mass effect occurs in 4.8% of patients with stroke treated with rt-PA within 3 hours after symptom onset and in up to 6.4% in patients treated between 3 and 6 hours. A major goal for stroke imaging is to identify patients at risk for post-thrombolytic intracranial hemorrhage.

Hypoattenuation on NCT or restricted water diffusion on MRI are associated with increased risk of thrombolytic-related hemorrhagic transformation. Clearly identifiable hypoattenuation involving more than one-third of the middle cerebral artery territory is currently being used as an exclusion criteria for tPA.

Although chronic microbleeds are an indicator of a hemorrhage-prone vasculopathy and are associated with an increased risk of spontaneous intracranial hemorrhage, their relationship with post-thrombolytic-related hemorrhage is still debated. MRI with spin gradient echo or susceptibility-weighted sequences is more sensitive than NCT for the detection of these small hemosiderin depositions.

Damage to the blood–brain barrier (BBB) is considered as one of the main contributing mechanisms to hemorrhagic transformation after reperfusion. Early detection of a damaged BBB could potentially be used to identify patients who are more likely to develop hemorrhagic transformation (HT) after reperfusion. Measurement of BBB permeability by using perfusion CT and MR is based on dynamic contrast-enhanced imaging of microvascular permeability that allows for quantification of BBB disruption. BBB disruption can also be identified as delayed gadolinium enhancement of the cerebrospinal fluid space on fluid-attenuated inversion recovery (FLAIR) images. This sign has been termed the hyperintense acute reperfusion marker (HARM). In recent investigations, it was found that defects in the blood–brain barrier predispose for both spontaneous and thrombolytic-associated hemorrhagic transformation in ischemic stroke (see Plate 23.4). Further clinical trials are required to elucidate if BBB imaging has a role in therapeutic decisions.

CT and MR Imaging for the Selection of Patients for Thrombolytic Therapy

Several clinical trials using MR perfusion imaging to extend the window for thrombolysis have demonstrated the safety and efficacy of this technique and strategy.

The DIAS and DEDAS trials, randomized patients within a 3–9 hour time window after stroke using a DWI/PWI mismatch of at least 20% to either placebo or escalating doses of desmoteplase, a new thrombolytic drug. Patients with early vessel recanalization and reperfusion showed a significant clinical benefit: 60% of the patients from the most effective dose tier had an excellent clinical outcome. Unfortunately, the recently published DIAS 2 phase III trial did not show any benefit in clinical outcome in either of the treatment groups.

The DEFUSE trial showed that baseline MRI findings can be used to identify groups of patients who are more likely to benefit from thrombolytic therapy. Patients with a baseline mismatch between PWI and DWI of at least 20% and a reduction in perfusion volume abnormality of at least 10 mL had a better clinical outcome. Data from this study suggested that a mismatch ratio (PWI volume – DWI volume/DWI volume) of 2.6 provided the highest sensitivity and specificity for identifying patients with whom reperfusion was associated with a favorable response. This study emphasized the importance of combining the information obtained from perfusion and vascular imaging. No relationship between early recanalization and favorable clinical outcome was seen in patients without a mismatch. On the other hand, no benefit could be expected if early recanalization of the occluded vessel failed, even in the presence of a large mismatch.

Although MRI has been used to extend the time window for reperfusion, there are as yet no published prospective multicenter perfusion-CT trials that can help to define how to best use this technique in acute ischemic stroke patients. Multicenter clinical trials using a validated perfusion-CT software package to select acute ischemic stroke patients are needed.

Conclusion

An increasing number of studies support the role of advanced neuroimaging techniques in selecting patients for acute stroke treatments, including reperfusion therapies in an extended time window. Physicians taking care of stroke patients should be familiar with the different components of advanced multimodal stroke imaging, the information provided by each component, and how this information influence management decisions.

Bibliography

Albers GW, Thijs VN, Wechsler L, et al. Magnetic resonance imaging profiles predict clinical response to early reperfusion: the diffusion and perfusion imaging evaluation for understanding stroke evolution (DEFUSE) study. *Ann Neurol* 2006; **60:** 508–517.

Astrup J, Siesjo BK, Symon L. Thresholds in cerebral ischemia - the ischemic penumbra. *Stroke* 1981; **12:** 723–725.

Davis SM, Donnan GA, Parsons MW, et al. Effects of alteplase beyond 3 h after stroke in the Echoplanar Imaging Thrombolytic Evaluation Trial (EPITHET): a placebo-controlled randomised trial. *Lancet Neurol* 2008; **7:** 299–309.

Fiebach JB, Schellinger PD, Gass A, et al. Stroke magnetic resonance imaging is accurate in hyperacute intracerebral hemorrhage: a multi-center study on the validity of stroke imaging. *Stroke* 2004; **35:** 502–506.

Hacke W, Furlan AJ, Al-Rawi Y, et al. Intravenous desmoteplase in patients with acute ischaemic stroke selected by MRI perfusion-diffusion weighted imaging or perfusion CT (DIAS-2): a prospective, randomised, double-blind, placebo-controlled study. *Lancet Neurol* 2009; **8:** 141–150.

Kidwell CS, Chalela JA, Saver JL, et al. Comparison of MRI and CT for detection of acute intracerebral hemorrhage. *J Am Med Assoc* 2004; **292:** 1823–1830.

Tan JC, Dillon WP, Liu S, et al. Systematic comparison of perfusion-CT and CT-angiography in acute stroke patients. *Ann Neurol* 2007; **61:** 533–543.

Wintermark M, Flanders AE, Velthuis B, et al. Perfusion-CT assessment of infarct core and penumbra: receiver operating characteristic curve analysis in 130 patients suspected of acute hemispheric stroke. *Stroke* 2006; **37:** 979–985.

Wintermark M, Reichhart M, Thiran JP, et al. Prognostic accuracy of cerebral blood flow measurement by perfusion computed tomography, at the time of emergency room admission, in acute stroke patients. *Ann Neurol* 2002; **51:** 417–432.

Wintermark M, Thiran JP, Maeder P, Schnyder P, Meuli R. Simultaneous measurement of regional cerebral blood flow by perfusion CT and stable xenon CT: a validation study. *AJNR Am J Neuroradiol* 2001; **22:** 905–14.

Advanced Monitoring of Brain Oxygenation and Metabolism

Bharath R. Naravetla[1] and J. Claude Hemphill III[2]

[1]Department of Neurology, Neurovascular Service, University of California, San Francisco, CA, USA
[2]Department of Neurology, University of California, San Francisco, CA, USA

Introduction

Current neuromonitoring techniques involve a range of tools that focus on the measurement of cerebral physiologic and metabolic parameters with the goal of improving the detection and management of primary and secondary brain injury in patients who have suffered traumatic brain injury (TBI), stroke, or subarachnoid hemorrhage (SAH), or have had neurosurgical procedures. Established methods have included measurement of intracranial pressure (ICP) and maintenance of cerebral perfusion pressure (CPP) or electroencephalography (EEG) monitoring for the detection of seizures.

Recognition of underlying disturbances of cerebral oxygen delivery and cellular metabolism in acute brain injuries has led to a strong interest in the development of techniques that would enable continuous, quantitative, and real-time measurement of brain metabolism in the neurocritical care unit. New tools that are currently available for advanced cerebral monitoring in brain-injured patients include devices that can measure the brain tissue oxygen tension ($P_{bt}O_2$), the jugular bulb venous oxygen saturation ($SjvO_2$), the cerebral blood flow (CBF), and the concentration of extracellular metabolites (cerebral microdialysis). Given the complexity of metabolic changes in acute brain injury, the concept of multimodality monitoring is also emphasized, in which information from multiple different monitoring modalities is integrated by the clinician in order to provide a more complete picture than could be obtained using just a single monitor.

Brain Tissue Oxygen Monitoring

Direct measurement of brain tissue oxygen tension ($P_{bt}O_2$) utilizes a microelectrode placed in the parenchyma of the brain (Figure 24.1). It has become the most commonly used advanced neuromonitoring technique and allows quantitative measurement of tissue oxygen tension in a focal region of the brain. Previously incorrectly considered as primarily an ischemia monitor, $P_{bt}O_2$ is probably more representative of the interplay between cerebral blood flow and oxygen diffusion.

Equipment and Technique

At present, the only commercially available tool for $P_{bt}O_2$ monitoring is the LICOX system (Integra Neurosciences, Plainsboro, NJ), which uses a polarographic Clarke-type microelectrode for

Emergency Management in Neurocritical Care, First Edition. Edited by Edward M. Manno.
© 2012 John Wiley & Sons, Ltd. Published 2012 by John Wiley & Sons, Ltd.

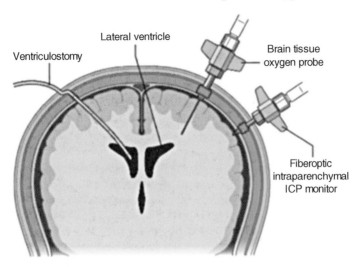

Figure 24.1. Drawing of a coronal section through the brain at the level of the third ventricle, demonstrating a ventriculostomy drain inserted into the lateral ventricle, an intraparenchymal brain tissue oxygen probe, and an intraparenchymal intracranial pressure monitor. (Reproduced from Fauci, AS, et al., *Harrison's Principles of Internal Medicine*, 17th edn, p. 1722; © 2008, McGraw-Hill with permission from The McGraw-Hill Companies.)

oxygen tension measurement and includes an integrated temperature probe. The $P_{bt}O_2$ probe is placed directly into the brain parenchyma usually with a fixed cranial bolt, approximately 2–3 cm below the dura. The frontal white matter is the area most commonly targeted for placement.

The location of probe placement remains a point of debate and various investigators have suggested that placement should be targeted to pericontusional or penumbral regions or to relatively normal regions of the brain. Our approach is to place the probe in the ipsilateral hemisphere in patients with nontraumatic intracerebral hemorrhage, the frontal lobe that is presumed to be at highest risk for vasospasm after aneurysmal SAH, and in the least injured hemisphere in the context of diffuse injury such as with head trauma.

Measurement

The probe is connected to an external monitor for a continuous reading of $P_{bt}O_2$ (expressed quantitatively in mmHg) and brain temperature. Generally, the initial readings during the first 2 hours after placement are considered unreliable. The oxygen microelectrode measures the tissue oxygen tension in a focal region approximately 17 mm^3 in volume. $P_{bt}O_2$ values are obtained continuously and in real-time. Proper functioning of the catheter can be confirmed using an "oxygen challenge" in which the F_iO_2 is temporarily increased to 1.0 in order to demonstrate a significant rise in $P_{bt}O_2$.

Relationship with Other Physiological Parameters

$P_{bt}O_2$ may vary with a number of physiological parameters. $P_{bt}O_2$ measurements have been shown to positively correlate with arterial oxygen tension, inspired oxygen concentration (F_iO_2), mean arterial pressure, CPP, CBF, hemoglobin concentration, and inversely with oxygen extraction fraction on positron emission tomography (PET) imaging and mean transit time on dynamic CT perfusion (CTP) imaging.

There is a linear correlation between $P_{bt}O_2$ and changes in end-tidal carbon dioxide measurements or CBF, and a sinusoidal correlation with mean arterial pressure, suggesting that $P_{bt}O_2$ is strongly influenced by factors that regulate the CBF and cerebral autoregulation. In general, acute hyperventilation decreases $P_{bt}O_2$. This is presumably mediated through a primary reduction in the CBF due to cerebral vasoconstriction. Of the various physiologic parameters studied in brain-injured patients, F_iO_2 and MAP (or CPP) have had the strongest and most consistent effect.

Clinical Utility and Prior Studies

Several studies in patients with TBI have shown that patients with $P_{bt}O_2$ levels less than 10–15 mmHg for extended periods of time, or on multiple occasions, have a worsened outcome. There appears to be a dose–response relationship in which longer durations and lower levels of $P_{bt}O_2$ are associated with an increasing mortality risk. Lower $P_{bt}O_2$ levels have also been associated with poorer performance on neuropsychological and cognitive testing after head trauma. Although there have been no randomized clinical trials assessing the efficacy of $P_{bt}O_2$-directed therapy, an observational study found that patients with severe TBI who were managed with $P_{bt}O_2$-guided therapy (goal $P_{bt}O_2 > 25$ mmHg) had a lower risk of mortality than historical controls managed with conventional ICP and CPP monitoring. Based on clinical and experimental studies, a $P_{bt}O_2$ level below 15 mmHg is now considered abnormal. Notably, one study using PET identified a $P_{bt}O_2$ of 14 mmHg as the threshold at which critical oxygen extraction occurs.

It is likely that the parameters influencing absolute $P_{bt}O_2$ levels are more complex than identifying a threshold parameter. $P_{bt}O_2$ is probably more closely representative of the relationship between CBF and $AVTO_2$ (the difference between the partial pressure of oxygen in the arterial and venous circulations: $P_aO_2 - P_vO_2$). $AVTO_2$ is probably an indicator of oxygen diffusion and thus the relationships between CBF and oxygen extraction are important to consider when investigating the causes of low $P_{bt}O_2$. Experience is varied regarding the relationship between $P_{bt}O_2$ and ICP; in general, $P_{bt}O_2$ decreases with increased ICP only when the CPP is concurrently decreased.

Practical Aspects of Patient Management

A low $P_{bt}O_2$ reading should prompt further investigation into a potential underlying cause. Because $P_{bt}O_2$ is a marker of CBF and oxygen diffusion, a reasonable first step is to obtain an arterial blood gas in order to determine if the patient's lung function has deteriorated or if the patient has a decreased CBF due to hyperventilation. Steps should then be undertaken to determine if cerebral perfusion is inadequate. In this circumstance, a CBF monitor may be useful as part of multimodality monitoring. Otherwise, consideration should be as to whether the CPP is too low, the ICP is too high, or the patient has disturbed cerebral autoregulation. A brief trial of more aggressive cerebrospinal fluid drainage or increased mean arterial pressure using fluids or pressors may undercover a cerebral perfusion deficit.

In general, we do not advocate simply increasing the F_iO_2 as this may correct the $P_{bt}O_2$ without actually fixing the underlying perfusion failure that led to the low reading. Limited data exists, however, to suggest that hyperoxic therapy might improve some aspects of pericontusional cerebral metabolic function. Thus, this remains an unproven option if all reasonable aspects of inadequate oxygen delivery have been ruled out and the $P_{bt}O_2$ remains critically low.

Available data suggests that red blood cell transfusion has only a very modest effect on the $P_{bt}O_2$.

⚠ CAUTION

$PbtO_2$ reading is

- Unreliable initially during stabilization/ calibration of the probe (~2 hours)
- < 15 mmHg is considered abnormally low

- Low reading should prompt assessment of P_aO_2 and CBF
- May be low due to hypometabolism from primary brain injury

Drawbacks

Brain tissue oxygen monitoring is an invasive procedure, although reported rates of complications are exceedingly low. $P_{bt}O_2$ provides a focal measure of tissue oxygen partial pressure and therefore may not be representative of processes occurring in other focal regions of the brain.

Jugular Bulb Venous Oxygen Saturation (SjvO₂) Monitoring

Assessment of the venous oxygen saturation in the jugular bulb as blood is exiting the brain provides a measure of global cerebral oxygen delivery and a way to estimate the global relationship between the CBF and cerebral metabolism. SjvO₂ monitoring can provide information on global cerebral hypoxia and indirectly on cerebral hypoperfusion or hyperperfusion.

Equipment and Technique

One simple method is to cannulate the internal jugular vein and advance a catheter cephalad until the tip resides above the level at which there is flow from the external jugular supply (usually above the C3 level). Blood can then be drawn and sent for venous blood gas measurement, including the partial pressure of oxygen (P_vO_2) and the venous oxygen saturation. Most described methods also use an oxymetric catheter that has a lumen for blood draws as well as a sensor (usually fiberoptic) that can measure the blood oxygen saturation continuously. There is currently no commercially available kit designed specifically for SjvO₂ monitoring. Thus, equipment that is used is borrowed from critical care monitoring tools designed for other uses. We use an Edwards 4 French size fiberoptic oxygen sensing catheter (with blood draw lumen) attached to a Baxter–Edwards Vigilance Continuous Oximetry Monitor. For placement, the dominant jugular vein (based on the size of the

jugular foramen on CT or cross-sectional lumen on ultrasound) is cannulated, usually under direct ultrasound guidance in order to avoid carotid puncture. Using the Seldinger technique, a 6 French pediatric introducer (5.5 cm in length) is placed. The oxymetric catheter is then advanced through the introducer until the catheter tip is placed at or near the jugular bulb to decrease blood contamination from the extracranial circulation.

Measurement

The catheter is connected to the external monitor for a continuous reading of SjvO₂ expressed as a percentage. Blood is sampled for venous blood gas testing to allow the catheter to be calibrated at the time of insertion and once or twice daily. By calculating the venous blood oxygen content (C_vO_2) and subtracting this from the arterial oxygen content (C_aO_2), the cerebral arteriovenous oxygen difference ($AVDO_2$) can be calculated. $AVDO_2$ is the amount of oxygen used by the brain.

Relationship with Other Physiological Parameters

SjvO₂ is influenced by parameters that relate to the cerebral oxygen delivery and metabolism. SjvO₂ is inversely related to the $AVDO_2$. If the cerebral $AVDO_2$ increases because the brain is extracting more oxygen, then the SjvO₂ decreases, and vice versa. If the arterial oxygen content being delivered to the brain drops significantly because of very low hemoglobin levels or F_iO_2 (thereby decreasing arterial oxygen saturation), then the SjvO₂ may decrease if the brain extracts the same amount of oxygen as before. If the brain extracts less oxygen because of large areas of brain infarction or cerebral metabolic depression due to either disease or the effects of sedative or anesthetic agents, then the SjvO₂ may increase. Low cerebral perfusion due to inadequate CPP, elevated ICP, or hyperventilation may be reflected in lower SjvO₂ values.

Clinical Utility and Prior Studies

Normal SjvO₂ is approximately 60%, although in brain-injured patients it may be higher. While the precise SjvO₂ threshold for cerebral ischemia may vary depending on the brain's ability to extract oxygen, an $SjvO_2$ of < 50% for greater than 10 minutes has generally been considered to represent an ischemic desaturation. Previous studies in TBI patients have found that ischemic desaturations are associated with worsened outcome in a dose-dependent manner. High $SjvO_2$ levels (typically > 80%) may reflect hyperemia or an inability of the brain to extract oxygen due to metabolic depression from sedative agents, poor oxygen unloading (e.g. sickle cell disease), or severe brain injury. Importantly, both abnormally high and low $SjvO_2$ levels have been associated with poor clinical outcome in TBI patients. However, it remains unclear whether this is causative (especially in those with high $SjvO_2$ levels) or whether this is principally a marker of the severity of brain injury.

$SjvO_2$ monitoring was used in a pivotal trial of CBF-directed therapy (to maintain a CPP $\geq$ 70 mmHg) versus ICP-directed therapy (to maintain an ICP < 20 mmHg). This trial demonstrated a dramatic reduction in ischemic desaturations in the patients undergoing CBF-directed therapy. However, there was no difference in 6 month outcome. This was thought likely due to a four-fold increase in ARDS in the CBF-directed therapy patients. The results of this study have been used to suggest that advanced neuromonitoring might be useful in targeting optimal cerebral oxygen delivery while limiting systemic complications imposed by aggressive use of fluids and pressors.

SCIENCE REVISITED

$SjvO_2$ is inversely related to cerebral oxygen extraction; $AVDO_2 = Hgb \times 1.34 (S_aO_2\text{-}SjvO_2) + 0.0031 \times (P_aO_2 - P_vO_2)$

- Both low and high $SjvO_2$ values are associated with poor outcome
- Causes of low $SjvO_2$ include low CBF, low CPP, fever, and seizures
- High $SjvO_2$ levels may reflect hyperemia or inability of the brain to extract oxygen from sedatives, poor oxygen unloading (e.g. sickle cell disease), or severe brain injury

Practical Aspects of Patient Management

The principal value of $SjvO_2$ monitoring lies in its ability to help clinicians to determine the global oxygen delivery to the brain principally by assessing whether cerebral blood flow is resulting in a normal, oligemic, or hyperemic state.

A drop in $SjvO_2$ should prompt an evaluation of $AVDO_2$ by assessing the arterial oxygen content in an arterial blood gas. If C_aO_2, is sufficient, then an assessment turns to the adequacy of the cerebral blood flow. Assuming that the arterial blood gas does not suggest hyperventilation, then the adequacy of the cerebral perfusion pressure should be of concern. Measures to lower the ICP or raise the CPP should be undertaken. Additionally, the possibility of an enlarging intracranial mass should be considered, especially if simple measures to treat the ICP or CPP do not quickly restore the $SjvO_2$. Given that a short duration (10 minutes) of ischemic desaturation is associated with a worsened outcome, continuous $SjvO_2$ monitoring is preferred over just checking jugular venous blood gases intermittently.

Conversely, an $SjvO_2$ value of more than 80% is generally considered as hyperemia or luxury perfusion. It may also indicate impairment of cerebral autoregulation. In this setting, especially if the ICP is high, consideration could be given to judiciously lowering the systemic blood pressure.

Drawbacks

$SjvO_2$ monitoring (Figure 24.2) is an invasive procedure and is associated with a small risk of infection, infiltration, hemorrhage, and carotid puncture. Because it functions as a global monitor, focal or regional ischemic changes might not be detected, and a relatively large volume of brain tissue must be affected before the $SjvO_2$ level drops significantly.

Cerebral Blood Flow Monitoring

Cerebral blood flow is considered as an important physiologic parameter in the setting of brain injury, as the CBF reflects the delivery of substrate to tissue. It was one of the first parameters to be measured, using various imaging

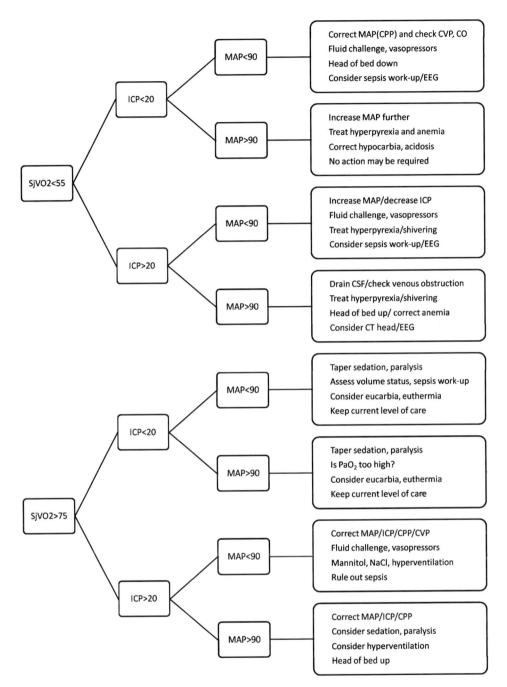

Figure 24.2. Flow chart representing a general approach to the management of abnormal SjvO₂ readings. Note that an abnormal value should be reconfirmed. The position and calibration of the catheter and light intensity are adjusted and if necessary a recalibration of the catheter should be performed before making any interventions for an abnormal value.

and vascular dilution techniques. Only recently has continuous monitoring in the neurocritical care unit become available. Monitors based on two basic methodologies are available: thermal diffusion flowmetry (TDF) and laser Doppler flowmetry (LDF).

Equipment and Technique

TDF is based on the principle of thermal conductivity of cortical tissue, where the temperature difference between two portions of a probe is detected and converted to quantitative CBF. Commercially available TDF microprobes include the QFlow 500 Probe and Bowman Perfusion Monitor (Hemedex Inc., Cambridge, MA, USA) and the Saber Cerebral Blood Flow Monitoring System (Flowtronics Inc., Phoenix, AZ, USA). The probe tip is placed 2–2.5 cm below the cortical surface through a burr hole and is usually secured using a bolt.

LDF involves a probe which is directly inserted into the brain parenchyma or over the surface of the brain. It is able to detect the density measurements of moving blood, thereby providing momentary percentage changes in local CBF. LDF provides relative information but not absolute quantitative values of CBF, thus limiting its utility.

Measurement

The probe is connected to an external monitor for a continuous reading of CBF expressed as mL/100 g (of brain)/min (for TDF probes). Values are dependent on the position of the tip of the catheter as they vary widely across gray and white matter.

Relationship with Other Physiological Parameters

CBF is influenced by mean arterial pressure, ICP, as well as the arterial partial pressure of carbon dioxide and oxygen depending on the patient's injury and whether cerebral autoregulation is intact. These relationships bring forth the important principle of CBF and cerebral metabolic coupling, where $CMRO_2$ is directly related to CBF and $AVDO_2$.

☝ CAUTION

Quantitative continuous CBF monitoring

- Values are highly dependent on location of the tip of the catheter
- Brain-injured patients may still have intact CO_2 reactivity, but impaired pressure autoregulation
- CBF decreases by 3% for every 1 mmHg decrease in $PaCO_2$

Practical Aspects of Patient Management

Normal average CBF in the human is approximately 55 mL/100 g of brain/min, but actual values may vary widely across gray and white matter. TDF probe tips are usually placed in the white matter, with the generally accepted normal range as 18–25 mL/100 g/min. The ischemic threshold for CBF is usually considered approximately 18 mL/100 g/min. The threshold for irreversible injury is 10 mL/100 g/min; however, this may be lower in white matter.

Although brain-injured patients may have impairment of pressure autoregulation, CO_2 reactivity is usually retained and the CBF may respond to hyperventilation. The CBF is normally decreased by 3% for every 1 mmHg decrease in P_aCO_2. Necessary steps taken to improve the CBF include increasing the CPP by raising the MAP or lowering the ICP. Current TBI guidelines suggest that the autoregulation status should be considered when targeting a specific goal CPP, and continuous CBF monitoring may help with this assessment.

Drawbacks

Because these methods measure focal CBF, values may not reflect processes in other parts of the brain. Inaccurate values may occur if the tip is near large vessels or, in the case of loss of tissue contact or displacement of the probe. TDF probes may be non-operational during fever (in order to avoid possible additional tissue injury).

Table 24.1. Advanced neuromonitoring modalities

Modality	Measured parameter	Normal value	Remarks
Brain tissue oxygen monitoring (PbtO₂)	Focal partial pressure of tissue oxygen. Related to CBF and oxygen diffusion.	Acceptable normal: 20–35 mmHg "Abnormal threshold": <15 mmHg	Should be considered in the context of other variables and clinical condition
Jugular bulb venous oxygen saturation monitoring (SjvO₂)	Global (measures saturation from single jugular vein)	Normal: 55–75% Oligemia: < 50–55% Hyperemia: > 75–80%	May not detect focal ischemic changes
Cerebral blood flow monitoring (CBF)	Focal rate of blood flow	Normal (white matter): 18–25 mL/100 g/min "Ischemic threshold": <18 mL/100 g/min Irreversible ischemia: <10 mL/100 g/min	Indirect measure of adequacy of metabolic oxygen delivery
Cerebral microdialysis (CMD)	Focal measure of lactate-pyruvate ratio (LPR), glucose concentration, glutamate, glycerol, or other measured metabolites	Glucose <15, LPR >30 are considered critical LPR >40 indicates metabolic crisis	Mitochondrial dysfunction may also elevate LPR >40

Cerebral Microdialysis

Cerebral microdialysis (CMD) differs from the other described advanced neuromonitoring tools because it does not measure physiological parameters, but rather allows measurement of the concentration of chemicals found in the brain parenchyma. This may allow direct assessment of the metabolic consequences of primary and secondary brain injury (Figure 24.3).

Equipment and Technique

CMD utilizes the capillary technique to collect a sample of extracellular fluid from the brain (or other tissue being monitored). A CMD system comprises three basic components: the CMD catheter, perfusate pump, and analyzer. The catheter is a fine tube made with a semipermeable dialysis membrane that allows diffusion of molecules from the extracellular space; a commonly used version has a cutoff of 20 kD. A "mock" CSF or normal saline is instilled into the microdialysis catheter via a small pump at a rate usually ranging from 0.3 to 1.0 μL/min.

Microdialysate is then collected in a microvial which is placed in a microdialysis analyzer to obtain the concentration of specified metabolites such as lactate, pyruvate, glutamate, or glucose. The most commonly used commercially available system is made by CMA Microdialysis (Stockholm, Sweden). The CMD catheter is inserted through a burrhole in a manner similar to the placement of P$_{bt}$O$_2$ or TD-CBF probes, although it can be placed "freehand" without a bolt system if a specific area of the brain is targeted during open craniotomy.

Measurement

Numerous parameters can be measured, including glucose, glutamate, lactate, pyruvate, glycerol or even concentrations of drugs. There is an inherent delay between the collection of the fluid at the catheter and its eventual migration to the microvial. Current protocols often involve sample analysis hourly; thus, analyzed values represent events that occurred recently, but not in real time.

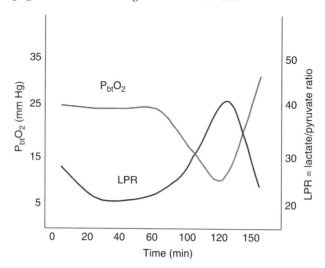

Figure 24.3. Advanced neuromonitoring in a 26-year-old woman with a GCS of 6 after severe TBI. Patient was inadvertently hyperventilated at the 60-minute mark, which caused secondary ischemia due to cerebral vasoconstriction and decreased cerebral blood flow. This was identified as a decrease in $P_{bt}O_2$ accompanied by an increase in the LPR. These abnormal cerebral metabolic parameters resolved when hyperventilation was discontinued.

Relationship with Other Physiological Parameters

Microdialysis values of brain metabolites such as lactate and pyruvate are generally considered to be indicators of the state of brain injury and aerobic metabolism. The results of CMD parameters may be challenging to interpret because they may demonstrate intrinsic tissue injury from the primary brain injury or secondary injury from additional insults such as hypoperfusion. Thus, direct correlation of lactate or lactate/pyruvate ratios with other common physiological parameters such as ICP or CPP may not be present unless there is a distinct and dramatic event resulting in tissue metabolic crisis.

Clinical Utility and Prior Studies

The most commonly measured values are lactate and pyruvate, with a lactate/pyruvate ratio (LPR) >40 generally considered to represent a metabolic crisis of brain tissue. Increases in this ratio may represent ischemia or mitochondrial dysfunction. Pathologic alterations in cerebral microdialysate concentrations have been correlated to changes in other physiological parameters, including $P_{bt}O_2$, $SjvO_2$, ICP, blood

pressure, hypoxia, and CBF as measured by xenon CT or oxygen extraction fraction as measured by PET. Metabolic crisis has also been reported during nonconvulsive seizures and hypoglycemia. TBI and SAH patients with poor clinical outcome have been shown to have elevated levels of excitatory neurotransmitters, elevated LPR, and abnormal lactate and glutamate levels. In a study of patients with severe TBI, increased lactate/glucose ratios and lactate levels correlated with $SjvO_2$ desaturations and an increased risk of death.

⚙ SCIENCE REVISITED

Cerebral microdialysis

- Intensive insulin therapy may be associated with cerebral hypoglycemia despite serum normoglycemia, and this may be associated with poor outcome
- Consensus statement recommend lactate-pyruvate ratio (LPR) as primary marker in TBI
- LPR > 40 considered as cerebral metabolic crisis

Practical Aspects of Patient Management

A recent consensus statement recommended the use of LPR as the primary marker for ischemia in TBI. Microdialysis glucose, glycerol, and glutamate are additional markers of impending ischemia. Because of the variability in values related to tissue injury and the inherent delay in values, the use of microdialysis targeted therapy has been challenging. However, CMD has helped to provide insight into the impact of other events on cerebral metabolic crisis and permanent tissue injury. For example, the use of insulin infusions to target normoglycemia has been found to lead to cerebral metabolic crisis and low cerebral glucose in some cases. Nonconvulsive seizures may lead to an elevated LPR and cerebral metabolic crisis. Nonconvulsive seizures have also been found to correlate with later brain atrophy. At present, CMD is reasonably considered as part of a multimodality monitoring approach, but not exclusively as a single neuromonitor.

Drawbacks

Because of the inherent delay in microdialysate transport through the catheter, values are not real time. As a focal monitor, it may demonstrate only local changes in metabolism. Another important limitation is the variability of results based on the location of the probe (in injured tissue, normal tissue, or areas of penumbra), bringing into debate the ideal location for catheter placement. Table 24.1 provides a summary of several advanced neuromonitoring modalities.

Conclusion

The ultimate goal of neuromonitoring in severe brain injury is to assess neurological function and help to predict as well as improve outcome by providing the ability to intervene while brain tissue is still viable and the patient is still salvageable. New neuromonitoring tools that allow the assessment of brain oxygen delivery, blood flow, and metabolism provide a new window into the acute management of brain injury. Because of the complexity and heterogeneity of processes occurring in brain-injured patients after trauma and stroke, no one monitoring method provides complete information. Thus, the above described invasive monitoring tools should be considered in the context of a multimodality monitoring approach. Newer monitors can complement the traditional measurements of ICP and CPP, findings on neuroimaging, as well as clinical neurological assessment. Future approaches to integrating this complex bedside data into user-friendly clinical treatment paradigms are challenging, but are likely to bear fruit in the long term.

Bibliography

Fauci, AS, et al., *Harrison's Principles of Internal Medicine*, McGraw-Hill 2008.

Hemphill JC 3rd, Knudson MM, et al. Carbon dioxide reactivity and pressure autoregulation of brain tissue oxygen. *Neurosurgery* 2001; **48**: 377–383.

Marcoux J, McArthur DA, et al. Persistent metabolic crisis as measured by elevated cerebral microdialysis lactate-pyruvate ratio predicts chronic frontal lobe brain atrophy after traumatic brain injury. *Crit Care Med* 2008; **36**: 2871–2877.

Oddo M, Schmidt JM, et al. Impact of tight glycemic control on cerebral glucose metabolism after severe brain injury: a microdialysis study. *Crit Care Med* 2008; **36**: 3233–3238.

Robertson CS, Gopinath SP, et al. SjvO$_2$ monitoring in head-injured patients. *J Neurotraum* 1995; **12**: 891–896.

Robertson CS, Valadka AB, et al. Prevention of secondary ischemic insults after severe head injury. *Crit Care Med* 1999; **27**: 2086–2095.

Rosenthal G, Hemphill JC 3rd, et al. Brain tissue oxygen tension is more indicative of oxygen diffusion than oxygen delivery and metabolism in patients with traumatic brain injury. *Crit Care Med* 2009; **37**: 379–380.

Rosenthal G, Sanchez-Mejia RO, et al. Incorporating a parenchymal thermal diffusion cerebral blood flow probe in bedside assessment of cerebral autoregulation and vasoreactivity in patients with severe traumatic brain injury. *J Neurosurg* 2011; **114(1):** 62–70.

Stiefel MF, Spiotta A, et al. Reduced mortality rate in patients with severe traumatic brain injury treated with brain tissue oxygen monitoring. *J Neurosurg* 2005; **103**: 805–811.

Stocchetti N, Canavesi K, et al. Arterio-jugular difference of oxygen content and outcome after head injury. *Anesth Analg* 2004; **99**: 230–234.

van den Brink WA, van Santbrink H, et al. Brain oxygen tension in severe head injury. *Neurosurgery* 2000; **46**: 868–876.

Index